The Director's Circle Book for 2008

The Johns Hopkins University Press gratefully acknowledges members
of the 2008 Director's Circle for supporting the publication of works
such as *Mary Elizabeth Garrett*.

Darlene T. Anderson

Anonymous

Dominic and Helen Averza

Alfred and Muriel Berkeley

John and Bonnie Boland

Darlene Bookoff

Sylvia Bookoff

Frank and Marie Cappiello

William and Charlotte Cronin

Jack Goellner and Barbara Lamb

Willard Hackerman

Charles and Elizabeth Hughes

Kristina M. Johnson

James D. Jordan and Angela von der Lippe

John and Kathleen Keane

Peter J. Klassen

Frank Mondimore and Jay Rubin

Ralph S. O'Connor

Peter Onuf

Eric R. Papenfuse and Catherine A. Lawrence

Braxton and Margaret Mitchell

Peter Devereux Nalle

Anders Richter

Jean B. Russo

David Ryer

Dorothy McIlvain Scott

R. Champlin and Debbie Sheridan

Murray and Janet Steinberg

Winston and Marilyn Tabb

Daun and Patricia Van Ee

Robert L. Warren and Family

MARY ELIZABETH GARRETT

*Society and Philanthropy
in the Gilded Age*

KATHLEEN WATERS SANDER

The Johns Hopkins University Press
Baltimore

© 2008 Kathleen Waters Sander
All rights reserved. Published 2008
Printed in the United States of America on acid-free paper

2 4 6 8 9 7 5 3 1

The Johns Hopkins University Press
2715 North Charles Street
Baltimore, Maryland 21218-4363
www.press.jhu.edu

Library of Congress Cataloging-in-Publication Data

Sander, Kathleen Waters, 1947–
Mary Elizabeth Garrett : society and philanthropy in the Gilded Age /
Kathleen Waters Sander.
p. cm.
Includes bibliographical references and index.
ISBN-13: 978-0-8018-8870-0 (hardcover : alk. paper)
ISBN-10: 0-8018-8870-0 (alk. paper)
1. Garrett, Mary Elizabeth, 1854–1915.   2. Women philanthropists—
Maryland—Baltimore—Biography.   3. Medical education—Maryland—
Baltimore—Endowments—History.   4. Women medical students—
Maryland—Baltimore—History.   5. Women in medicine—Maryland—
Baltimore—History.   6. Johns Hopkins University. School of Medicine.
I. Title.
HV28.G28S26 2008
361.7'4092—dc22
[B]   2008006555

A catalog record for this book is available from the British Library.

*Special discounts are available for bulk purchases of this book. For more
information, please contact Special Sales at 410-516-6936 or
specialsales@press.jhu.edu.*

The Johns Hopkins University Press uses environmentally friendly book
materials, including recycled text paper that is composed of at least 30
percent post-consumer waste, whenever possible. All of our book papers
are acid-free, and our jackets and covers are printed on paper with
recycled content.

To
Sam and Anne Hopkins,
James Rea Garrett and Edith Hoyt Garrett,
and, always,
John and Libby

You can never imagine what it is to have a man's force of genius in you, and yet to suffer the slavery of being a girl.

GEORGE ELIOT, *Daniel Deronda*

Contents

ooking today at the sprawling Johns Hopkins Medical Institutions, where twenty thousand students, faculty, staff, and visitors converge daily on a bustling, fifty-two-acre campus, it is hard to imagine a time when the famous medical school struggled mightily to get off the ground—and nearly did not. At a critical moment, when all seemed lost, Mary Elizabeth Garrett, a shy, thirty-eight-year-old Baltimorean, who believed in the potential greatness of American medicine and the need to educate women equally to men, risked much in her personal life to assure that the Johns Hopkins University opened the most advanced medical school in the country. Her gift did no less than forever change American medicine and medical philanthropy.

Sadly, like so much of women's history, the story of this remarkable woman— whose significant philanthropic involvement in education, medicine, and suffrage spanned three decades at the turn of the twentieth century—has been largely lost to the historical record. Who was she? How did she come to have such a fortune—nearly $100 million in today's currency—in an era when women seldom controlled their finances? What were her motivations for contributing to such a range of issues?

Certainly, I assumed, the answer would prove simple enough. Mary Elizabeth Garrett would turn out to be a rabid feminist warrior bent on tearing down gender barriers in a male-dominated society. Or a kindly, altruistic aristocrat with money to spare. Or a feisty woman intent on provoking tradition-bound trustees of male-run institutions. Or a woman scorned.

The answer was all of the above—and much more.

Mary Elizabeth Garrett first slipped into my life very quietly, unobtrusively, in the early 1990s. As I researched women's philanthropy and voluntarism of the nineteenth century for my doctoral dissertation and later a book on the Woman's Exchange Movement, I often came across short—very short—references to her in the historical archives. Always abbreviated and unembellished but nonetheless tantalizing, the notations usually stated just the bare facts: "Mary Elizabeth Garrett of Baltimore in 1893 gave $354,000 to start the Johns Hopkins University School of Medicine." The sheer amount of her philanthropy was only the beginning of the appeal—and her story. This mystery woman stayed with me for years until I had the chance to probe deeper. Soon enough I was hopelessly seduced into telling the untold story.

As a historian, I was drawn by many elements of Mary's life. Her life span, 1854 to 1915, covered the time period of most interest to me. It included the turbulent years leading up to the Civil War, which tested the principles of the young nation, and the subsequent aftermath of the anything-goes Gilded Age. Her philanthropies, activism, and personal life featured a captivating cast of characters and a fascinating panorama of topics, not least of which was her family's involvement in the commercial destiny of Baltimore and the development of the country's first major railroad, the Baltimore and Ohio.

Having worked in higher-education development and communications for twenty-five years, many of them spent with major donors whose gifts have made a great impact in education and medicine, I was interested in learning more about the woman who became one of the country's great philanthropists. Writing Mary Elizabeth Garrett's story would merge my scholarly interest in women's history with my professional work in the philanthropy of higher education.

An unexpected bonus during the ten years of my research for and writing of this biography has been meeting others who share my passion for bringing Mary Elizabeth Garrett's story to life, particularly the Hopkins and Garrett families. I am indebted to Anne and Sam Hopkins for their many years of encouragement and gracious hospitality. Sam is a great-great-nephew of Johns Hopkins. I first met Sam in the mid-1990s, and we have since spent many pleasant hours in his living room, sipping tea and talking about the need to give Mary Elizabeth Garrett the recognition she deserves. Over the years, Sam showed an uncanny sense for when my energies were flagging and I needed a hearty pep talk to jump-start the project. He never failed to call with a much-welcomed invitation for lunch, often hinting at an intriguing tidbit of history that would once again pull me back to task.

Jim Garrett, a great-great-nephew of Mary Elizabeth Garrett, and his wife, Edie, eagerly supported the project from the first moment. Jim welcomed an examination of his family and was always on hand to answer questions and provide otherwise unattainable documents. He offered a present-day family touchstone to the long-ago subject of the biography.

I thank the staff of the Johns Hopkins University, who were instrumental in bringing the story together. In the mid-1980s, Nancy McCall of the Alan Mason Chesney Medical Archives rescued long-forgotten documents and with Elizabeth M. (Rooney) Peterson began to compile what is now a substantial Mary Elizabeth Garrett collection. Nancy, Rooney, and I spent long hours brainstorming about Mary, delving into the intricacies and nuances of her life. Also of great assistance at the medical archives were Andrew Harrison and Marjorie Winslow Kehoe, who designed a beautiful website, "Celebrating the Philanthropy of Mary Elizabeth Garrett."

Many faculty members of the Hopkins School of Medicine find Mary's perseverance and determination an inspiration to their work in medicine today and prominently display her portrait in their offices. I have greatly enjoyed getting to know them over the years and learning about the challenges they face in the awe-inspiring profession that they have chosen for their life's work. They have initiated several programs in the School of Medicine that work toward the improvement of women in medicine and recognize Mary's legacy, notably the Women's Leadership Council, overseen by Janice E. Clements, PhD, as vice dean of the faculty, and the Department of Medicine Task Force on Academic Careers of Women in Medicine, under the consultation of Emma Stokes, PhD. In 2005, the School of Medicine in collaboration with the Fund for Johns Hopkins Medicine started the Mary Elizabeth Garrett Leadership Fund to raise money to advance women in the medical profession.

Archivists and librarians are a researcher's best friend and I greatly appreciate many along the way who helped to track down important, hard-to-find documents: Layne Bosserman of the Enoch Pratt Free Library in Baltimore; Lorett Treese, Marianne Hansen, Barbara Ward Grubb, and Eric Pumroy of the Bryn Mawr College Special Collections Department; Peggy Woodward, former archivist, and Elizabeth Di Cataldo, archivist, of the Bryn Mawr School; Jackie O'Regan, former curator, and Cindy Kelly, former director, of Evergreen House; and Francis O'Neill of the Maryland Historical Society, H. Furlong Baldwin Library.

Helen Lefkowitz Horowitz played a vital role in shaping the manuscript from its first expansive draft to its leaner, more focused final iteration. She brought unique talents to the project as a renowned historian and authority on the Garrett-Thomas relationship and women's education. I am grateful for her close, critical scrutiny of the manuscript. Robert J. Brugger, history editor at the Johns Hopkins University Press, enthusiastically welcomed the manuscript and nurtured it along the way. Copy editor Susan Lantz expertly crafted the manuscript and smoothed the rough patches. I thank them both for their guidance and care.

I also appreciate several colleagues who read all or parts of the manuscript or offered their expertise, notably James D. Dilts, Courtney B. Wilson, John P. Hankey, Karen M. Footner, Doris Weatherford, Eric L. Holcomb, Judith Bair, and Robert I. Cottom. I thank Hasia Diner for being close at hand with insight and direction for twenty years.

Early in my research I had the good luck to communicate with Donald Garrett Dickason of Princeton, New Jersey. After retiring from a long career as a college administrator, Don began an ambitious project to document the extended Garrett clan through DNA testing and research. His work greatly helped to piece together elusive details of the Garretts' immigration to the United States in 1790 and their earliest years in Pennsylvania and Maryland. Don passed away in July 2006. I very much appreciated his enthusiasm in sharing his research.

Several artists have become part of the collective effort to bring Mary's story to a wider audience. Actors Yvonne Erikson and Kate Briante have poignantly portrayed her life in one-woman dramatizations. Brece Honeycutt's lovely sculpture *Silence*, first unveiled at Evergreen House and now permanently installed at Bryn Mawr School, captures the many restrictions imposed by society on Mary Elizabeth Garrett and women of her generation. In 2006, Fairfax County, Virginia, seventh graders Madeleine Stokowski and Elizabeth Yim took home second-place honors in the National History Day competition for their documentary film *Strings Attached: How Mary Elizabeth Garrett's Philanthropy Revolutionized the Study of Medicine.*

The Washington Biography Group, ably led for twenty-five years by Marc Pachter, director of the Smithsonian Institution's National Portrait Gallery, provided helpful monthly discussions and a roomful of sympathetic colleagues with whom to commiserate on the ups and downs of biographical research and writing.

In 2005, I was fortunate to travel to Russia to teach for a semester at St. Petersburg State University on a Fulbright grant. I thank the Council for International Exchange of Scholars and the Fulbright program for providing that once-in-a-lifetime experience. I frequently lectured on philanthropy and voluntarism, activities of critical importance in a democratic society but concepts that are only slowly gaining acceptance in Russia. As I lectured on grass-roots reform, I found myself gaining a greater appreciation of the vital role played by voluntarism in American culture and of how philanthropists such as Mary Elizabeth Garrett have been an exceptional force in building great institutions in the United States.

I am forever grateful for the support and patience of my husband of thirty-five years, John, who has lived through enough unsolicited dinnertime lectures about Woman's Exchanges and Mary Elizabeth Garrett to write sequels to the books. And always, I appreciate the encouragement provided by my journalist daughter, Libby Sander, Bryn Mawr College Class of 1999. She benefited—as have so many others—from the great generosity of Mary Elizabeth Garrett.

Mary Elizabeth Garrett

QUIET REVOLUTIONARY

" *I* wish Mary had been born a boy!" John Work Garrett, the nineteenth century's great Railroad King, often thundered about his only daughter and youngest child, Mary Elizabeth.[1] His was not the usual lament of a father wishing for a son to carry on the family name. He had sons to do that. Rather, his regret was that his daughter—his bright and capable child, his adoring devotee, who was well suited to become his heir apparent—was prohibited by social convention from following in his footsteps.

Yet Mary Elizabeth Garrett, every bit her father's strong-willed, resilient daughter, emerged triumphantly from the shadows of such restrictions to become one of the country's most influential philanthropists, reformers, and behind-the-scenes "railroad women." In the Gilded Age, when a woman's name rarely appeared in the newspapers—save for a titillating arrest report or a review of a fashionable gala—Mary's name often occupied the headlines. She was a favorite of the turn-of-the-century press, who were fascinated by her unique combination of wealth, activism, business expertise, and extraordinary philanthropy. She became one of the country's most publicized women, unselfishly using her money and status to transform women's lives and to break down the barriers that prevented women's equal participation in society.

Beginning in 1884, when she inherited one of the largest industrial fortunes of the time—the *Chicago Tribune* reported she was the "wealthiest spinster in America"—and continuing until she died in 1915, her name was associated with the most important women's movements of the day. She pushed beyond woman's traditional sphere, inching her way into the inner sanctum of the male-dominated world of railroading. In an era when women could not sit at the corporate table as equals to the captains of industry, Mary used her railroading knowledge to covertly manipulate control and influence. "But that she is a woman," a commentator wrote of her business savvy, "she would to-day be President of that road" (the Baltimore and Ohio Railroad). "She is probably better posted on railroads and their intricacies than any woman in the world," the New York Times noted of her often-concealed intrigues inside the family-directed B&O. She "possessed business capabilities ranking among the financiers of America," the Baltimore News concurred.[2]

Mary Elizabeth Garrett used her status and skills not to run a railroad but to advance an uncompromising vision for women's place in the expanding United States. Many of her contemporaries, such as settlement-house founders Jane Addams, Ellen Gates Starr, and Florence Kelley, and reformers Mabel Hoadley Dodge and Josephine Shaw Lowell, worked to improve the lives of wage-earning women and immigrants. Mary, instead, focused on elevating women through groundbreaking preparatory and higher education, graduate medical education, and suffrage. Through her philanthropies, she boldly expressed her vision of women's equal status in society as skilled physicians, well-educated leaders, and professional career women. "Miss Garrett [is] the most progressive woman of wealth our country has produced," asserted Frances Willard, president of the nation's largest women's organization, the Woman's Christian Temperance Union.[3]

For all of her stature and influence, Mary was a quiet revolutionary, never seeking attention or celebrity for herself. "She hated the limelight," the Baltimore News explained.[4] She did not give public speeches or write notable treatises. She forbade newspapers to run photographs of her. She preferred to work behind the scenes and let others take the credit for what she made possible.

Despite her reluctance, fame found and elevated her. During her lifetime, Mary was recognized as one of the country's most influential philanthropists at a time when such activities were identified primarily with wealthy men—Carnegie, Peabody, Vanderbilt, Rockefeller, and Hopkins. When large-scale philanthropy was just emerging, and few philanthropists dared to invest in the nascent, still unproven, field of academic medicine, Mary set a precedent. In 1893, she gave the money to start the Johns Hopkins University School of Medicine. "Gives Away a Fortune," the Baltimore American proclaimed of the gift that ended the two-decade struggle to open the nation's first graduate-level medical school.[5]

But it was not how much she gave, but rather how she gave her money that made her a pioneer. Mary fine-tuned the art of "coercive philanthropy."[6] She did not just give money away; she carefully controlled how it was spent. She used her wealth as a bargaining chip, often a blatant bribe, forcing policy change at male-run institutions to equal the playing field to women's advantage.

Little did anyone suspect that the new, all-male Johns Hopkins University would become a battleground for women's advancement. When making her gift to Hopkins, Mary insisted on the unheard-of condition that women medical students be admitted "on the same terms as men." Her revolutionary gift marked a milestone for women. "American women have scored another significant victory," a Chicago newspaper proclaimed.[7] As important was that her gift created a new, elevated academic model bridging American medicine from a backward nineteenth-century profession to the modern age of scientific enlightenment of the twentieth century.

Mary continued her unique style of philanthropy by infusing Bryn Mawr College in Pennsylvania with extraordinary amounts of money, once again with a rigid requirement: that her intimate friend and companion, Martha Carey Thomas, be appointed president. Through her largess, Baltimore's Bryn Mawr School, which she had helped to found in 1885, gained prominence as a pioneering preparatory school for girls. Her final years were spent with longtime friends Susan B. Anthony and Anna Howard Shaw, working tirelessly on suffrage and continuing her work toward equal rights for women.

While Mary's life story provides a colorful example of opulent Gilded Age material wealth and extravagance, it also reveals much more about the restrictions and frustrations many women endured. In an era of unbridled runaway capitalism, extremes of great wealth and abject poverty, and unparalleled greed and guile, how did women, who ranked as second-class citizens—even wealthy women like Mary Elizabeth Garrett—respond? Then, as now, philanthropy allows us to examine those issues of most concern to individuals and society. Mary fully understood, through personal disappointments and setbacks, the impediments women faced in a male-dominated society. She watched as her brothers and men around her enjoyed opportunities and visible signs of success, while women often were left behind in a society that allowed such disparities. Mary's philanthropies were motivated by the opportunities that had been denied her. By looking at her activism, we can better understand the barriers she and her contemporaries hoped to break down.

Mary's philanthropies have left a lasting legacy on American culture and, similarly, were of central importance to her own life. Like many women of her era who reinvented themselves in highly creative ways, Mary's activism allowed her to break free of Victorian-era expectations of matrimony and motherhood. She forged her life's work through philanthropy, transforming herself from a shy girl into an innovative reformer—and one with clout. She finally found the voice that had been silenced in her early years.

But like many women who broke through Gilded Age expectations, she paid an extraordinarily high price for her nonconformity. Her singular vision to fulfill her philanthropic convictions, to advance women in the public sphere, caused her once-valued relationships with family and friends to fracture and fall away, often leaving her tragically lonely and ill. In the roller-coaster economy of the late nineteenth century, her great fortune ebbed and flowed. She often lived on the financial edge to fulfill her philanthropic commitments.

Mary embodied a host of contradictory traits. She was painfully shy in public, yet lively and enthusiastic with friends. She often was swayed by others' powerful personalities, yet stood firm when negotiating a deal. She could be comically frugal in mundane matters, yet extravagantly generous with her philanthropies. She was chronically incapacitated with real or psychosomatic illnesses, yet bore the tremendous, almost unimagined, weight of her financial commitments on her own. She could be fiercely loyal to her causes but compromised longtime relationships when they impeded her goals.

Although Mary's life was one of great personal accomplishment and, often, despair and disappointment, it can only be told within the historical context of her powerful and visionary family and the role they played in shaping the nation. Baltimore, the city that nurtured her, and the Baltimore and Ohio Railroad, which her family directed for three decades, also figured prominently in her life. Situated precariously between North and South during the turbulent years of the nineteenth century, Baltimore combusted with ideas, innovation, and divisiveness. Polarized between old Southern traditions and restless "New Women," it percolated as a hotbed of feminist and anti-feminist activism.

Mary hailed from a long line of great institution builders. The Garretts of Baltimore reigned as one of the most influential mercantile families on the East Coast through much of the nineteenth century. Mary's paternal grandfather, Robert Garrett, a poor Irish immigrant, prospered in the commercial abundance of antebellum Baltimore. He looked to the West, to the lucrative interior of the new United States, for Baltimore's commercial future and made a fortune hauling valuable goods in his Conestoga wagons over the National Road.

Mary's father proved even more legendary. John Work Garrett ruled the Baltimore and Ohio Railroad, the nation's first major railroad, with an iron, often brutal, hand, steering it through the perilous years of the Civil War and serving as a valuable advisor to President Abraham Lincoln. In the war's tumultuous aftermath, he helped struggling Baltimore to get back on its feet. It was said that "no one could commence a business venture from New York to Washington without his approval."[8] In post–Civil War America, Mary's family rose to national prominence and unimagined wealth.

In this larger-than-life epic drama of wars, politics, railroads, and commercial expansion across the country, Mary emerged an unlikely candidate to bear the family's legacy. She struggled to find herself among male ambition and success. Like all well-to-do young girls of the antebellum era, she was expected to be inconspicuous and obedient and to learn her future obligations as a proper upper-class woman. But the Civil War changed life for all Americans. The postwar years offered exciting, undreamed-of opportunities for women. The world for which Mary had been carefully prepared no longer existed.

It was no accident that this quiet young woman would make a lasting impact on American culture. Her beloved, powerful father was the most dominant force in her life. As she grew to maturity in the years after the Civil War, her father exemplified the possibilities that lay beyond the Victorian-era expectations of female domesticity. She was exposed to the world of high finance and railroading as few women were. She became her father's personal secretary, accompanying him on railroad business and meeting the great men of the era. She enjoyed an unorthodox education under his guidance and learned how to be a shrewd negotiator, a skill that would serve her well as a philanthropist. She won her father's hard-earned respect. "During her father's lifetime, she was his close friend and confidante," the *Baltimore Sun* noted. "He relied a great deal upon her judgment."[9]

Her father's trust validated her worth as a woman. She was not an invisible daughter. He valued her. In return for her father's confidence, she devoted her life to enshrining his memory and promulgating his legacy. She relished carrying the Garrett family name and imprimatur, often expressing the sentiment, "I have my father's name and pride."[10]

Nineteenth-century American women's history is replete with examples of the power of the father-daughter relationship. Louisa May Alcott died, heartbroken, on the day of her father's funeral. Jane Addams, bereft at her father's untimely death, dedicated her life's work and *Twenty Years at Hull House* to his memory. Lucy Stone's activism was, in part, fueled by her father's refusal to pay her tuition at Oberlin College, even though he had the means to do so. Elizabeth Cady Stanton spent her life avenging the abused and broken women who came in tears to her father's law practice.

Mary also drew strength from a lifetime of strong female friendships, starting first with close companions in Baltimore, her lively, inquisitive "Friday Night" group of young women, and later through a national network of prominent activists, including writer Sarah Orne Jewett and physicians Mary Putnam Jacobi and the famed Blackwell sisters, Elizabeth and Emily. In the Victorian era, female friendships often were an integral part of a woman's life, providing emotional and social support in a society in which men and women were highly segregated.

For the most part, Mary's friends and associates were women who chose, for various reasons, not to marry. They did not want to center their lives on husbands and children. With the brilliant and charismatic Carey Thomas, Mary forged a lifelong emotional bond and a powerful working relationship. Thomas's undisputed position as the nation's leading advocate and spokeswoman for women's higher education combined with Mary's wealth, family status, and business skills to form a dominant and complementary force for women's advancement.

We are fortunate that Mary was not "born a boy," as her father had wished, for we would have been denied one of the nation's most effective philanthropists, reformers, and visionaries. Today, her legacy pervades our lives. In the academic year 2003–04, more women than men were enrolled in American medical schools.[11] They are educated at coeducational medical schools with exacting academic standards—thanks in large part to Mary's far-sighted gift to open the nation's first coeducational, graduate-level medical school at the Johns Hopkins University. Young women attend college preparatory schools with high scholastic requirements—thanks to the innovative thinking of Mary Elizabeth Garrett and the other founders of the Bryn Mawr School. A highly selective doctoral degree–granting women's college, Bryn Mawr College, continues to educate women leaders for the future—thanks to the largess of Mary Elizabeth Garrett a century ago. Women have the right to walk into a voting booth and enjoy other advancements that evolved from the suffrage movement—thanks to the dogged determination of thousands of women nationwide and the much-needed financial assistance of women like Mary Elizabeth Garrett.

As important, Mary Elizabeth Garrett helped to set the stage for contemporary large-scale philanthropy, not only in medicine but also for women. Today, women wield enormous power through their philanthropic giving. Whether through inherited or self-made wealth, women represent a dominant force in the American voluntary sector. A century ago, Mary broke through prevailing stereotypes, showing how one woman, politically disenfranchised and socially marginalized, could dramatically change society through large-scale gifts. In the Gilded Age, when wealthy men exerted power through philanthropy, Mary exemplified how the purse could serve as an alternative power source for women. She showed how women, too, could be institution builders through their philanthropy.

Perhaps Mary Elizabeth Garrett's greatest legacy is her generosity of spirit to give other women what she had been denied. She might have kept her great wealth for herself. Yet she chose to share her fortune for generations to come, dedicating her life to help women live "on the same terms as men."

—◦◦◦—

CHAPTER 1

GARRETT'S ROAD

ROBERT GARRETT AND SONS

Had Mary Elizabeth Garrett's arrival into the world at 3:30 A.M. on March 5, 1854, been announced in the newspapers—a convention not yet fashionable—Baltimoreans more than likely would have taken little notice. They had far more serious matters to think about. Baltimore, a thriving, polyglot port city, the third largest in the nation and founded in 1729 on the principles of benevolence, tolerance, and philanthropy, now festered with divisiveness and unrest. Nativist Know-Nothings, with their campaign of hatred and bigotry, controlled City Hall. Secession was a word heard all too often in Maryland, the slave-holding state that precariously straddled North and South. By 1854, the saber-rattling over slavery and states' rights that had consumed North and South for decades had intensified, as Baltimore increasingly felt the effects of dangerous, discordant events that were unfolding daily throughout the country. The fraying nation, with Maryland at its explosive epicenter, inexorably moved one step closer toward complete conflict.

But on that early March day, political hostilities and the specter of war must have seemed far removed from the Garrett home. Mary's father, John Work Garrett, dutifully noted in the well-worn family Bible that his fourth child, the first Garrett daughter in three generations not to be assigned the first name of Elizabeth, was "born on the Sabbath." The happy parents presented their infant daughter with a coral necklace. Her three older brothers—Robert, born in 1847; T. Harrison, nicknamed Harry, born two years later; and Henry, born in 1851—were on hand to greet the newest member of the family.[1] (Henry Garrett, named after his paternal uncle, Henry Stouffer Garrett, suffered from an undisclosed malady in infancy and remained an invalid for life. Very little is known about him.)

Mary had the good fortune to be born to parents who shared a passionate, highly compatible marriage. Theirs was a match made in heaven, a warm and loving relationship. "No hint of scandal" marred the Garretts' lives. A family friend once remarked, "I have never seen in all my life an instance where man and wife were more completely a unit." John Work Garrett and Rachel Ann Harrison had married eight years earlier, in 1846, at the bride's home on Cathedral Street near Centre Street, where Rachel had been born twenty-three years earlier. The twenty-six-year-old groom gave his bride a ruby and diamond wedding ring, and her father presented her with a gold bracelet and matching necklace set with emeralds and pearls.[2] The newlyweds settled into a three-story house on the south side of Fayette Street, between Howard and Eutaw streets, not far from Baltimore's busy harbor.

The Garretts and the Harrisons were prominent Baltimore mercantile families that had prospered for a half century. Rachel, often called Rit or Ann, was one of ten children of Ann Maria and Thomas Harrison, a successful merchant and a member of Baltimore's city council. She was "a charming lady, gentle and kindly in manner and bright and interesting in conversation," an observer noted, "active and vivacious." Already well established as one of Baltimore's grande dames by the time she gave birth to Mary, Rachel was "one of Baltimore's most gracious ladies."[3]

Like her contemporaries of the upwardly mobile merchant class, Rachel had been raised with proscribed, inflexible expectations for her place in life — to be an attentive, nurturing mother and a steadfast helpmeet to her busy, beleaguered husband. In the antebellum years, an entire industry of popular culture, including such publications as William Alcott's 1837 book *The Young Wife* and the magazine *Ladies' Garland*, advised a dutiful wife to assure that her home was "a refuge from the vexations and embarrassments of business, an enchanting repose from exertion, a relaxation from care by the interchange of affection" for her husband. According to most accounts, Rachel lived up to such lofty expectations. She was her husband's "companion of all his hours — those given to business as well as to home life."[4]

Mary's father, scion of a wealthy merchant family, would have needed a supportive wife and able "companion of all his hours." Thirty-four years old when Mary was born, John Work Garrett was already making his mark on Baltimore commerce and proving to be a sound successor to his father, Robert Garrett. John Work Garrett had come a long way since Robert's humble, impoverished beginnings in the United States sixty years earlier.

Robert Garrett's early life captures the poignant story of countless immigrants at the turn of the nineteenth century. At the age of seven, in 1790, Robert, his Scots-Irish parents, John and Margaret MacMechen Garrett, and his siblings had sailed with 210 brave souls aboard the brig *Brothers* from Lisburn in County Down, near Belfast in Northern Ireland, to Pennsylvania. They set out for their new life with only a few meager farm tools in hand, eager to "devote themselves to the culture of the earth." But despite their hopeful start, like many immigrants who made the hazardous Atlantic crossing, Robert's forty-year-old father did not survive the journey to see his adopted homeland. "Before reaching the destined port, the hand of disease rested on the patriarch of the band after but a few hours of severe illness," the ship's captain noted of John's sudden death. "His mortal remains were committed to the deep."[5]

Young Margaret, only twenty-nine when left husbandless on the high seas, carried on, her fatherless children in tow, entering through the Port of Wilmington, Delaware. They quickly found help among family friends in Baltimore, where a "fatherly Mr. Morris prepared the Garretts for a more permanent location in Cumberland County," near Harrisburg, Pennsylvania.[6] Margaret's brother-in-law, Andrew Garrett, already was established there on a modest farm that included one horse and two cows.

The young widow and her clan joined an energetic population of settlers scattered on homesteads and in hamlets in the interior of William Penn's former Quaker colony. The lush, rolling land must have looked familiar to the weary travelers. It closely resembled the fertile, verdant fields of Northern Ireland they had left behind. Energetic and eager to provide for her young family, Margaret took well to the land and "cultivated the farm successfully." The Garretts stayed in central Pennsylvania for eight years, before moving west in 1798 to a farm near the newly incorporated village of West Middletown, in Washington County, Pennsylvania.[7] The busy little hamlet lay a few miles southwest of Pittsburgh, not far from the Ohio River.

West Middletown, known in Robert Garrett's time as West Middle Borough, with its hodgepodge of brick and wooden buildings of no particular architectural style and smelling of barnyards and stables, was not unlike countless little commercial crossroads sprouting up across rural America. Nonetheless, it left an indelible mark on young Robert. Like many such cauldrons of diversity, the little town festered with religious animosity. Thomas Campbell, an Irish immigrant disgruntled with the local Presbyterians, spun off his own heated brand of Calvinism, whose followers were eventually known as Cambellites of the Christian Church. As an adolescent, Mary's grandfather thrived in West Middletown's spiritual bickering. He threw himself squarely into the religious frenzy of the little village and soon found himself "warmly attached to all the peculiarities of Presbyterianism."[8]

During his years in Pennsylvania, Robert, like most Americans at the time, did what he could to patch together a livelihood. He joined up with a teamster, Captain Alexander Sharp, not far from the toll road soon to become the National Road, which would shape his own destiny and that of the young nation. Sharp put Robert to work in his tannery and "on his wagons," changing the huge wheels on the endless parade of rickety wagons that traversed the always-busy, raucous road. It was dangerous and punishing labor, and it did not take long before Sharp found that his ambitious new employee "showed an extraordinary capacity for business." He encouraged Robert to move on and seek his fortune in Baltimore by opening a trading business. Sharp promised to use his influence to send Robert "all the patronage to be had." Reluctant at first, Robert soon took the boss's advice. As a "mere lad" of seventeen, he moved on to better prospects in Maryland.[9]

Settled by a Roman Catholic—Cecil Calvert, Lord Baltimore—Maryland, the "middle colony" named for its mid-Atlantic location and the hybrid nature of its culture, opened its doors to immigrants and progressive ideas unwelcome elsewhere. Maryland's Religious Toleration Act of 1649 had codified the colony's commitment to diversity and acceptance. By 1828, Jews had attained the right to vote. The Society of Friends, or Quakers, scorned and persecuted in New England, found refuge in Maryland, just south of their heartland in Pennsylvania. After Quakerism's founder, George Fox, visited Maryland in 1672, the sect, with its liberal progressivism, flourished in Baltimore and Annapolis.

Baltimore took its name from an ancient fishing village in southwestern Ireland in County Cork, "the parish nearest America." Founded to export the colony's most valuable commodity, tobacco, the Baltimore of a century later "throbbed with all of its business," trading with the Far East, Europe, the West Indies, and South America.[10] At the time of its charter, Baltimore had faced steep competition from its more senior neighbor to the southeast on the Chesapeake Bay, Annapolis, the "Athens of America," where wealthy tobacco planters and merchants lived in baronial splendor and had for nearly a century garnered political, social, and economic clout for the robust colony.

But Baltimore stole the crown and soon gave New York and Philadelphia a run for their money as well. With its deep harbors and idyllic mid-Atlantic seaboard location two hundred miles farther inland than its northern competitors, it did not take long for Baltimore to edge closer to omnipotent New York. In a situation similar to that of New Orleans, an almost-equal mixture of free and enslaved blacks, around ninety thousand of each, coexisted in Baltimore, often working in similar occupations with European immigrants. African Americans created an invaluable labor force for Baltimore and a rich culture that thrived within a diverse, heterogeneous population.

There could not have been a better place than Baltimore for an ambitious young frontier merchant to strike it rich. A "gay, brave town famed for its progress," as one admirer described Baltimore at the turn of the nineteenth century, would have welcomed an enterprising merchant such as Robert Garrett to ensure its prosperity and financial status on the highly competitive eastern seaboard. More than seventeen hundred wagons, carts, and fishing boats brought prized goods into the bustling city each day to trade. Baltimore boasted "tall church spires and a new cathedral, neighborhoods of genteel civility and boisterous activity," and, not least, a theater lighted by "aeriofoam gas," as the newspapers delighted in advertising.[11]

Starting as a clerk in the produce and grocery commission house of Patrick Dinsmore, Mary's grandfather soon established the commercial partnership of Wallace and Garrett. Successful from the start, in 1820 he opened his own wholesale grocery business at 34 North Howard Street, aptly naming it Robert Garrett and Company. Setting out on a new, solitary venture seemed a tenuous proposition at the time. The country had plunged into its first major economic depression after the onset of industrialism. The Panic of 1819 would last nearly three years, striking both rural and urban Americans with equal ferocity. Banks and businesses failed at an alarming rate. To make matters worse, a yellow fever epidemic raged through Baltimore, forcing many businesses to temporarily close. Although competing with some of Baltimore's oldest and most established firms, Robert Garrett and Company held its own.

Bright, ambitious, and, most important, familiar with the potentially lucrative hinterlands, Robert Garrett knew well the riches that lay beyond the Allegheny Mountains. The seemingly endless interior of the vast continent had long seduced him. As a boy living near Pittsburgh, he often had paddled down the Ohio River as it snaked its way south between Ohio and Virginia, turning west at the mouth of the Muskingum River near Marietta, into what in 1803 would become the seventeenth state, Ohio. From there, he had made his way into the bountiful interior to trade with the Shawnee and Delaware tribes, returning each spring to West Middletown laden with furs and other valuable goods to sell through a network of nearby towns and villages. Knowledge of this area would prove crucial for the Garretts' and Baltimore's later commercial success. While other Baltimore merchants in the early decades of the nineteenth century traded in worldwide markets, Robert Garrett instead looked to the region of his childhood in Western Pennsylvania and beyond to the vast stretches of the expanding, abundant nation.

Boisterous and bawdy Howard Street, where Mary's grandfather opened his business, was the commercial hub of the prosperous port city, with its huge warehouses and lively taverns serving whiskey at three cents a glass. Inside the spacious, three-story warehouse of Robert Garrett and Company, precious goods, either coming from or going to the West, accumulated. No matter from which direction the goods came or went, they all passed through the Garrett warehouse, "solid, broad, [with] three floors and a garret, with deep cellar."[12] Out front, on the dirt street, teams of huge "six-in-hand" Pennsylvania farm horses stood adorned with jingle bells, anxiously waiting to pull the bulky blue and white, boat-shaped canvassed Conestoga wagons along the National Road and across the mountains. The National Road, "America's Main Street" as it often is called, traversed the country's easternmost mountains, connecting the overcrowded Atlantic seaboard with the unlimited possibilities and wide-open land that lay to the west. As the horses impatiently snorted and chomped, workers at the Garrett warehouse piled prized eastern manufactured goods and raw materials into the massive wagons. When all was made ready, the Conestoga caravan, reminiscent of an ungainly trading procession on the ancient Silk Road, plodded out of downtown Baltimore, slowly making its way west through the village of Frederick, Maryland. It then turned northwest onto the National Road to make the dangerous trek over the Alleghenies. Ahead lay the intimidating, hazy, blue mountains, unfolding one three-thousand-foot peak after another. On a good day, Robert's convoy might trudge ahead twenty miles on the bumpy, noisy, two-lane thoroughfare, which passed a few miles south of the Garrett farm in West Middletown.[13]

Mary's grandfather held sway over his rapidly expanding mercantile empire of Robert Garrett and Company from the tiny counting room of the warehouse. Abandoning the frontier garb of his rural Pennsylvania boyhood, the successful young Baltimore merchant epitomized "the *gentleman debonair*, wearing only black clothes, sometimes with a white necktie and the low-quartered, well-blacked shoes in which he dressed his shapely feet suggested he had given up pumps and silk stockings."[14]

In the early years of the nineteenth century, Robert Garrett joined a dynamic group of young men who were similarly seeking their fortunes in Baltimore, men such as Johns Hopkins, William Walters, Enoch Pratt, and George Peabody. Garrett, Hopkins, and Peabody established business and social ties that would continue through future generations and would shape Baltimore's commercial fortunes and cultural prominence.

Hopkins, named Johns from the maternal side of the family, was born in 1795 at Whitehall, a tobacco farm fifteen miles from Annapolis, the second of eleven children. His devout Quaker parents, Samuel and Hannah, freed their slaves, preferring instead to put their own sons to work in the fields. Hopkins came to Baltimore in 1812, a few years after Robert Garrett had arrived, to join his uncle's grocery business, helping to keep it financially afloat during the war with the British. "Buy goods and do the best thee can," Hopkins's uncle had enthusiastically advised his ambitious young nephew.[15] And he did. Hopkins started his own wholesale company, Hopkins Brothers, and soon earned the first of his fortunes selling "Hopkins Best" whiskey, for which, it was said, the Quaker gentleman later expressed regret.

George Peabody, born in South Danvers, Massachusetts, also in 1795, entered into partnership with Marylander Elisha Riggs to form a prosperous trading house. After two successful decades in Baltimore and making the first of his many fortunes, in 1837, he opened one of the first American financial firms in London. He expanded the interests of booming American companies, such as Robert Garrett and Company, through his vast European commercial contacts and started the company that later in the nineteenth century would become the famed financial House of Morgan.

Drawing on his friends and contacts from his early trading years in Western Pennsylvania, Robert's new business pushed ever westward. News of the success of Robert Garrett and Company and its extensive trading network moved quickly up and down the National Road by word of mouth. Distribution centers and trading houses as far away as Indiana soon struck partnerships with the enterprising young merchant.[16]

By the 1820s, Mary's grandfather had risen to commercial primacy. The once-penniless Irish immigrant, "by nature affable and courteous in his intercourse, either as a man of business or socially," became a "venerable citizen." Robert Garrett's vision to channel the goods of western farmers through the port of Baltimore and out to the wider world proved valuable to Baltimore's commercial ascendancy. "Mr. Garrett was among the foremost in insisting upon Baltimore's looking for the future mainly to the West, and taking her position in the vanguard of the western march of American enterprise," an observer wrote.[17]

Continuing his earlier Presbyterian "peculiarities" from his boyhood in West Middletown, Robert presided over the board of Baltimore's Associate Reformed Presbyterian Church and financed the church's new edifice. Civic-minded, philanthropic, and eager to improve his adopted city, he served on the boards of the Baltimore Water Company and the Baltimore Gas Company and started the Western National and the Eutaw Savings Banks.[18]

And he married well. On May 19, 1817, he wed twenty-six-year-old Elizabeth Stouffer, daughter of a Baltimore merchant who traded with the West Indies. Their marriage produced five children, with Elizabeth enduring three pregnancies in as many years. Henry Stouffer was born in 1818; Robert Close, in 1819; John Work, Mary's father, in 1820; and Elizabeth Barbara, in 1827. Robert Close died at age five in 1824, and little is known of the fifth child, James, who apparently did not survive infancy.[19]

As a mature elder statesman, Mary's grandfather struck a dashing figure, a "tall gentleman, erect, largely framed, not corpulent, with white hair, a kindly eye, a firm, yet sweet mouth and his smooth-shaven skin hale with the uniform roseate tint of healthy old age." He hospitably greeted customers, "holding his spectacles in one hand and the newspaper in the other."[20] In 1833, the fifty-year-old Irish immigrant became a citizen of the country whose future he was helping to shape.

Education became a priority for Robert's sons. Unlike their immigrant father, who had little formal education, Henry and John benefited from the best education of the day. Both attended Boisseau Academy in Baltimore. Henry went on to Belair Academy in Harford County, north of Baltimore. At age fourteen, John attended a preparatory school operated by Lafayette College in Easton, Pennsylvania, and later matriculated to the college.[21]

Like many sons of the merchant class, the fates of Mary's father and uncle were sealed at birth. They would follow their father into the family business. By 1839, Robert Garrett and Company was so prosperous that its owner welcomed his two sons as partners, conferring their rising status in the rechristened Robert Garrett and Sons. With the addition of his bright, capable sons, Robert's company slowly transformed from a successful trading company to a powerful, influential financial house.

There was no ascending easily to top management for the two junior partners. Henry and John were expected to learn the family business from the bottom up. They settled into their respective duties and began a grueling apprenticeship under their father's guidance. They learned to tan leather, as their father had done forty years earlier with teamster Alexander Sharp. They mastered salting pork and packing madder and Spanish whiting. Henry stayed in Baltimore, while John headed west to expand the business over the mountains. Like his father before him, John's firsthand travels through Virginia and into Ohio, Kentucky, Indiana, and beyond would prove valuable, reaffirming Baltimore's advantageous location to trade with the interior. From the start, Mary's father displayed a sixth sense about Baltimore's most profitable commercial direction, and, like his father, believed that Baltimore's prosperity lay to the west. An observer noted that he "obtained a thorough business education and a practical knowledge of the vast resources of that Western country to which he was afterwards to contribute so largely in brains and money."[22]

Mary's father and uncle proved hardy enough for their formidable roles as Baltimore's new antebellum merchant princes. Both were large men, about six feet in height. John was described as "handsome, impressive and vigorous." He was "a man of large, commanding frame, more portly than his father; his face, full with large forehead, heavy eyebrows and a firm mouth." The *Baltimore Sun* found him "large, with strongly marked features indicative of great will power and immense capacity for endurance. His face was kindly as well as intelligent." While physically resembling his younger brother, Henry had a different temperament, more flamboyant and mischievous. Those who knew him described his "manly, massive form" and his "playful words."[23]

Both sons showed natural entrepreneurial flair. They caught on quickly, expanding Robert Garrett and Sons in innovative directions: buying new warehouses, building hotels—notably the Howard House and the Eutaw House—and securing new international trade routes and business associations. At the end of the Mexican War, in 1848, Robert and his sons turned their attention to the American Southwest and the lucrative markets of California. They built the *Monumental City*, the largest steamship in Baltimore. It made regular runs between Baltimore, New Orleans, and San Francisco. The company added to its fleet and expanded business to South America and Europe.

By the mid-1850s, with a wife, four young children, and a profitable family business to his name, John Work Garrett began his move up, away from the Garretts' first home on Fayette Street near the center of town. John and Rachel joined the procession westward, a mile away, to Baltimore's newly created suburb near Lexington and Fulton Streets, an area that eventually became known as "Garrett Park." Horse-drawn trolleys easily connected the well-to-do residents from their new suburban homes to downtown. The *Baltimore Sun* pronounced that Baltimoreans could "reside at a distance from the places of business in more healthy locations without loss of time and fatigue of walking."[24]

The tranquility of the neighborhood was shattered one night when the Garrett house caught on fire. Mary's brothers, Robert and Harry, just youngsters, were dramatically rescued and "carried to the house of neighbor, General George H. Steuart."[25]

By the time she was two years old, Mary's family moved again, not far away, to a larger, semi-detached mansion on "Delaware Place" facing fashionable

Franklin Square, with expansive townhouses selling at $10,000.[26] The upscale neighborhood gained fame "as the most inviting place of rural beauty in the city . . . attracting numerous companies of ladies and gentlemen to its pleasant walks and shady bowers."[27] Fortunate Franklin Square residents enjoyed the newest urban amenities of indoor bathrooms and freshwater reservoirs. The square's elegant mansions surrounding a bucolic park were set back from the noisy street and featured large windows and French doors, iron balconies and finely carved mantels. A sampling of Baltimore's elite lived nearby: dry goods magnate R. M. Sutton, Judge Henry Stockbridge, and Governor Augustus Bradford.

The Garretts frequently escaped to Landsdowne, their country home in Baltimore County, a few miles south of Franklin Square, not far from the Patapsco River.[28] There, they converted an old farmhouse into an enjoyable rural retreat, allowing the children boundless room to play and Mary's father to indulge his avocation of husbandry.

Despite the luxury that surrounded her at Franklin Square and the country comforts of Landsdowne, Mary's earliest memories were of a dismal and lonely childhood. First, there was the matter of her preoccupied brothers, Robert and Harry, who seemed to want nothing to do with their little sister and proved to be of little use as companions. "I was 5 yrs. younger than my second brother," she later wrote of the age differences, "and had no sisters and knew few children."[29]

More serious, though, were Mary's health problems. Yellow fever and typhus frequently swept through the busy port city. The chilling record of disease and death were published regularly by the city's Health Office in the Baltimore newspapers, a testament to the ineffectiveness of the medical profession to fight off infectious disease. The list included "dropsy and diphtheria, organic diseases of the heart, inflammation of the bowels and lungs; and convulsions and consumption." Mary and her brothers, living safely away from the pestilence of the harbor, escaped the ravages of the all-too-common nineteenth-century childhood diseases. Even if a child survived infancy, a plethora of infectious microbes could strike at any moment. Despite the availability of the country's fifth medical school at the College of Medicine of Maryland just a few blocks away from the Garrett home on Franklin Square, scientific medicine and medical education, still in their embryonic stages, could do little to fight calamitous disease.[30]

Mary's problems were of another, more chronic nature. "When I was about eight months old," she later wrote, "a very serious trouble with the bone of the right ankle developed, which seriously affected my general health."[31] The family physician, Dr. Nathan Smith, attributed the trouble to a careless nurse, who had let Mary fall. When all hope of mending the injury was nearly exhausted, Rachel took her youngest child to the fashionable Victorian spa of Cape May, New Jersey, where Mary "took the treatments." She improved, but very gradually.

By the time most children start walking around the age of one, Mary was confined to leg braces, which she wore for several years. "For some years," she recalled, "I wore [a brace] with irons, and then one with whalebones." She did not have the stability to walk without braces until she was four years old and did not wear what she described as "ordinary" shoes until about the age of ten. For many years, until she was twelve or thirteen, she depended on the braces. This ankle injury, which would in one form or another plague her for life, only served to strengthen her physical fortitude and mental stamina. "I became a very strong child," Mary later wrote of her childhood ordeal.[32]

Despite the best medical care and treatment at the spas of Cape May, there was little doctors could do to correct an injury that would certainly affect the growth of the leg. The inactivity in her childhood caused weight gain and awkwardness, making her feel unattractive and shy. "I was heavy and the lameness made me less active than ordinary children and also more solitary," she later recalled.[33]

Photographs of Mary at this young age do not reveal an injury or unattractiveness. Her calf-length dresses and high-top shoes concealed her ankle infirmity. With an oval face that revealed pleasant features and dark, pulled-back hair, she was a pretty child. She was every bit her father's daughter, already displaying the Garrett propensity for fullness, the "heaviness" that she described. At a young age, six or seven, she wore the fashionable, but rigid, clothing of an adult woman: full, stiff dresses supported by layers of petticoats required of proper young ladies, even those just barely out of the nursery.

But other, far graver concerns than Mary's ankle injury gripped the Garrett family. By 1854, the year Mary was born, the once-powerful Baltimore and Ohio Railroad, on which Baltimore and the expanding Garrett commercial empire had depended for more than two decades, faced dire financial problems. The B&O sputtered and threatened to stall. The financial instability of the all-important railroad sent shock waves through the city—and the Garrett family.

A MAN OF VAST POWERS

More than likely, Mary's father, then eight years old, joined several hundred other onlookers on the cool, brisk Independence Day in 1828, for the grand celebration when the cornerstone of the Baltimore and Ohio Railroad was laid at Mount Clare Shops. The festivities took place less than a mile from John Work Garrett's

boyhood home on Fayette Street. The crowd cheered as ninety-year-old Baltimorean Charles Carroll, the only surviving signer of the Declaration of Independence a half century earlier, vigorously turned the first spade of dirt to set the cornerstone in place. "I consider this to be among the most important acts of my life,
second only to signing the Declaration of Independence, if even second to that,"
the elder statesman noted prophetically of the significance of the day. "The result
of our labours will be felt not only by ourselves, but by posterity—not only by Baltimore, but also by Maryland and the United States."[34] The gala event marked the
centennial celebration of Baltimore's founding.

That day also signified the beginning of what would become a decades-long,
highly complex, and mutually beneficial financial relationship among the Garretts, Baltimore, and the nation's first major railroad, the B&O.

The inauguration of the B&O could not have happened a minute too soon. The
railroad was "born as much out of fear as out of high ambition," an observer noted.
Baltimore's lucrative trade with the interior suddenly faced fierce competition.
After the War of 1812, other eastern seaports, particularly New York, increasingly el-
bowed their way into the vast resources of the West. By the 1820s, Baltimore and its
critical lifeline to prosperity, the National Road, came face-to-face with a formidable obstacle. The Erie Canal, two hundred miles to the north, with its more efficient means of shipping goods to the interior through a seamless network of canals
and rivers, threatened to render the National Road obsolete and boost New York's
trading dominance. Transporting goods by mule-drawn barges on the canal slashed
transportation costs between New York and Ohio by as much as 90 percent.[35] The
"Big Ditch," as the canal came to be called, became a big problem for Baltimore.

Hand-wringing Baltimore merchants and bankers gathered in early 1827 to
form a committee to debate "the best means of restoring to the City of Baltimore,
that portion of the Western Trade which lately has been diverted from it by the introduction of Steam navigation."[36] The committee faced a conundrum. Trying to
replicate the Erie Canal by building a proposed 340-mile canal from Baltimore
and across the Allegheny Mountains to the Ohio River was out of the question.
The cost was staggering: $22 million. The idea was quickly quashed.

The committee soon found an unlikely candidate to save their city, a seemingly awkward and very peculiar mode of transport: a horse-drawn wagon on
tracks. "Railroads," recently developed in England, were just in their embryonic
stage, but were proving to be efficient and cost effective. Pennsylvania had tried a
short-haul railroad, the Portage Railroad, to run between Hollidaysburg and
Johnstown. Farther north, in Quincy, Massachusetts, the modest but successful
three-mile Granite Railroad had opened in 1826, hauling granite blocks.

The Baltimore committee turned to the State of Maryland for financial backing, applying for a bill to incorporate a joint stock company. By March, the legislature complied and newspapers announced the first public sale of fifteen thousand shares of stock. No one could have imagined the wildly enthusiastic response. Within four hours on the first day, all but about a thousand shares were sold. "Excitement had gone far beyond fever heat and reached the boiling point," a commentator wrote of the buying frenzy. By the twelfth and final day of stock sales, forty-two thousand shares, valued at more than $4 million, were sold to twenty-three thousand shareholders, some scraping together enough money to buy only a fraction of a share. The railroad "is bringing an empire to our doors," the *Baltimore American* boldly pronounced.[37] The B&O, which inaugurated America's transportation revolution, had been formed and financed within two short months. It represented the first public-private partnership in corporate America.

The founders dreamed no small dreams. They proposed to construct a railroad that would essentially run parallel to the National Road, traverse a formidable mountain range, and span major rivers and gorges. Such a daring and financially extravagant plan had never been tried before in the United States. They aimed to stretch and connect their new railroad across the vast continent, through the newly incorporated states and loosely confederated territories, and out to the Pacific within three decades.

In 1830, after the line's second year, inventor Peter Cooper modernized the B&O, and all of railroading, with his steam-driven "Tom Thumb" locomotive. Over the next decades, the B&O pressed ever forward, slowly winding its way across the Allegheny Mountains near the timeworn paths of the National Road, where Robert Garrett's Conestogas had hauled beeswax and kegs of powder a few years earlier.

But fulfilling the B&O founders' dreams proved difficult. The inauguration of the B&O opened a floodgate of competition. The line was continually burdened with too much debt and too little capital to keep up with its fast-growing northern rivals. Enormous engineering obstacles faced the B&O with each new river to cross and each new mountain to scale.

By the B&O's third decade, the Garretts had become integral to its survival and, in return, greatly profited from the relationship. Johns Hopkins, similarly, was quick to see the potential of the railroad and enthusiastically invested in it, eventually becoming the company's largest stockholder and most powerful board member. In 1853, Robert Garrett and Sons sold bond issues to help finance the railroad's westward expansion, using company investment outlets to raise the money. The company advanced $1 million to construct the crucial 131-mile line to connect Bellaire, a few miles south of Wheeling, to Columbus, Ohio, opening the B&O to the lucrative markets of the West. Although private funding, such as that provided by Robert Garrett and Sons, helped to expand the B&O, the city and state went into debt to build the line. Marylanders were taxed to support the railroad, from which only a handful of major stockholders greatly profited.

Mary's uncle, Henry Garrett, served as a B&O director and, in 1854, Mary's father also joined the board. John Work Garrett craftily engineered a scheme to increase dividends to 30 percent, a move that would greatly benefit the Garretts and Johns Hopkins, the major stockholders. But the board split on the idea.

The debt of the line continued to mount. In 1854, the Baltimore City Council extended a $5 million emergency loan to relieve some of the B&O's enormous debt, but the last-ditch attempt was not enough. Worse, the Panic of 1857, another of the country's economic depressions that ferociously struck every two decades "fell with a force upon the struggling Baltimore & Ohio."[38] The railroad faced calamity.

On November 17, 1858, the B&O board called a special meeting to decide the future of the struggling line and, by association, the fortunes of Baltimore. "All members of the board were present, in view of the fact that the meeting was held especially for the election of a president," the *Baltimore Sun* reported.[39] Johns Hopkins, a director since 1847 and chairman of the financial committee, represented stockholders who hoped to keep the line in private hands. Chauncey Brooks, the B&O's incumbent president, was renominated and represented the State's interest to control the railroad. Dissension and divisiveness filled the meeting room on that November day.

Hopkins stepped forward to nominate Mary's father, his thirty-eight-year-old protégé and son of his friend and associate for half a century, Robert Garrett. Hopkins had lobbied long and hard for Garrett's candidacy, wining and dining opposing directors to convince them of Garrett's ideal traits for the demanding job. Johns Hopkins's nephew, Joseph, later recalled, "We knew that Uncle Johns wanted Mr. John Work Garrett to be president of the Baltimore and Ohio Railroad. There was a great deal of opposition to it among the directors of the road; but I knew that Uncle Johns had determined to put it through. He told me he was going to have a dinner for the directors of the road and [he] wanted me to get some frogs from the pond at Clifton [Hopkins's country home]. We had a great deal of curiosity to see how Uncle Johns would get his way with the opposing directors. Champagne and wine flowed freely during the dinner."[40]

The vote was finally cast. The results were close: sixteen for Garrett and fourteen for Brooks. By a vote of two, the B&O remained in private hands. Johns Hopkins's lobbying had worked.

The board asked the new president to address the group. The *Baltimore Sun* reported that, "Mr. Garrett was conducted to the chair by Johns Hopkins, Esq., and being called upon for an explanation of his view addressed the board." Garrett emphasized his unquestionable loyalty to the railroad and to Baltimore, recalling his family's long-standing interest in Baltimore's prosperity. "My ancestry have been identified with Baltimore for many generations and I, born in your midst, have all my interests, my affections and my future here," the new president affirmed in his acceptance speech. "I have no higher pride—no greater ambition, than to lend my humble efforts to promote the advancement and prosperity of my native city and my native State."[41]

He reiterated the Garretts' financial support of the railroad and their struggle to keep the company successful. "When this great road was opened to the Ohio River, and the disappointment in the extent of business from that source was felt by all, in common with others I spared neither personal efforts nor private means to aid in completing connections virtually essential to Baltimore to the great centre of the western railway system—and those efforts have resulted in securing a communication with the West by which a stream of prosperity has been continually poured upon us that must be appreciated by all." Like the B&O founders thirty years earlier, John Work Garrett dreamed big. He assured the board he would promote "all commercial, mechanical, manufacturing, mineral and agricultural interests traversed by the road." He concluded his address by asking "the cordial cooperation of the board in accomplishing the results equally desirable to all."[42]

It was as if by divine providence that Mary's father stepped in on that day to rescue the rapidly failing railroad. He was the right man for the job, a charismatic visionary who would lead the company in highly imaginative, entrepreneurial ventures in the years ahead. The new president would prove to be tactful, persuasive and, most importantly, financially generous with legislators; autocratic, almost tyrannical in his management; and brutally forceful and uncompromising with the wage earners who kept the railroad running. Perhaps most imperative in the bloodthirsty railroad business, he could be as ruthless and driven as his competitors. He was "a man of vast powers and abilities. Of huge size, he usually dominated the men around him, both physically and mentally. He possessed all the great qualities of leadership. He had, when he needed it, real charm. He was the personification of firmness itself," an observer noted.[43]

Over the next quarter of a century, Mary's father would rise to become the most powerful man in Maryland. Like a handful of other railroad giants, Garrett would yield "near-absolute power with a skill that bordered in recklessness." In an era when a railroad could make or break a city's fortunes, Garrett would keep Baltimore in the running. "[T]o the day of his death, the word of the President of the Baltimore and Ohio was law to the Governors, all state officials, including senators and members of the House of Representatives," a commentator wrote.[44] Within just a few years, Garrett, in effect, gained complete control of the B&O.[45]

Garrett's election to the B&O presidency began an unprecedented reign that soon earned him national celebrity as "the Railroad King." From that point forward, the history of the country's first major railroad would be characterized simply as "Before Garrett, Garrett, and After Garrett."[46] The words of loyalty to the railroad and Baltimore that Mary's father spoke following his election on November 17, 1858, would resonate in every action he took as president over the next twenty-six years. Garrett, along with his guide and mentor, Johns Hopkins—the two most important men involved with the B&O—would steer the railroad and Baltimore through the next, even more perilous chapters.

The new president inherited a fractious and fragmented board, demanding stockholders, labor unrest, and the largest number of workers—eight per mile—of any railroad. Like for most railroad tycoons of the day, the well-being and safety of the B&O workers was of little concern to Garrett, as long as they kept the trains running on time, full, and profitable. Garrett's new domain included one of the most expansive railroads of the day, with a $26 million capital investment, 4,500 employees, 236 locomotives, 3,668 freight cars, 124 passenger cars, and an annual operating budget of more than $2 million.[47] Agreeing on an annual salary of $4,000—a pittance compared to the value of the B&O stock the family already owned—the new president faced the almost insurmountable challenge of trying to keep his influential investors happy with a robust dividend, while remaining competitive in the country's most cutthroat and vicious industry.

What set the B&O apart from its competitors and propelled it to national prominence in the waning days of the 1850s was its domain. Its 514 miles of track ran through both slave-holding and non-slave-holding states in what would soon be the epicenter of the coming war. The railroad was caught figuratively and geographically in the middle. It originated in a slave state, but did most of its business with the North. Although profiting from Northern commerce, the B&O had Southern leanings. The *Wheeling Intelligencer* likened the B&O to "the amphibious animal that could not live on land, and died in the water." In his 1855 book on the first decades of the B&O, *Rambles in the Path of the Steam-Horse*, Ele Bowen explained: "The B&O is to all intents and purposes a Southern improvement, identified with Southern interest and built by Southern capital. It is, in fact, the only route by which Southerners can reach the Atlantic cities with

their servants unmolested by the wily 'underground' interference of crazy abolitionists, now swarming along all the great lines of travel in the State of Illinois,
Ohio and New York."[48]

Mary's father set out not only to restore the B&O to its glory days, but, as important, to transform his beloved Baltimore into a world entrepôt. "He was going
to make Baltimore a great ocean port, a world port," an observer noted. "That
would mean not merely improved docks and warehouses for his road at the wa-
terside of his chief town, but a Baltimore and Ohio steamship line, whose vessels
would find their way to all the important ports of the seven seas." Like his father
before him, John Work Garrett dreamed of connecting the riches of overseas markets with the thriving towns of the vast United States and the B&O, "Garrett's
Road" as it would soon be called, would serve as the pivotal link. From his earliest days as B&O president, Garrett, reaffirming his father's business sentiments,
"repeatedly confirmed and emphasized that Baltimore possessed remarkable
advantages of location as a port of shipment and market for the West."[49]

By 1860, the new president paid the lucrative 30 percent dividend he had
maneuvered earlier and continued extending the railroad westward. Garrett had
momentarily rescued the rudderless B&O. With the election of a vigorous, competent and aggressive new railroad president, the fortunes of Baltimore were
looking up. So were the Garrett coffers. The extravagant stock dividend set the
precedent for others that would follow, making Garrett and his major stockholders very rich men. It was, however briefly in the beginning of the foreboding decade of the 1850s, "an era of fine pickings," as one commentator noted.[50]

Mary's family enjoyed the fine pickings that John Work Garrett's new stature
and prosperity conferred. With his position as president of the B&O solidified,
Garrett's young family rose to prominence. The Garretts had come a long way
since Robert Sr.'s Conestoga wagons lumbered across the National Road to the
hinterlands fifty years earlier. The Garretts had outgrown Franklin Square. The
railroad president and his family were ready to begin their reign among Baltimore's royalty. There was no better place to show their ascendancy than at Mount
Vernon Place, Baltimore's most prestigious address.

AN AIR OF ARISTOCRACY

In the antebellum age of gentility and civility reserved for a rarefied few, Baltimore proudly displayed its rising prosperity at elegant Mount Vernon Place. Located a mile north and a world away from the noisy and foul-smelling waterfront
and factories, where the workers who contributed to the city's wealth lived in

shanties and crowded wooden row houses, sedate, stylish Mount Vernon Place by midcentury had become the preferred address of the city's new mercantile elite.

It was here, beginning in the early 1860s, living among Baltimore's successful and visionary leaders, that Mary learned how to be a proper young Baltimore lady—and an innovative philanthropist and activist. Mount Vernon Place would provide Mary's geographical and social grounding throughout most of her life.

A generation earlier, the tree-lined square had been the southern tip of Belvedere, a sprawling estate owned by Baltimore's Revolutionary War hero John Eager Howard. In 1809, Howard donated the land, the highest point in the city, to erect a monument to his friend and the former commander-in-chief of the Continental Army, George Washington. On July 4, 1815, thirty thousand people gathered at the site to watch the laying of the cornerstone of the monument. Fourteen years and $200,000 later, the nation's first Washington Monument was completed. Robert Mills, who would later create a similar memorial to the first president in Washington, D.C., designed Baltimore's 178-foot obelisk. Herman Melville catapulted Baltimore's monument to national stature in 1851 when he wrote in *Moby Dick; or the Whale* that "Great Washington stands aloft on his main mast in Baltimore and like one of Hercules' pillars, his column marks that point of human grandeur beyond which few mortals will go."[51] The fame of the monument sent residents into such a frenzy of monument building that Baltimore soon earned celebrity as "The Monumental City."

One-by-one, the city's well-to-do merchants and industrialists moved to residences lining Mount Vernon Place's four adjacent small parks, laid out in the form of a Greek cross that converged at the foot of the towering Washington Monument. Mount Vernon Place showcased the nineteenth century's most notable American architects, each outdoing the other to build larger and grander townhouses for Baltimore's elite class. The famed architects created an eclectic mix of then-fashionable Italianate, Greek, or Renaissance Revival styles that up-and-coming industrialists favored to replicate Old World classicism. Many of the grand three- and four-story mansions boasted ten-foot-high marble fireplaces, sturdy, classical columns on ornate facades, intricately detailed interiors, hot water and the greatest extravagance of all—indoor water closets.

Mount Vernon Place left no doubt about its residents' place in society. A visitor to Baltimore in 1848 observed that "the houses are fine, spacious and elegant. There is, moreover, an air of aristocracy, which is seldom to be met with. It is clear enough that aristocrats live in this place, and although Americans decry this class of men constantly, there is certainly something about a people and institutions, of the aristocratic caste, which gives the impression of superior dignity."[52]

Mary's family soon joined the aristocratic caste. Her grandparents were the first to establish a Garrett presence on Mount Vernon Place. In 1856, Robert and Elizabeth Garrett commissioned architect Louis L. Long to build a mansion at 101 West Monument Street, on the southwest corner of West Monument and Cathedral Streets.[53] Long, who had recently completed the stylish "Brownstone Row" on the other side of the square, designed one of the grandest of the Mount Vernon mansions for the Garretts.

Unfortunately, Mary's seventy-four-year-old grandfather could not enjoy his sumptuous new home, so far removed from his hardscrabble Pennsylvania childhood of a half century earlier. He died suddenly on February 4, 1857, at the Eutaw House Hotel, where he and Elizabeth had been living during the construction of their Mount Vernon Place mansion. "He had retired in his usual good health (which had been uncommonly good for one of his age) on Monday evening," the *Baltimore Sun* reported the next day. "At about two o'clock the next morning he was taken suddenly very ill." The doctor was summoned and determined that Robert suffered "an attack of paralysis." All was done to revive him, "but he lay in his condition until life was extinct."[54]

The *Baltimore Sun* concluded, "his life, which has been one of usefulness . . . passed as to command the good will of all who knew him."[55] The funeral, attended by "a very large number of the old friends of deceased and prominent businessmen," was held at Robert's beloved Associate Reformed Presbyterian Church, which had been his spiritual mainstay since his earliest days in Baltimore.[56] He was buried in the family plot at nearby Green Mount Cemetery, at the northern line of the city.

Mary's Uncle Henry moved into the newly finished Garrett mansion, where he lived with his unmarried sister, Elizabeth Barbara, nine years younger, and their widowed mother, Elizabeth. The mansion was valued at $600,000 — an extravagant amount at a time when a laborer on the B&O might spend one dollar a week for boarding-room rental.[57]

Facing north on Monument Street, the Garretts' home was a thirty-room, three-story, Italianate brick mansion. It featured an imposing entrance portico supported by fluted Doric columns and tall French windows with surmounting brackets on the first two floors. A double flight of exterior marble stairs converged at the front door. The Washington Monument, a beacon of the area's affluence and stature, stood just a block away.

Inside the mansion, the black-and-white marble-floored foyer led to a grand staircase that gracefully wound its way to the upper floors. The top floor housed the servants. Like similar Victorian Age mansions, the Garrett mansion's dark, wood-paneled rooms displayed the finest furniture gathered from exotic parts of the globe. Heavy armoires, possibly mahogany or rosewood, overstuffed chairs, sofas, marble-topped tables, portieres, and bookshelves crowded the rooms. Rich damask draperies shielded the wealthy residents from the tumultuous outside world and the dirt and dust of the unpaved streets. Expensive hand-woven carpets covered the marble and parquet floors, and landscape paintings, portraits, and tapestries — along with clocks, gilded mirrors, and brass ornaments — covered every square inch of wall space. By midcentury, most homes of the wealthy used gas lighting, an improvement over the oil lamps and candles of the average family.[58]

The mansion had little yard for strolling or reposing. The private Mount Vernon Park outside the doorstep served those purposes. Like the green at Franklin Square, the small park enveloped by stately homes had been fenced in 1845 to maintain its exclusivity to nearby residents.[59]

The John Work Garretts left Franklin Square and followed the rest of the family to Mount Vernon Place. They moved to 50, now 12, East Mount Vernon Place, into a Federal-style, three-story townhouse, next to "Brownstone Row" on the north side of the park.[60] They could look diagonally across the park, past the Washington Monument, to Henry Garrett's mansion, two blocks away. The alley behind the house's stables became known as "Garrett Alley."

From either end of Mount Vernon Place, the Garretts, Mary's Uncle Henry at 101 and Mary's family at 12, commanded full view of the graceful square and its grand buildings. Just a stone's throw away from Henry, at 11 West Mount Vernon Place, in 1853 Samuel K. George built a stylish townhouse. Two decades later, John Work Garrett would buy this house for Mary's brother Robert as a wedding present. Nearby, Latrobe's Basilica of the Assumption, called "North America's most beautiful church," stood as a symbol of Maryland's founding principle of religious tolerance.[61]

Diagonally across the park from Mary's house, One West Mount Vernon Place, built for Dr. John Hanson Thomas and his family, gained fame as "one of the most elegant and princely specimens of architectural taste" on the East Coast. The twenty-two-room mansion concealed a secret chamber, a wine cellar, a conservatory, and a terrapin bin to store the succulent Maryland culinary delicacy. Nearby, merchant William Tiffany, a cousin of the New York Tiffanys, in 1842 built an impressive late Georgian mansion with British Doric columns on a double lot. A few doors west of Henry Garrett's mansion another successful merchant, Enoch Pratt, who made a fortune selling mule shoes, horseshoes, and nails, built a three-story Greek Revival mansion for $250,000 in 1847. Its unembellished facade reflected the no-nonsense owner. It was said that if Pratt, who hailed from a frugal old New England Puritan family, spotted a salable nail lying on the street, he would stop his carriage to pick it up and sell it.[62]

William Walters lived at 5 West Mount Vernon Place, where he assembled Baltimore's finest art collection. He earned his first fortune as a grain merchant. But, like fellow Baltimorean Johns Hopkins, who lived in a more modest townhouse a few blocks south on West Saratoga Street, Walters soon discovered that Marylanders liked whiskey as much as they did their Chesapeake Bay crabs and oysters. By the 1850s, he owned the country's largest wholesale liquor business. Walters later acquired lucrative banking and railroad interests, where he made an astronomical fortune. In later years, his son, Henry, reputed to be the wealthiest man in the South, spent an estimated $1 million annually to expand the Walters' famed art collection.

Despite suffering from the dual blows of a childhood leg injury and uncompanionable, disinterested older brothers, Mary's life on Mount Vernon Place took on the same routine followed by other daughters of wealthy East Coast families. In her earliest years, she watched as her older brothers Robert and Harry went off to school and enjoyed independence in the wider world, while she remained closer to home. Robert attended the Dahl School in Baltimore and later was sent to the Friends School in Providence, Rhode Island.

Unencumbered by household chores, young girls of Mary's well-to-do class were expected to join literary clubs and to socialize within a small circle of similarly elite friends. Records do not indicate if Mary had a tutor in her early childhood, although it is likely she did. She immersed herself in the world of literature, first the primers required of a young girl and later the classics and novels that were becoming popular in midcentury. This led to her lifelong quest for self-education. She became an avid reader. "I read fluent Eng. [English] before I was six & read everything I could lay my hands on from that time on, good, bad, & indifferent, by sunlight, lamplight or firelight as long as I could see the paper," she later wrote.[63]

Mary also would have been expected to learn etiquette and the fine art of making social rounds, as her mother had learned a generation earlier. While men gathered at their clubs well away from feminine interference, wealthy antebellum women "called on" each other in their homes. And one had to be properly dressed to make social rounds. Charles Street, the main boulevard connecting Mount Vernon Place to the center of the city, gained fame, according to one commentator, as "the thoroughfare of our best society . . . which on a fine afternoon is thronged with the fashion and elite of our city." Living in a busy port city, Baltimore women were accustomed to the latest fashions from the capitals of Europe, whose styles they imitated. Ships arrived daily in Baltimore's harbors stocked with "silks, satins, millinery and other choice materials to delight the feminine heart."[64] To help sort it all out, by the 1850s, a plethora of women's magazines regularly pronounced the latest fashion to eager and always anxious readers.

But just as Mary was mastering the art of endless social rounds and instructions on fashion, there were other occupations that Baltimoreans, particularly the Garretts, took quite seriously: philanthropy and reform. As they ascended the social ladder, supporting civic programs through monetary contributions and helping to improve their city was as integral to the Garretts as managing the B&O and steering Baltimore's commercial future. At an early age, Mary was immersed in her family's civic activism, absorbing instructive lessons not only of how men could change the urban landscape but also how otherwise disenfranchised women could leave their mark through voluntarism. For this education, Mary's home on Mount Vernon Place was in exactly the right place.

By midcentury, Mount Vernon Place acquired the reputation not only as one of the wealthiest and most elegant urban areas on the East Coast, but also a center of innovative philanthropy in the United States. Through much of the nineteenth century, Baltimore counted the highest number of millionaire philanthropists in the country.[65] The city's penchant for philanthropy and reform could be attributed to a unique combination of factors: industrial wealth, religious idealism, Quaker progressivism, and not least, its unique geographical location between North and South, with its festering political issues and a diverse blend of free and enslaved workers. Baltimore became an incubator of activism and philanthropy.

Baltimore, like most urban areas, was sorely in need of philanthropists' good deeds in midcentury, and the city's wealthy patrons would not have had to look far to do good. Few Baltimoreans enjoyed the "good buildings and spacious streets" of the better neighborhoods described by a visitor to Baltimore in 1843.[66] Instead, the needy lived all around the grand houses of Mount Vernon Place, in attics, in alleyways, and in the ethnic neighborhoods that characterized the diverse city. Their presence was not nearly as visible as the titans whose massive mansions lined Mount Vernon Place.

While immersed in the innovative reform and philanthropy all around her in Baltimore, Mary's model of good works was much closer to home: her family. Mary's grandparents, Robert and Elizabeth, established the Garrett model of philanthropy that would come to define the family in the generations ahead. Robert continued his long-standing support of the Associate Reformed Church for half a century. Mary's grandmother, Elizabeth, set the example for the Garrett women by throwing herself into charitable work. She started the Society for the Relief of the Indigent Sick and the Baltimore Orphan Asylum, in which she remained active for fifty years. She also established the Union Protestant Infirmary. Her influence on Baltimore philanthropy laid the foundation for a later charity, the Association for the Improvement and Condition of the Poor.[67]

Mary's father, too, learned early to carry on the family tradition. His favorite organization was Baltimore's Young Men's Christian Association, an organization he enthusiastically supported throughout his life. The YMCA movement had started in England, and it did not take long for its ideas to cross the Atlantic. Like England, the United States was in the midst of rapid social and economic change brought on by industrialization and urbanization. YMCA founders offered examples of acceptable, Christian behavior by steering unmarried male wage earners away from the temptations of "the theater, the saloon, the ballroom, the gaming table, and prostitutes, whose 'feet go down to death, and whose steps take hold on hell.'"[68]

By the 1850s, Baltimore's wealthy philanthropists started other innovative, often secular, institutions. In 1852, Moses Sheppard founded the Sheppard Asylum; upon his death five years later, his bequest of $570,000 funded the institution. A decade earlier, in 1844, city leaders had formed the Maryland Historical Society to bring together the city's business, cultural, and philanthropic interests. Two years later, Baltimoreans raised $35,000 to build an elegant Athenaeum building to house the new historical society. By midcentury, residents of all ethnic and religious backgrounds were actively engaged in running orphanages, asylums, alms houses, and industrial schools.

As men left their mark of benevolence and reform, so, too, did Baltimore's women. All around her, Mary saw examples of how women used their voluntary organizations to improve their communities and push beyond societal restrictions to open opportunities for themselves in the public sphere. Cultural and charitable activities allowed women to carve a niche outside of the home, to break free of the rigid expectations of domesticity espoused in the popular press, and to do more than simply provide "a refuge from the vexations and embarrassments of business" for their overworked husbands. Antebellum women, instead, often found other, more visible and vocal means to make their presence felt. Through their voluntary groups, women connected locally and laid the groundwork for impressive nationwide networks that would explode in numbers and influence during and after the Civil War. They enthusiastically swapped ideas about their charities and along the way created a vibrant and powerful feminine culture, all the while leaving their indelible mark of reform on American culture. And best, such activity was acceptable, even expected. "The cause of benevolence is peculiarly indebted to the agency of women," a minister eagerly proclaimed in his Discourse on Female Influence. "She is fitted by nature to cheer the afflicted, elevate the depressed, minister to the wants of the feeble and diseased, and lighten the burden of human misery."[69]

Women, even wealthy women, generally did not control large amounts of money. Instead, they improved their communities and did their good deeds through old-fashioned elbow grease and, often, grinding hard work in their charities to help the needy. Morally charged women intent on perfecting an imperfect society waged a constant battle against poverty and what they perceived to be moral disintegration all around them. In Baltimore, brigades of benevolent women regularly made their way into the city's most blighted areas on their "friendly visiting" to the poor, to do what they could to ameliorate the misery of abject poverty—much of it caused by their industrialist husbands and fathers. They freely dispensed advice, perhaps not always welcomed, to poor women on healthful living, industrious habits, and most important, middle-class standards of morality and behavior. The Female Moral Reform Society, with energetic chapters across the country and a mission to convert "fallen women" into "true women," became one of the most widespread and popular women's groups in the antebellum years.

The names of Baltimore's charities left little doubt about their mission: the Corporation for Relief of the Poor and Distressed of Every Religious Denomination Whatsoever, the Humane Impartial Society for Poor and Needy Women, the Orphaline Charity School for Girls, the Female Association for the Relief of the Sick Poor and for the Education of Such Female Children as Do Not Belong to or Are Not Provided for by Any Religious Society, the House of the Friendless, and the Home for the Incurables.[70]

The wide circle of Garrett friends and acquaintances was similarly occupied. In 1857, Quaker Mary Whitall Thomas, whose daughter would one day become president of Bryn Mawr College and Mary's companion, along with another Baltimore activist, Margaret Elliott, opened a sewing school for needy girls in Federal Hill near the harbor.

But there was another issue that galvanized Baltimore's philanthropists and reformers, particularly the large and influential population of Quakers: slavery. The presence of slaves often most jolted visitors, particularly travelers coming from Europe or traveling south of the Mason-Dixon line for the first time. Baltimore often was their first experience with "the peculiar institution," as slavery was euphemistically called. Although slavery waned in Baltimore by the 1850s, its presence was palpable. Located in a border state next to the free-labor North, Baltimore's slavery was more fluid. Baltimore slaves often hired out to do skilled labor and infrequently saw their owners. They often mixed freely with free blacks.

Mary was surrounded by slavery, at Mount Vernon Place, throughout Baltimore and Maryland—and in her own family. In 1860, her father owned one male slave and employed a free black male and three white servants, two of whom were Irish females, a typical combination of free and enslaved household labor for well-to-do antebellum Baltimoreans. Across the street from the Garretts, in the Thomas mansion, a French governess worked with four free African Americans and two slaves.[71] Mary did not leave behind any account of her childhood encounters with slaves.

Abolition thrived in the slave-holding city. But the diligent efforts of Baltimore's philanthropists and abolitionists could do little to subdue the increasing rancor between North and South. The country waited uneasily for the triggering event that would bring the issues of slavery, states' rights, and most importantly, secessionism, to a boil.

The event that ignited the national conflagration occurred on the B&O. The rail line, which three decades earlier had promised riches to the struggling city, now embroiled Baltimore in the coming war. Mary's father and the B&O—"Garrett's Road"—moved to center stage for the prelude to the nation's greatest conflict.

The spotlight shifted to a federal arsenal in Harpers Ferry, Virginia, where in October 1859, John Brown and his ragtag band of insurgents waited to ambush an approaching B&O train and take control of the U.S. arsenal, with the intent of arming the South's enslaved labor force and inciting rebellion. John Work Garrett, notified quickly of the trouble, alerted Secretary of War John B. Floyd. A young officer, Colonel Robert E. Lee, was sent to lead the Marines to quell the insurrection. Justice was swift. Within two months, John Brown and his compatriots hung from the gallows. Lee, the conquering hero, and Garrett, the confident railroad president, rode victoriously, side by side, into the throngs of cheering crowds in Baltimore.

Within a year, the course to war was irreversible. John Brown's martyrdom had achieved the desired effect. It became, as one observer noted, "the curtain raiser" for the bloodiest of American events.[72] Battle lines were being drawn across the nation, as Maryland became a barometer of hatred between North and South. The state's predominantly Southern traditions and sympathies would eventually clash with its Northern economic dependency and political ties.

Mount Vernon Place, known for its tranquility, refinement and good deeds, would similarly break apart and come to symbolize Baltimore's anguished separation. The Garretts, who had spent a half century uniting and connecting the young country by trade and rail, now faced division within its own ranks. Like many families in the border state of Maryland, the Garretts would soon become a family torn by divided loyalties. Mary, the little girl, who considered herself to be "a very strong child," would need to call on every bit of that strength over the coming years.

—◦◦◦—

CHAPTER 2

ASCENSION

THE BROTHERS' WAR

Perhaps nowhere were personal vendettas and political animosities of the Civil War felt more keenly than in Maryland, the border state that lay geographically between North and South and politically on the fault line of the vitriolic rhetoric over states' rights, secession, and slavery. "It was a terrible time for all on the border," Mary later wrote as she looked back at that tumultuous era. For young Mary, the war years provided a poignant lesson in loyalties—political, economic, and familial. The "Brothers' War," as the Civil War was often called for the divisiveness it caused within families, took on personal meaning as it divided her nation, her city, and eventually her family. "When this war is over," English writer Anthony Trollope wrote during his visit to the city in the spring of 1861, "every man in Baltimore will have a quarrel to the death on his hands with some friend whom he used to love."[1]

Trollope's prophecy played out tragically on the Garrett stage. From ages seven to eleven, Mary watched as her father, as president of the B&O, increasingly wielded national influence with President Lincoln and the War Cabinet in Washington to help keep the fractured Union together. She often looked back to the excitement of that time when her father seemed to be a pivotal player in the great national drama. "The Baltimore and Ohio played a very conspicuous part and my father through his connection with it a very important part," she later recalled.[2] Unfortunately, despite his national stature, Mary's father could do little to prevent his own family from disintegrating into disunity and despair.

John Work Garrett—Southern Democrat, family patriarch, and railroad president—in 1860 staunchly affirmed the Baltimore and Ohio's role as "a Southern railroad." Although the line depended on Northern commerce, Garrett often made mention of "our Southern friends."[3]

He soon had to choose one side or the other. He made an economically sound decision, an about-face from his Southern stance. "His heart gave in to his head," a commentator noted.[4] Garrett made the essential 514 miles of B&O rail lines running through both slave and free states available to the former congressman from Illinois who would soon occupy the White House: Abraham Lincoln. Garrett knew that his own personal fortunes and those of Baltimore and the B&O would be better served by joining forces with the North, which could not hope to win the war without the indispensable B&O tracks that connected Washington, D.C., to its Union core. Garrett and the strategically placed B&O became crucial to the Union, demonstrating for the first time that in war, railroads were as essential as weapons. Over the next four years, the B&O would earn yet another moniker: "Mr. Lincoln's Road."

Lincoln liked Garrett from the start, dismissing rumors of the Garretts' pro-Southern sympathies. "I know Mr. Garrett and I like him very much," the president commented. "I don't believe all the things people say about his secessionist principles." Mary recalled that Lincoln offered her father "a major generalship . . . but he preferred to keep his own position."[5]

Not all the Garretts shared John Work's enthusiasm for Lincoln or preserving the Union. The house of Garrett soon became a house divided. Throughout her life, Mary remembered this time quite vividly as the turning point of familial relationships, particularly between her father and his brother and between her father and her own brothers. "My father was of course a Union man, but with very strong Southern sympathies, but he was alone in his family," she wrote.[6]

Mary's earliest years had been spent in isolation and illness in her secure and comfortable surroundings, first at Franklin Square and, by the early years of the Civil War, at Mount Vernon Place and the family's country estate of Landsdowne. But the war, with its dramatic events so inevitably linked to her father and the B&O, expanded her world, providing the first glimpse of the dangerous, yet exhilarating, prospects that lay beyond the shaded, gated park outside her sheltered home.

Life in the Garrett household suddenly turned upside down. "Our life was irregular, to the last degree," Mary remembered, "as we always waited for my father. His hours were very uncertain." But that uncertainty also brought excitement. It was during this time, as the impressionable young daughter sat at her father's knee, listening intently as he talked of the war and railroads, that Mary first experienced the intoxication of power, deal making, and celebrity. This was the masculine side of life, one much different from her mother's and her own projected paths. Her socialization during the turbulent war was far different from that of previous generations of young, well-to-do girls. "There was a good deal of excitement about my childhood," she later wrote, "for it was the war time and my father was in the thick of the struggle."[7]

Amidst the swirl of turmoil, young Mary watched and absorbed. The "good deal of excitement" she had noted unfolded daily in her house, as her father met with businessmen and politicians about the war. No longer did Mary feel isolated and lonely. "Interesting men from all over the country were coming and going all the time about all sorts of things," she remembered.[8] When not in consultation with Secretary of War Edwin Stanton or the financier of the war, Treasury Secretary Salmon P. Chase, Mary's father would be inspecting the B&O's tracks or meeting with military generals and state officials. Mary enthusiastically took every bit of it into her young mind. She liked to inconspicuously eavesdrop on her father's meetings whenever she could, under the guise of being immersed in one of the books she so loved to read. When the "interesting men" met with her father, she would sit, "curled up in a big chair in the library with a book and listening to all I could hear."[9]

Her father *was* in the thick of it, as Mary described. Well before the controversial sixteenth president of the United States took office in Washington, D.C., on March 4, 1861, Mary's father once again found himself pulled into the "theater of conflict" as he had been with John Brown's 1859 raid at Harpers Ferry.[10] This time, the spotlight shifted to Baltimore. Within five weeks of Lincoln's inauguration, the new Confederate States of America boldly announced the seriousness of their mission to sever ties to the Union by firing on the federal troops at the massive, still-unfinished Fort Sumter in Charleston Harbor, South Carolina, on April 12. Lincoln responded by calling up seventy-five thousand volunteers to quash the "secesh" rebellion.

A week after the firing on Fort Sumter, on the morning of April 19, Mary's father anxiously prepared for the arrival of a thirty-five-car train from the North bearing the first eager, Rebel-hating troops who had responded to Lincoln's call to arms. The train carried seven hundred armed troops from the Sixth Massachusetts Volunteer Militia of Concord and Lexington, along with unarmed volunteers from seven Pennsylvania companies. As the train slowly chugged its way toward "Mobtown," as Baltimore had been named just a few years before during the nativist Know Nothing riots, the men were told to load their rifles in preparation for entering the unpredictable city. They arrived at seven in the morning at the

President Street Station on the Philadelphia, Wilmington, and Baltimore Rail-road. A longstanding Baltimore City ordinance that prohibited locomotives in city streets forced the troops to disembark at the President Street Station on the east side of Baltimore's harbor and to make their way on foot across town to the Camden Station a mile away to board the B&O train for Washington. Within minutes, an angry, rock-throwing mob surrounded them. Police department mar-shal George P. Kane frantically telegraphed for military assistance, exclaiming: "Streets red with Maryland blood!"[11]

In Washington, Lincoln anxiously waited. "Why don't they come?" he asked as he paced, looking out the White House window.[12] He sent reinforcements to Baltimore, all the while wondering about the fate of the southward-bound Union troops.

At the B&O's Camden Station, Mary's father hurriedly worked to subdue the mob, marshalling the embattled troops onto the Washington-bound train one by one as they struggled their way through the treacherous crowd. "By his presence and influence," a commentator noted, Garrett helped to suppress the riot.[13] As the troops rode out of town, safely on board the B&O southbound for Washing-ton, some vengeful soldiers continued shooting out the windows, taking down a Maryland farmer along the way.

Before the skirmish ended, a dozen people, soldiers and citizens alike, lay dead and Baltimore earned the distinction as the first battleground of the Civil War. The *Baltimore American* earlier had predicted the day's tragic events: "Baltimore is to be the battlefield of the Southern Revolution," setting an ominous tone for the city's role in the quickly escalating war.[14] The first blood of the war that would eventually claim more than six hundred thousand lives was spilled in the heart of Baltimore, on the border ground symbolizing the fracture between North and South.

Although many would later claim that the riot represented but a fraction of Maryland citizens, the episode had lasting effects, forever branding Marylanders, particularly Baltimoreans, as pro-Southern, pro-slavery rabble-rousers and trou-blemakers. The April 19th riot reaffirmed John Work Garrett's support of the Union. He called the melee "misguided." "Rebels," instead of "Southern friends," increasingly punctuated his speeches.[15]

As Mary's father increasingly threw himself into the Union's effort to win the war—being summoned at a moment's notice to meet with Lincoln and the War Cabinet, passing along vital intelligence about Confederate movements, or mov-ing Union troops on the B&O to the first battles of the war—Mary's Uncle Henry stepped up his support of the war as well. But Henry chose different loyalties. The

Garretts' long-standing, yet tempered, pro-Southern sympathies were displayed prominently in Henry's enthusiastic support of Baltimore's secessionist movement. His reckless actions cost the family dearly in fear of public scandal and embarrassment.

Notwithstanding their very different personalities—Mary's father being the more serious and steadfast, her Uncle Henry the more flamboyant and affable—the two brothers enjoyed a close, comfortable relationship. Although two years apart in age, in their mature years they resembled twins, both large-framed with round, friendly, whiskered faces. They had developed a productive and complementary business relationship after working together for twenty years in Robert Garrett and Sons, with Mary's father often climbing on horseback to tend to business in the westernmost reaches of the Garrett commercial empire while Henry stayed nearer to home, solidifying business in Baltimore. John had married and produced four children. Henry remained unmarried, a Baltimore *bon vivant*. John had named his youngest son, born in 1851, in honor of his brother.

Yet, it was John, the younger brother, who chose the family's public affirmation to side with the Union. It was this issue that divided the brothers and the Garrett family and set Henry on an entirely different road during the Civil War.

When Mary's father ascended to the presidency of the B&O in 1858, Henry took over the family business of Robert Garrett and Sons, occupying a solid position in Baltimore with a reputation as a fair and skilled businessman. President James Buchanan and his secretary of the treasury often sought Henry's advice on banking and related financial issues. Henry was publicly described in glowing terms: "genial, full of pleasantry, and most companionable" and "having a mind accustomed to observation and sound reflection." He took a special interest in his church and had hoped to build a small parish in the mountains near the family's summer vacation retreat, Oakland, in Western Maryland. He loved classical literature and art and was especially devoted to Mary, her brothers, and the family business. He lived a companionable life with his younger, unmarried sister, Elizabeth Barbara, and their widowed mother in the spacious thirty-room mansion at 101 West Monument Street on Mount Vernon Place. "Towards that aged Mother . . . his filial devotion was such as is rarely seen and could not be surpassed," a commentator recalled.[16]

But Henry's familial devotion abruptly ended when it came to his brother's support of the Union. In direct and often dangerous counteraction to his brother, Henry threw his support behind perilous plots to undo Maryland from the Union. Mary wrote of the anxiety and rebelliousness in Baltimore and in her own family. She particularly remembered her uncle's secretive secessionist occupations during this time: "My father's only brother was always doing things that put him in danger of arrest."[17]

Henry Garrett was not alone. Far beneath superficial, everyday rebellions—women's Confederate-inspired dresses, Baltimoreans displaying anti-Union signs—lay far more sinister secessionist plots to free Maryland from Union ties and keep the Confederate Army armed. Baltimore secessionists developed an elaborate network to covertly ship arms to their comrades across the Potomac River. Dr. John Hanson Thomas was reputed to have stashed arms for the South in the concealed hideaway of his elegant mansion at One Mount Vernon Place. Even the city's police marshal, George P. Kane, hid an arsenal of Confederate-bound cannons, ammunition, muskets, and rifles in his warehouse. Many secessionist schemes were hatched at the outwardly sedate Maryland Club, where Henry ruled as a ringleader, at the northwest corner of Cathedral and Franklin Streets, a minute's walk from Henry's home on Mount Vernon Place.

Ironically, as they sequestered themselves from the increasing confusion of the outside world, Maryland Club members were, themselves, plotting their own brand of disorder. They cheered at the firing on Fort Sumter and applauded the rapid secession of Southern states from the Union in the following weeks. The daring steps by the rebellious Southern states only served to strengthen members' resolve to push Maryland in the same direction. Soon their ovations turned to action as they strategized and implemented their own "underground railroad"—far different from the underground network that secreted slaves out of Southern bondage—stockpiling warehouses with arms to ship to the Confederacy.[18]

The activities of the Maryland Club could not remain forever clandestine, and soon news of its members' treasonous tactics seeped outside its doors. Early in the war, federal troops grew suspicious and raided the club. Union General Benjamin F. Butler threatened that at the first sign of trouble, he would "put a bullet through it." Inevitably, Henry was arrested. Simon Cameron, secretary of war, gave the Garretts much-needed, discreet assistance, writing on September 1, 1861, "Learning that Henry Garrett has been arrested for some supposed want of loyalty to the government of the United States, I hereby order his release until this department shall have investigated the subject." The Garretts' attorney, Reverdy Johnson, also intervened for John Work Garrett. "Your brother Henry's case will not be reached for several days yet. When it is reached, if all the witnesses are here, as I do not suppose they will be, it will be postponed or continued," Johnson assured the anxious family. Henry's case was never heard.[19]

Such discoveries only tightened the federal reins on Baltimore and made the Garretts even more anxious about Henry's activities. Although many Baltimore business leaders eventually subdued their secessionist sympathies in favor of maintaining their commercial ties to the North—and staying out of jail—Henry remained openly rebellious and embroiled in the movement, continuing to put himself and the family in peril. Luckily for the Garretts, Henry escaped serious punishment for his treasonous activities, more than likely because of the valuable contribution his brother was making to the Union's survival. As Mary recalled, her uncle "would have certainly been in prison if it had not been for their confidence in my father at Washington."[20]

By the first months of the war, as his brother plotted to send arms and supplies to the Confederacy, John Work Garrett's visits to Washington to meet with Lincoln became more frequent. Lincoln did not need to be convinced of the importance of the Iron Horse—the railroad—in commercial or military ventures. Like his presidential predecessors Washington and Jefferson, who had endorsed building the National Road to connect the farthest reaches of the expanding nation, Lincoln was committed to building a national network of railroads.

Despite their importance, rail lines were vulnerable. Even before the first "official" battle of the war at Bull Run on July 21, 1861, Mary's father felt the wrath—and the vigor—of the competently led Confederate Army as the B&O faced some of the earliest confrontations of the war. Thomas "Stonewall" Jackson became expert at destroying key junctions of the B&O near the critical area of Harpers Ferry. Idiosyncratic and mediocre as a professor at Virginia Military Institute just months before, the fiercely religious Jackson transformed himself into a formidable foe on the battlefield, earning a generalship in the first year of the war. He successfully closed down much of the B&O for the first ten months of the war, destroying four hundred cars, forty-two engines, and shops, depots, and machinery. By 1863, before Jackson was accidentally killed by his own troops at Chancellorsville, Confederate troops had captured 150 miles, nearly 30 percent, of B&O tracks.[21] Jackson's vengeful destruction of the B&O reinforced Garrett's decision to back the Union.

Garrett complained to Lincoln in the early months of the war that the B&O lines were not adequately protected. He suspected that federal troops, under the control of Secretary of War Simon Cameron, were lax in defending the B&O, since Cameron sat on the board of the B&O's major competitor, the Pennsylvania Railroad, which would greatly benefit with the B&O sidetracked. Relief was soon in sight, however, when Garrett's longtime ally and friend Edward Stanton replaced Cameron, who decamped to Russia as U.S. minister.

Another former acquaintance moved into Garrett's world, but in a far more menacing way. General Robert E. Lee, who had so brilliantly led the Marines in capturing John Brown and his insurgents at Harpers Ferry in 1859, now wore a military stripe of another color as the Confederacy's premier commander of the Army of the North Potomac. Lee proved to be an even greater threat to the Union and the B&O than was Stonewall Jackson. By 1862, on his seemingly unstoppable march north into Pennsylvania, Lee repeatedly pillaged the B&O lines and the lush farmlands of Western Maryland. On his retreat from the Battle of Antietam on September 17, 1862, the bloodiest single day of the Civil War, with four thousand men killed and eighteen thousand wounded, Lee avenged the brutal battle by burning everything in sight. A B&O official wrote to Mary's father that the railroad lines could be traced "by a continuous line of fire" in the Confederates' wake.[22]

Despite Union losses, Antietam offered enough of a glimmer of hope for the Union that Lincoln soon drafted the Emancipation Proclamation, which was made public on January 1, 1863. But Lee's successful retreat back across the Potomac in a slow seventeen-mile procession alarmed Lincoln, who grew increasingly impatient with the timidity of Union general George B. McClellan. Many speculated that had McClellan stopped Lee in his tracks and finished the job at Antietam, the war might have ended there. McClellan, former president of the Ohio and Mississippi Railroad and a West Point graduate, was a friend of Garrett's. Shortly after the battle, Lincoln summoned Mary's father to accompany him to visit McClellan at Antietam. By the end of the meeting with Lincoln and Garrett, McClellan had been relieved of his duties. McClellan would remain a lifelong friend of the Garretts.

There was one force that Mary's father found much harder to conquer and control than Lee and Jackson combined: his own family. The war's divisiveness was dividing yet another generation of Garrett brothers beyond John Work and Henry: Robert and Harry, Mary's brothers. Two years into the war, the tedium of the classroom and life on Mount Vernon Place held little interest for Robert, Mary's restless, adventurous sixteen-year-old brother. In 1863, the lure of combat, youthful exuberance, the impassioned calls to arms—temptations that have lured countless young men off to war since the beginning of time—finally ensnared young Robert. Robert might have been seduced by the exciting, dangerous espionage of his Uncle Henry. Or perhaps the romantic notion of the legendary Lee, the indomitable Confederate hero, sitting astride his beloved mount Traveller, proved to be irresistible to yet another generation of Garrett men. Or possibly Robert was enticed by the adventures of another Maryland son, scion of an old, aristocratic family, who already had gained notoriety as a dashing Confederate hero. Harry Gilmor, raised in splendor in a castle-like mansion north of Baltimore and nurtured on the romantic chivalrous tales of Sir Walter Scott, slipped south across the Potomac and into legend as a swashbuckling, self-styled Southern warrior, enchanting the ladies and inspiring young men as he cut a swath of destruction.

For whatever reason, Robert stole away from home, from under his father's watchful eye, through the federal barricades that encircled Baltimore and ran off to join his father's old friend and now adversary Robert E. Lee's determined northward march. Lee had found many such enthusiastic Confederate recruits in Maryland. Mary recalled the night that Robert simply "disappeared."[23] John Work Garrett's son had joined forces with the man who was systematically trying to destroy the nation—and the B&O. Knowing their son had joined Lee sent John Work and Rachel into apoplectic rage and worry—and for good reason. Their child joining Lee's forces at any time in 1863 would have struck terror into the heart of any parent. Mary later wrote that Robert joined Lee in "the Valley of Virginia," which would have been especially frightening.[24]

After retreating to Virginia in the wake of the bloody Battle of Antietam in September 1862, Lee refortified his troops and carefully strategized his next attacks. Baltimoreans waited anxiously, fearing their city might be Lee's next target. Within a few months, Lee's forty-five thousand Confederate troops struck with a fury, not in Maryland, but in Virginia. Once again, the Rebel troops proved to be a fearsome force by sorely defeating Union troops of double that number at Chancellorsville, Virginia, in early May 1863. Now fully in control, Lee headed North with a vengeance, toward a sleepy little college town in southern Pennsylvania, Gettysburg. Overly confident, Lee sent his men into a suicidal attack, Pickett's Charge. At the end of the three-day battle in early July 1863, fifty-one thousand troops—twenty-eight thousand Confederates and twenty-three thousand Union— lay dead or wounded. The battle was, according to a Union bugler, "the work of the very devil himself."[25]

As it did many families in Baltimore, Gettysburg took a tragically personal toll on the Garretts. Rachel's brother was killed fighting for the Confederates. The family was enveloped in anxiety and anguish. Although only nine years old, Mary fully understood the chaos in her family and the impact of Robert's actions. She recalled when her father discovered Robert had run away. "It was that dreadful night," she wrote. Her father broke down and sobbed uncontrollably. That great bear of a man, so strong and steadfast in the public eye, had watched as his brother, Henry, had carried on treasonous activities and been arrested. Now his son, too, was in harm's way, aligning himself with the enemy. Perhaps the full enormity of the schizophrenic nature of the war and the toll it was taking on his family and the nation came crashing down on him at this instant. Mary remembered, "There was anxiety for all at home."[26]

Mary's father sent some of his men to retrieve Robert, who managed to elude his pursuers for a week. At last word came that he had been found. He was brought home. We can only imagine the scene at the moment when the captured young runaway was brought before his enraged father to answer for his transgression. Mary referred to this time as the "unhappy days of Robert's dissipation."[27]

Robert was not the only brother who had fallen from grace in their father's eyes. Garrett was also "dismayed with Harry's behavior," Mary wrote, although the details of the fourteen-year-old's misconduct are not known.[28] Before the war's end, Robert was packed off to Princeton College, well above the Mason-Dixon line and out of temptation's way. Harry soon followed. Her miscreant brothers' misfortune proved to be Mary's great chance, as her relationship to her father grew closer. In her brothers' absence, Mary increasingly began to perceive her role as a stabilizer in her father's tumultuous life, her "father's confidante," as she described their relationship.[29]

Mary was not the only one hoping to give succor to the embattled railroad president. Through the hectic years of the war, Rachel provided comfort and ballast for the splintered family. She protected her beleaguered husband from the pressures of his demanding job, often taking lunch to him at the B&O offices. When he worked at home, which he much preferred to do, Rachel stood "as a buffer between him and the outside world," an observer wrote. "She received callers; in most cases, not merely received, but dismissed them. If they managed to convince her of the necessity of talking to her husband, she generally sat in on the conversation and frequently joined in it. Her comments and questions were apt and to the point."[30]

As the war came to a close, Lincoln commended Garrett for being "the right arm of the federal government in the aid he rendered the authorities in preventing the Confederates from seizing Washington and securing its retention as the capital of the Loyal States." Garrett provided other forms of aid to the president. Shivering in the White House during the frigid winter of 1864–65, Lincoln sent a hurried dispatch to Garrett in January: "It is said we shall soon all be in the dark hour unless *you can* bring coal to make gas," Lincoln urgently implored Garrett. "It is very important to us."[31] Mary's father immediately complied with the president's request.

In his Second Inaugural Address, delivered on March 4, 1865, in the waning days of the war, Lincoln urged conciliation and healing between the two fractured regions. "With malice toward none; with charity for all; with firmness in the right," he implored the wounded nation to "finish up the work we are in; to bind up the nation's wounds."[32] But by that day, neither side felt charitable toward the other. The South lay in ruins—farms, plantations, cities, and livestock laid to waste. The population was demoralized. The North, although victorious, felt little benevolence toward the rebellious southern half of the nation.

Lincoln perceived his Second Inaugural Address as a beginning of the last half of his presidency and a rebirth for the reunited nation. Instead, his end was but a few weeks away. On April 14, 1865, the B&O paymaster escorted triumphant Gen. Ulysses S. Grant and his wife to Philadelphia. They had declined an invitation to accompany President and Mrs. Lincoln to Ford's Theatre that evening for the fateful performance of "My American Cousin," during which John Wilkes Booth's bullet put an end to the president's life.

Lincoln's funeral was held at the Capitol on April 19, four years to the day after the first blood of the Civil War had been spilled on the streets of Baltimore by the mob riot, foretelling the tragedy of the coming war. On the day after the assassination, Mary's father was called upon for a somber assignment: to plan the funeral procession that would carry the president's remains back to his final resting spot in his home of Springfield, Illinois. Garrett, who had arranged Lincoln's clandestine ride through Baltimore and unceremonious entrance into Washington four years earlier, now arranged for the slain president's final ride on the B&O.

At eight in the morning on April 21, Lincoln's long black and silver coffin, draped with "flags and funeral black," was placed on a dark-garlanded train in the B&O's Washington station. Mary's father accompanied the inconsolable Mary Todd Lincoln. Slowly, the funeral train, preceded by a "pilot engine," trudged north out of Washington and arrived in Baltimore at ten. A huge crowd waited at Camden Station on the cold, drizzly spring morning. An observer wrote, "The coffin was slowly unloaded and taken to the waiting room of the station to the hearse outside, which carried it to City Hall, where a vast number of people passed by it and gazed upon the features of the martyred president."[33]

In the five hours that Lincoln's coffin rested in Baltimore, the city stopped all motion and church bells continuously tolled. In the still-divided city, thousands of shocked mourners filed past the coffin. Many Baltimoreans draped black bunting from their windows. The Baltimore Sun reported that Baltimore's "streets were completely deserted and the city bore a solemn stillness," adding "Mr. Lincoln has had no equal since the days of Washington in all those traits of character which adorn the human mind."[34] At three in the afternoon, the train departed Baltimore for Philadelphia, the next stop on the funeral procession's sixteen-hundred-mile journey to Springfield.

After the president's assassination, "Mr. Lincoln's Road" played one more important role in the war it had so valiantly helped to win. In the summer of 1865, a constant parade of B&O railroad cars once again carried troops, not to bloody combat, but to their homes. In all, more than a quarter million men and twenty-seven thousand horses and mules were transported in 1865 on the B&O, this time to happier destinations.[35]

The unthinkable war was finally over. It had stretched across most of the continent and brought an end to the all-powerful slave economy that the South—and the North—had depended on for more than two centuries. By the war's end, death, despair, and disunity had entered almost every American home. More than 623,000 men had died—one out of eleven service-age men; another half million were wounded.[36]

Baltimore's "quarrel to the death," as prophesized by Anthony Trollope as the war erupted in the spring of 1861, did, indeed, continue well after Lee's surrender to Ulysses S. Grant at Appomattox in April 1865. Unlike Henry Garrett, many Baltimoreans had suppressed their outward expression of Southern sympathies during the war. At its conclusion, they unleashed and renewed their anti-Union venom with vigor. They enthusiastically contributed to the Southern Relief Fund, quickly raising $100,000 for impoverished Confederate soldiers. They threw off all pretense of Unionism, regaining Democratic Party control and renewing Deep South sentiments that would last for generations. Most egregious to many pro-Southern Baltimoreans was the treatment of their sons and husbands who had been killed in battle. Many dead soldiers lay unburied by their Union victors. Often families were imprisoned as they tried to claim their fatally wounded Confederate sons and husbands.

Mary's father, who had seen his family and nation torn apart by the conflict, publicly called for a truce between the two feuding regions. "His voice was the earliest, as it was the boldest, on behalf of reconciliation and peace," a commentator noted.[37]

The Civil War had a profound effect on all Americans. At its conclusion, nothing would be the same. Although women's experiences varied across class and race lines, many women found the war opened up opportunities and allowed them to move more freely in public activities. The war years bridged women's restricted expectations of the antebellum era with new opportunities and expanded public roles that would unfold in the coming years.

In Maryland, women had performed heroic and adventurous deeds during the war and were publicly acclaimed. Barbara Fritchie, who gained fame from the John Greenleaf Whittier poem with the first line "Shoot, if you must, this old gray head," defiantly defended her Frederick home from the marauding Confederates. Rosie O'Neal Greenhow gained notoriety as a spy. Clara Barton, the "Angel of the Battlefield" who risked her life tending to the wounded and dying on both sides, opened the doors for nursing as an acceptable profession for women. Even women who wanted no such displacement from traditional roles often found themselves, in the absence of husbands and fathers sent off to combat, running farms and family businesses, ministering to wounded soldiers in makeshift battlefield hospitals, and pounding the pavement, tirelessly raising money for the "glorious cause" of North or South. The U.S. Sanitary Commission galvanized and politicized women across the nation, as they astutely and effectively organized relief societies in large urban areas and small hamlets alike. The head of the commission, Rev. Henry W. Bellows, commented that the war had sparked "an uprising of women of the land."[38]

For young Mary, the war's impact was just as profound, as she absorbed the changing dynamics of her family and her nation. As she watched and eavesdropped on the father she adored conduct business and command the attention of prominent national leaders, she was being transformed. "He talked as free to me as to anyone else, even my mother," Mary wrote. He talked about business, politics, family affairs—"all his hopes and dreams for the future."[39]

Certainly one of John Work Garrett's dreams must have been for the great expansion and dominance of Baltimore and the B&O after the war. To this end, as a commentator later noted, Garrett's "aim was always to dedicate every possible resource to the advancement and efficiency of the road."[40] This singular determination, so idealized by his young daughter, would in the years following the Civil War earn Mary's father distinction as a fierce competitor to be reckoned with.

His impressionable daughter adored his ambition—and the undreamed of status and privilege it would soon confer.

I BECAME VERY SENSITIVE

John Work Garrett's loyalist decision to support Lincoln and the Union soon produced major paybacks, not only for the B&O and Baltimore, but also for the family coffers. In the two decades following the war, Mary's father amassed one of the great fortunes of the day and rose to the pinnacle of East Coast power. "Of all the old order of the large men of the Baltimore and Ohio, he was the last. And the greatest," a commentator wrote of Garrett's influence. By 1867, John Work Garrett owned 14,500 shares of B&O stock, valued at $1.7 million. In an era when the average male factory worker might earn $500 annually, Garrett's combined assets totaled more than $2 million. And he was just getting started. In the war's profiteering aftermath, Garrett upheld the covenant made on the day he took office as B&O president in 1858 to keep Baltimore and the B&O economically viable at all costs, "to promote the advancement and prosperity of my native city and my native State."[41]

In early October 1867, Mary's Uncle Henry, the defiant Confederate sympathizer who had caused the family untold anguish during the war, was stricken with typhoid fever while vacationing at the family retreat in Western Maryland. He had gone there to escape his annual bout of hay fever. He died on October 10 in his Monument Street house at the age of fifty. Before gasping his dying breath, the once robust and often rowdy Henry, perhaps disbelieving of his own imminent, untimely mortality, whispered his favorite William Cowper couplet, expressing what all around must have been thinking: "God moves in a mysterious way, his wonders to perform."[42]

With the Confederacy a lost cause, Henry had found new occupations after the war. He immersed himself in the work of the Associate Reformed Church, where his father had served on the board years earlier. Henry purchased a new organ for the church. He took the church's pastor, the Reverend Jonathan Leyburn, under his wing, spending countless hours debating religious doctrine, while generously contributing to the church's treasury. He had "an unostentatious concern for religion and charity," an observer noted.[43]

"A large concourse of sorrowing friends" attended Henry's funeral in the parlor of his home on West Monument Street on October 12. The grateful pastor returned his patron's kindness with gracious tributes, attesting to Henry's habitual, almost heroic, church attendance and piety. "He was always in his place, no matter what the weather. Through sunshine and through storm, amid heat and cold he came; and one night, when it was so tempestuous that I myself did not even go, I found on meeting him the next day that he had been there," the young pastor told the gathered mourners.[44]

The newspapers were equally generous in their assessment of Henry's life. "He was favorably known for many years here and abroad . . . [and] has been connected with some of the largest financial transactions which have taken place in our midst during the past twenty-five years," The *Baltimore Sun* reported the day after Henry died. "In his character of merchant, he was regarded as accurate and upright. He possessed a benevolent and kindly nature and was without ostentation. He was a bachelor."[45] No mention was made of Henry's treasonous activities during the war.

That Christmas, a bereft John Work Garrett presented Mary and Rachel with traditional keepsakes of his departed brother: pearl-encrusted brooches with lockets of Henry's hair. Mary's father immediately set out to fulfill the wish his brother had made before the war to build a church in Oakland in Western Maryland. Henry had spent many pleasurable days in the "Glades region," the beautiful mountains of Maryland, visiting farms with such idyllic names as Milk and Honey and Kindness.[46]

In his brother's memory, John Work Garrett designed a church of sandstone transported from a nearby quarry at Rowlesburg, West Virginia. Completed the year after Henry's death, the Garrett Memorial Church soon became known as the "Church of Presidents," as future presidents Ulysses S. Grant, Benjamin Harrison, Grover Cleveland, William Taft, and Theodore Roosevelt worshipped at the church while vacationing in the Maryland mountains.

With his brother, lifelong business partner, and, as Mary described, "my father's closest friend," now gone, Garrett turned to the two most likely successors to carry on the family's business, Robert, known by then to his friends as Bob, and Harry.[47] Mary's brothers were twenty and eighteen, about the same ages her father and uncle had been when they joined the family firm nearly three decades earlier. Robert had graduated with honors in 1867 from Princeton. Both he and Harry were absolved of their earlier adolescent misdeeds during the Civil War and brought back to Baltimore to take their adult positions in Robert Garrett and Sons.

Baltimore had taken an economic beating during the war, losing its primacy among East Coast port cities. Although Maryland did not secede with the eleven Confederate states, it, like its more southern neighbors, suffered the great economic calamity brought on by the ravages of the war. Baltimore, once among the nation's top three industrial cities, dropped to sixth in the number of wage earners, population, and industrial output.[48]

For Mary's father, Baltimore's economic decline only meant it was ready to rebuild. Teaming with the B&O's other major stockholder, Johns Hopkins, Garrett positioned the B&O and its feeder industries to receive abundant federal patronage. Baltimore began its slow but steady industrial climb back up. The city once again stirred with profitable activity. Within a few years of the war's end, the city was soon labeled the "Liverpool of America" for its robust commerce.[49]

Baltimore's postwar rebirth was no accident. Mary's father carefully engineered the B&O's role in it, sparing no cost—even if it meant keeping the state legislature in his pocket. For the next twenty years, no governor, state senator, congressman, or judge stood a chance of election without Garrett's approval and

Maryland's powerful political bosses were his closest allies. Not surprisingly, during Garrett's presidency, the B&O never lost a legal suit. As one observer noted of Garrett's financially persuasive tactics: "Mr. Garrett realized he must have a dominant influence in the State Government, and that, most important, he must have a Governor who would be guided by him in all matters pertaining to the great property . . . To that end, his agents were busily engaged in politics from one end of the state to the other."[50]

During the war years, the B&O, with its mandate to transport federal troops and supplies, had been held back from expansion. Mary's father watched as his powerful competitors to the north extended in all directions, firmly planting themselves in lucrative commercial markets in the Northeast and West. Once the war was over, Garrett took off with a vengeance, rebuilding the B&O's war-damaged tracks and aggressively extending the line to Pittsburgh, Chicago, and New York. Wherever railroad tracks ran, the Garrett name was well known. In 1876, Garrett, Indiana, an important junction on the B&O's Chicago line, was incorporated in honor of John Work Garrett's role in bringing the railroad westward. Many of the main streets of the thriving town were named after the officers of the B&O and its Midwestern subsidiaries.[51]

Once again focused on the B&O's entrepreneurial, commercial expansion, Garrett built the Locust Point compound, an enormous sprawl of wharves, railroad lines, and immigration and industrial buildings on Baltimore's main harbor. It soon bustled with business day and night. European immigrants arrived daily on an endless stream of B&O steamships, the "Baltimore to Bremen line," Mary's father started in association with North German Lloyds Company in 1868. Baltimore soon ranked as the country's third largest immigration port, after New York and Boston. Over the next decades, nearly 1.5 million immigrants would enter through Baltimore's port.[52] At "Immigration Pier," travelers were quickly processed, transferred onto B&O trains, and whisked westward to find employment in the hinterlands. Many hardly touched Maryland soil. Others stayed, forming vibrant neighborhoods and contributing to Baltimore's growing prosperity.

Never forgetting its Southern roots, after the war the B&O carried relief goods to devastated Southern states and helped to rebuild the former Confederacy's struggling markets. Baltimore became a prime supplier of wholesale goods to the South. The B&O offered sleeping cars, dining cars, and its own express freight company. These profitable enterprises earned additional, very sizable chunks of revenue for the ever-expanding railroad.

Mary's life, for a time filled with the excitement and exhilaration, the terror and dissension of the war, soon transformed into a life filled with world travel, opulent weekend retreats, mingling with the country's wealthiest families—and her first taste of independence. The year after the war ended, at age twelve, Mary started attending school, more than likely at Miss Kummer's School for Young Ladies. Records do not indicate exactly where Mary attended school, and her correspondence never mentions the school by name. However, later Mary recorded owning a "gold locket with an MEG monogram with a lock of Miss Kummer's hair."[53] "Mademoiselle Kummer," as she was known, occupied the Tiffany Mansion on Mount Vernon Place from 1865 until 1875. This would have been a big step for Mary, an emotional weaning, as it was for any sheltered, adolescent girl. For the first time, she was outside the direct influence of her family.

At the fashionable school, Mary met her first two longtime friends, Julia Rebecca Rogers and Elizabeth King. Both were the same age as Mary and their families traveled in the same circles. Julia, whom Mary nicknamed "Dolly," was the daughter of a prosperous Baltimore steel magnate. "Bessie" King, an aspiring artist, hailed from one of Baltimore's most prominent Quaker families, and her widowed father was a longtime associate of Mary's father. Bessie suffered from chronic bad health, possibly the all-too-prevalent "consumption" (tuberculosis) of the nineteenth century and frequently spent her winters in the South with relatives. Despite her frail health, Bessie was the most outspoken of the group, often arguing with Miss Kummer about the controversial new subject of women's rights.[54]

The three girls became inseparable at Miss Kummer's. When apart they wrote newsy, confessional, inquiring letters, testing each other's fidelity and allegiance in their brave new world of intimate adolescent female friendships. Mary had longed for such female companionship in her otherwise male-dominated life. By 1870 the three inquisitive, intellectual kindred spirits formed a reading group, gathering in each other's homes to debate their favorite authors and fictional characters. Julia, who became a legal ward of John Work Garrett's after her widowed father died, quickly moved to the forefront of Mary's budding emotional attachments to female friends, forging an intimate bond of friendship and affection that would intensify over the next decade.

Off Mary would go each day, equipped with the usual staples of the classroom of the time: a slate, a quill pen, a writing book, and her texts. More than likely, Mary studied those subjects mandatory for the daughters of the elite classes. Nearby on Lexington Avenue near Monument Square, Miss Kilbourn's Academy offered "mental culture," which helped a young girl "to think, understandingly, upon her daily task . . . to compare one step with another, forming a regular chain of thought." Young girls were also drilled in "moral instruction and discipline," in which they learned "in simple language, the meaning of obedience to parents . . . in every shade of coloring, the sin and ingratitude of disobedience." Above all else, Mary would have learned selflessness, "to regard the character and feelings of others and that carelessness in this respect is inexcusable."[55]

The Franklin Square Female Seminary, located not far from where the Garretts lived before the war, offered painting, music, and language, as well as lectures on philosophy, physiology, astronomy, and hygiene "delivered by professional gentlemen." Teachers were always mindful to not offer too much academic instruction, fearing that such intellectual exertion would create in a young girl "mental inactivity or mental dependence." The young students might be encouraged to contribute to a literary journal to share their thoughts about "The Power of Beauty," "The Advantage of Resisting Temptation," or "The Wonderful Water Lily."[56]

At first, Mary's experience at Miss Kummer's was invigorating, and she savored every minute of it. She described the principal as "a very attractive and a very stimulating woman."[57] Mary soon became one of the principal's favorites, a status that allowed her free reign of the school's library. She often stayed after class, poring over her beloved books, and would be sent home across Mount Vernon Park only reluctantly at day's end. But it was not long before Mary grew bored with the school's traditional curriculum and the once-stimulating principal, whom she ultimately found to be "very conservative about girls' education, believing in cultivation, not in college." Mary, far more interested in discussing the great philosophers and character development in the Brontë sisters' novels than the finer points of the latest Parisian fashions on Charles Street, soon tired of what she considered the "low standards and poor teaching." Disinterested by dreary instruction in moral discipline and resisting temptation, Mary, Julia, and Bessie instead gave in to temptation and rebelled against Miss Kummer's restrictive curriculum. They formed their own biology class to study science. To the complete horror of friends and family, the girls dissected a rat.[58]

During her years at Miss Kummer's School, Mary developed personality traits that would continue through life. She had been a shy child, and in adolescence her introspection continued. Perhaps she felt overshadowed by Robert and Harry's rising social stature in the family and the community or self-conscious from the lameness caused by her childhood ankle injury. Her writings at this age do not reveal the source of her difficulty. She became self-critical and sensitive. It is likely that many of her traits were exacerbated in adolescence by what she later recalled as teasing at school, writing that she suffered from "attacks of hysteria wh. [which] my school mates often amused themselves by trying to produce by making me laugh while I lost control of myself." She was anxious and nervous—probably the "hysteria" she mentions—developing a "habit of jumping at any unusually loud sound or sudden [movement]." Her behavior, she wrote, "was so much commented upon that I became very sensitive."[59]

She left school by the time she was seventeen, from disillusionment with the uninspiring curriculum and, possibly, because of the taunts from her classmates. Once again, she was tutored at home, either alone or with "two friends," most likely Julia and Bessie, and did not continue with formal education. As before the war, during her isolated and lonely earliest years on Franklin Square, Mary pieced together her own self-education, immersing herself in the literary classics. Her diary of 1870, written when she was sixteen, reveals an early interest in the writers whom she would follow throughout her life. In the summer of that year, she listed her favorites: Dickens, Thackeray, Macauley, Ruskin, Morris, Tennyson, Emily Brontë, Byron, and a host of others she, no doubt, vigorously discussed with Julia and Bessie in their reading group. She learned to speak fluent Italian and French and practiced German and Greek, carefully mastering the grammar of the languages in her meticulous script in tidy notebooks.[60]

Despite her lingering shyness, Mary's physical health slowly improved. She was finally able to throw off the leg braces that had encumbered her practically since birth and began to enjoy the freedom of movement once prohibited to her. She developed "the bad habit of squinting" and was taken to an "oculist," who found her to be nearsighted and prescribed what were then called "spectacles." Robert and Harry, for some unexplained reason, disapproved of her glasses, forbidding her to wear them. It was only when she was older, when she could "no longer stand the suffering of not being able to see properly," that she persuaded her father that she should be allowed to wear the glasses.[61]

On her fourteenth birthday, Mary started her periods, an event for which she was totally unprepared. "My mother never mentioned the subject to me," she later recalled. In an era in which women were valued singularly for their reproductive and sexual capacity, it is not surprising that puberty caused such anxiety. Physicians, clergymen, and educators developed an elaborate set of explanations to define women's fragility and inferiority based on the female cycle of puberty and menopause. "Ovulation fixes woman's place in the animal economy," one doctor put forth, forever imprisoning a woman to her reproductive cycle.[62]

Puberty was the rite of passage into womanly behavior for Victorians. As a young girl's innocent, childlike body transformed into that of a curvaceous, seductive woman, she became a sexual being—a very unsettling time for all around her. A young girl was expected to take on the moral and emotional restraints of womanhood and to take to heart the lessons learned at school about selflessness and obedience to parents.

Mary was now expected to be demure, silent, and submissive, traits that would make her more attractive in the marriage market in but a few short years and would keep her safely within the confines of Victorian propriety. While her brothers displayed their strength and fortitude during puberty—Robert, after all, had run off to become one of Robert E. Lee's warriors when he was sixteen—Mary's path during puberty was expected to be far more circumspect. Doctors recommended that young girls confine their activities to the least exertion possible to preserve their scant amounts of energy. Limited outdoor activity was permitted, but more outward displays of strength required for social or educational or even charitable activities were ill advised, particularly during menstruation.

Mary later remembered her adolescence with great discomfort, for these years no doubt were awkward, perhaps even embarrassing to her in a family in which her mother did not talk of indelicate subjects relating to sex, and certainly, her brothers and father stayed as far away from the topic as possible. She had, as she described, very "irregular menstruation," a medical problem that would plague her throughout her life, but thought little of it, since she "had been brought up without the slightest attempt to teach me any of the laws of health."[63]

But she certainly picked up on other laws of the Garrett household. By adolescence, Mary began to display her father's business acumen and fiscal frugality. She began her lifelong love affair with keeping lists and accounts of every letter she wrote, every gift she gave, every penny she spent. Like her father, she became a stickler for business matters, particularly her own personal business matters. She saved every imaginable receipt—for soap, for jewelry, for lingerie—for every purchase she made.

It appears that in her adolescence, Mary was given a regular weekly allowance of five to ten dollars, the equivalent of two weeks' wages for a female factory worker in the 1870s. Upon receiving her allowance, she duly noted it under "accounts received" in her ledger. From that amount, she would deduct her expenses: a scarf (one dollar) here, a hat (three dollars) there, or a gift for her mother or a household servant. After each entry she carefully listed the "balance forward," thus giving a running account of the precise amount in her personal treasury.[64]

She logged incoming and outgoing letters in her journals. Her most frequent correspondents were Julia; Bessie; her mother's sisters, Rebecca Harrison and Florence Harrison; her father's sister, Elizabeth Garrett; and Jenny Walters, her neighbor on Mount Vernon Place and daughter of William Walters. But in one journal she wrote not a word—a lovely leatherbound diary given to her by her family's longtime friend and business colleague, financier George Peabody. On the first page, Peabody inscribed: "With the affectionate regards and best wishes of George Peabody, November 12, 1866."[65] The remaining pages of the journal are blank. Perhaps she wanted to preserve the treasured gift as a keepsake. That fall, George Peabody, the longtime European representative of Robert Garrett and Sons, had returned from London to Baltimore for the dedication of the new cultural institution on Mount Vernon Place that he had established before the war. Although by the time he returned to Baltimore in the fall of 1866 he had lived in London for three decades, his alliances to the country that had launched him remained steadfast. During the Civil War, his influence in London was indispensable to President Lincoln in maintaining England's often-wavering support of the Union. He had raised much-needed capital from international bankers to expand American railroads, including the B&O.[66]

Peabody had once relished the accumulation of wealth and its attendant power and influence. By his own admission, he was "extremely fond of money and very happy in acquiring it . . . I labored and struggled and economized continuously . . . and I have been proud of my achievements."[67] But by middle age, he had grown weary of riches and material possessions. He turned over management of his company to his business partner, Junius Morgan, and set out full time to distribute his enormous wealth, which he did with great passion and enthusiasm. His lifetime philanthropies eventually totaled more than $7 million, both in Europe and the United States.

Peabody spent his later years dispersing his grand fortune by establishing orphanages and cultural institutions on either side of the Atlantic. He significantly raised the philanthropic bar with the amount of his large-scale gifts. There had certainly been other notable philanthropic milestones in the United States—Stephen Girard's unprecedented gifts to fund public works throughout Philadelphia in the 1830s; John Harvard's bequest to establish a university in his name; and Englishman James Smithson's $500,000 bequest to start what in 1846 would become the Smithsonian Institution in Washington, D.C. But Peabody's philanthropy differed in a significant way that would influence American philanthropy in the years ahead. Peabody's gifts were not in the form of a bequest, to be given only after his death. Rather, he wanted to see his philanthropy put into action while he was still alive. This was a departure from the way in which most major institutions had been privately funded in the past. Peabody provided a model that later major American philanthropists, including Mary Elizabeth Garrett, would follow.

In 1851, as Baltimore simmered in its prewar animosities, Peabody initiated the idea of establishing a cultural institution in Baltimore. Five years later, he made his first trip back to the United States in nearly two decades. It was during this trip that he gathered together prominent Baltimoreans John Pendleton Kennedy, Reverdy Johnson, and Charles James Madison, among others, to form a board of trustees to develop his innovative concept. Peabody envisioned offering a library, an academy of music, a lecture series, an art gallery, and classes for the public, particularly for public-school children. He left the details of implementing his vision to the appointed trustees. His gifts to endow the Peabody Institute in Baltimore eventually totaled more than $1.2 million.

The sparkling white marble Peabody Institute opened on October 25, 1866. Thousands of eager onlookers crowded into Mount Vernon Place to see Baltimore's newest crown jewel and its tall, elegant, and very famous seventy-one-year-old benefactor. Children were given the day off from school and brought presents to the celebrity patron. Newspapers from around the world covered the festive event surrounding the famed philanthropist. Joseph Henry of the Smithsonian Institution delivered the inaugural address.

While in Baltimore, Peabody stayed with the Garretts. Mary's father asked a favor of him. Johns Hopkins needed counsel about an important matter. Hopkins, with a financial estate that would soon reach $8 million, needed advice on how best to disperse his vast fortune. Like Peabody, Hopkins had never married and had no heirs. His lifelong love for his first cousin, Elizabeth, remained unfulfilled. Mary's father had often encouraged Hopkins to write a will, but to no avail. "Mr. Hopkins had on many occasions introduced the subject of the disposition of his estate," Garrett recalled, but he had never written a will.[68] Garrett felt that Peabody's philanthropic ideas might be useful to Hopkins. He took advantage of Peabody's visit to bring the two men together. He invited Hopkins to dine, so that Peabody "might give his experience and views" on philanthropic giving. Although Peabody modestly said that he "never gave advice" about such matters, he agreed to counsel his friend. Hopkins cordially accepted the dinner invitation.[69] Little did the participants suspect that the meeting Mary's father arranged in his home would have a profound effect on the future of higher education and medicine in the United States.

"After my family left the table at 8 o'clock," Mary's father later recalled, "I introduced the subject, and the conference continued until an hour past midnight. The conversation was remarkable." During the fateful meeting in the Garrett home, Peabody recounted his longtime association with Hopkins, whom he described as "the only man I have met in all my experience more thoroughly anxious to make money and more determined to succeed than myself." Peabody explained how he had transformed himself from financier to philanthropist: "When aches and pains made me realize that I was not immortal, I felt, after taking care of my relatives, great anxiety to place the millions I had accumulated, so as to accomplish the greatest good for humanity. I . . . formed the conclusion that there were men who were just as anxious to work with integrity and faithfulness for the comfort, consolation and advancement of the suffering poor as I had been to gather fortune."[70]

Peabody suggested that Hopkins pursue the same plan of action that he had taken a decade before when he chartered the Peabody Institute: "I called a number of my friends in whom I had confidence to meet me, and I proposed that they should act as my trustees . . . I then, for the first time, felt there was a higher pleasure and a greater happiness than accumulating money, and that was for giving it for good and humane purposes."[71] Johns Hopkins soon prepared his will. He followed Peabody's advice to appoint a board of trustees to fulfill its terms. Hopkins, too, hoped that one day his fortune would create a world-renowned institution.

And where was twelve-year-old Mary when this portentous meeting took place in her home? Unfortunately, she did not leave an account. She was in the house and had dined with the guests and, according to her father's explanation, had left the room with other members of the family so the men could talk. But did she quietly slip back into her father's library to listen in on the conversation, as she had so often done during the Civil War when her father plotted and planned with generals and politicians? Was the inquisitive young girl quietly, inconspicuously, curled up in her favorite chair, pretending to read a book, while listening to the celebrated men of her time discuss how wealth, vision, and philanthropy could be combined to create great institutions?

In the postwar years, men such as Garrett, Peabody, and Hopkins were among the privileged few in a position to discuss disposing of great riches. They had ascended to the stratosphere of Gilded Age wealth and power. And there was no better ride to the top than on the railroad. Railroads ruled in the aftermath of the war, in the Golden Age of Railroading. The symbol of their dominance was prominently displayed in the national frenzy that surrounded the laying of the Golden Spike, at Promontory Point, Utah, at the completion of the transcontinental railroad in May 1869. The United States, just four years before divided by civil violence, was now connected from coast to coast by a network of rail lines. The ambitious dream of reaching the Pacific, expressed forty-one years earlier by the founders of the country's first major railroad, the B&O, was finally realized.

The B&O, while not as big as its northern competitors, the Pennsylvania, the

Erie, or the New York Central, held its own in a vicious climate of competition and corporate one-upmanship. No sooner had Mary's father successfully brought the B&O through the rigors of the Civil War than he faced yet another formidable force: rate wars. Garrett's life became an endless round of meetings with other railroad presidents to iron out rate and turf battles. One commentator noted that undercutting competitors' passenger and freight rates occurred as frequently as "small pox or the change of season."[72]

In the late-century "Age of Social Darwinism," in which only the best and brightest were expected to climb their way to the top, there was a tacit understanding, at least among the reigning industrialists, that the reward for keeping a city or an industry financially prosperous was the right to live well—and large. Private industrial fortunes jumped ten to twenty times what they had been on the eve of the Civil War.[73]

After she left Miss Kummer's at age seventeen, Mary soon found a far more interesting companion than the schoolmates who had teased and taunted her. As his empire expanded after the war, John Work Garrett turned to an unlikely candidate to provide valuable assistance: his inquisitive and adoring daughter. The little girl who had once loved to eavesdrop on her father's meetings would soon learn firsthand from the master the business of the B&O—and how to drive a hard bargain.

PAPA'S SECRETARY

One by one, Mary's father brought his children into the family's vast commercial empire. While Robert and Harry assumed their places in the boardroom, Mary, too, found her place at the corporate table, albeit in a much less visible and financially lucrative position than her brothers. Like her father and now her brothers, the pressing needs of the B&O and with it, Baltimore's financial solvency, began to shape her life. In the post–Civil War years, the third generation of Garretts—Mary, Robert, and Harry—set out on paths dictated by their powerful father.

When Robert and Harry returned to Baltimore from Princeton in 1867 after Uncle Henry's death, they were welcomed into the family business of Robert Garrett and Sons. Robert's career path abruptly swerved. He soon found himself being groomed to succeed his father at the B&O. Four short years after graduating from college, Robert, at age twenty-four, catapulted to the top. He was elected to the presidency of the Valley Railroad, a short line in the Shenandoah Valley managed by the B&O. In a grand twist of historical irony, Robert succeeded Robert E. Lee, the famed general for whom he had run away from home eight years earlier. The former Confederate general, who became president of Washington College—soon to be known as Washington and Lee College—after the war, had once again allied himself with his former adversary, John Work Garrett. Lee advocated for a rail line to be brought to the college town of Lexington, Virginia, in the Shenandoah Valley, and served as the line's president for a few short weeks before he died in 1870. Mary's brother held the office of president until 1875.

By all accounts, Robert was inexperienced and unqualified, perhaps even disinterested, in such a coveted position. It did not matter. In the Gilded Age, young upper-class men often were as restricted in their life's options as women. Corporate primogeniture still ruled for firstborn sons of the elite. As the son of John Work Garrett, Robert had little choice but to follow in his father's footsteps. We can only speculate whether Robert might have chosen a different path for himself, given the opportunity to do so. Had his escapade in joining Lee's army in 1863 been an indication of a wish for a more adventurous, liberated life than that of a railroad president?

While John Work Garrett was always described in larger-than-life terms—vigorous, large, determined, autocratic—his oldest son was described as being much less forceful and aggressive. Robert had, perhaps, a more gentle nature, one not cut out for the rigors of the cutthroat railroad business. Good-looking and dapper, Robert was "average in height, always well dressed and never seen on the street without a flower in his buttonhole. He was affable and courteous in manner . . . a great lover of flowers."[74] The senior Garrett had served a demanding and strict apprenticeship in his early career, working his way up the corporate ladder of Robert Garrett and Sons and, later, standing firm against all odds to keep the B&O commercially competitive. Robert had led a far easier life. He was not as strong and determined as his father and not hardened to the realities of the ruthless world of postwar railroad rivalries.

Harry, a handsome young man with a dimpled chin and a nature and disposition similar to his brother's, similarly followed the prescribed family path as directed by his father. By 1871, he headed Robert Garrett and Sons' international banking division, negotiating overseas loans for the B&O. Like his brother, he developed a keen aesthetic sense, one that would flourish in the years ahead as he became one of the country's great collectors of art, coins, and rare books.

With their professional paths solidified, Mary's brothers next turned to the second most serious decision for young men: marriage—an economic undertaking of grave importance to the elite class in the Gilded Age. Both brothers married exceedingly well, forging unions with remarkable women from patrician families whose wealth and influence more than equaled that of the Garretts. The marriages solidified the Garrett social and commercial connections up and down the East Coast and beyond.

In February 1870, twenty-one-year-old Harry married eighteen-year-old Baltimorean Alice Dickerson Whitridge, whose first famous American ancestor had administered the oath of office to George Washington on his second inauguration. She was born in Baltimore on Saratoga Street, not far from Mount Vernon Place. Alice's pedigree was impeccable. Her father, Horatio L. Whitridge, hailed from an old, moneyed Rhode Island family and owned a vast fleet of clipper ships, earning a fortune for the family in the shipping business. Alice's family included Supreme Court justices, military heroes, financiers, doctors, and the first mayor of Baltimore, James Calhoun. The Whitridges owned Tiverton, a Newport estate named for a twelfth-century English castle built by Henry I for the Earls of Devon. The Whitridges lived at Tiverton before moving to Maryland and, later, continued to pass away idyllic summer holidays at the Rhode Island estate. Like Mary, Alice had attended Miss Kummer's School on Mount Vernon Place.

Two years later, twenty-five-year-old Robert made a similar match, marrying twenty-one-year-old Mary Sloan Frick, a daughter of one of Baltimore's most prominent lawyers. Like Alice, who was the same age, Mary Frick's lineage dated back to pre-Revolutionary heroes. The couple's fathers, John Work Garrett and William Frederick Frick, served on many Baltimore boards together. It is likely that Robert and Mary Frick knew each other from childhood. The wedding was a grand social event for Baltimore and particularly for eighteen-year-old Mary Elizabeth. She saved the gold ring decoration from the top tier of the wedding cake for the rest of her life.[75]

Both the Garrett and the Frick families bestowed lavish wedding presents upon the new couple. The bride's father presented the couple with Uplands, the family's ancestral estate near Catonsville in Baltimore County, where Mary Frick had been raised. Not to be outdone, John Work Garrett gave his son and new daughter-in-law a stylish townhouse built in 1853 by Samuel George at 11 Mount Vernon Place, just a half block east of the Garrett mansion at 101 West Monument. Along with the house, Garrett purchased items essential for any newlywed couple, such as the ancient armor displayed in the library.

The Garrett men had their work cut out for them. In 1873, the country plunged into yet another devastating economic depression. The stock market closed down for ten days—"a week of Sundays," as President Ulysses S. Grant insisted—to let things settle down. By the score, businesses across the nation went under, more than five thousand in the first year. The railroads were hit especially hard, with eighty-nine defaulting on their bonds.[76]

Through it all, as he had done so many times before, Mary's father kept the B&O on track and profitable—but precariously. Within a two-year period, the debt of the B&O shot skyward, from $11 million in 1871 to $19 million in 1873. Garrett borrowed liberally to offset the debt. In the midst of national economic hardship, he imposed strict—some observers saying unnecessarily cruel and unbearable—wage cutbacks on B&O workers. He had little to worry about. Labor was cheap and available in the postwar years, particularly during an economic depression. Wage earners were desperate to get any work they could, and a never-ending supply of immigrants eagerly lined up for work on the B&O. Garrett mandated two back-to-back 10 percent reductions on the workers' already-meager wages. He euphemistically was called a "severe economist" and "rigid disciplinarian" in his fiscal affairs, seeming to have little concern for the laborers who kept the lines running.[77]

Garrett lowered his own "wages" as well. He willingly cut his annual salary from $6,000 to $4,000, not too much of a dent in his fortune, valued at well over $2 million at that time. Other major B&O stockholders did not feel much of a pinch, either. Dividends, in fact, increased during the national economic downturn. The company raised dividends from 8 percent to 10 percent throughout the tenuous times. Junius Morgan, who succeeded George Peabody as the B&O's European representative, fretted about the line's debt load and disproportionate dividends. He continually advised Garrett to lower the dividend. His advice went unheeded. Garrett's first concern was to keep his stockholders happy.

By the 1870s, Mary's father was at the top of his game. After his success and national visibility during the Civil War, his name became a household word. In December 1872, Maryland's General Assembly passed an act naming the farthermost region of the state, near where Robert Garrett Sr.'s lumbering Conestoga wagons had trekked a half century earlier on the National Road, Garrett County in John Work Garrett's honor. That same year, rumors flew that Garrett was a serious contender for the Democratic presidential nomination, all former allegiances to Lincoln's Republican Party having died with the slain president in 1865. He made an unsuccessful run for the Senate. A brand of cigars was named in Garrett's honor, and a West Virginia volunteer militia christened itself the "Garrett Rifles." The B&O was by now commonly called "Garrett's Road." A commentator claimed that Garrett ran "the most important trunk line in the world."[78]

Garrett's national celebrity and corporate frugality made him a wealthy and powerful man. But, after more than fifteen years of heading a railroad—keeping the trains running during the Civil War, steering the line through economic depressions, going toe to toe with competitors such as the New York Central's Commodore Vanderbilt and the Penn's Tom Scott during endless rate wars—his health declined. In early 1873, he began to complain of extreme fatigue and occasional dizziness. The exact nature of Garrett's illness is not known, but in the years ahead he often would suffer from similar crushing debilitations. More than likely his health was greatly affected by, as one observer later noted, "the great enterprises in which he was engaged"—the tremendous strain of running the railroad.[79] He offered to resign the presidency, but the board refused. B&O vice president John King took over as interim president.

Garrett's doctor ordered what any good doctor of the Victorian era usually recommended for a wealthy patient: rest and relaxation during a grand and prolonged tour of Europe. In the midst of the devastating Panic of 1873, in which hundreds of thousands of workers nationwide slipped deeper into poverty, Mary set off with her parents on what would become an eighteen-month Grand Tour, the first of many trips they would take over the next decade to restore her father's frequent lapses of health. They sailed in July aboard the North German Lloyd steamer *Berlin* for Southampton. They looked forward to seeing the picturesque sights and luxuriating at therapeutic spas. Most of all, they hoped to leave behind the chaos of railroad rate wars and financial crises.

Keeping an eye on the family business were Harry at Robert Garrett and Sons and Robert at the Valley Railroad. Closer at hand, however, Garrett enlisted his daughter, now nineteen years old, to help in business matters on their travels. It seemed a natural evolution. A decade before, Mary, the self-described "confidante" to her father, had absorbed his every word, learning bit by bit about the intriguing world of railroads and commerce. But it was during the Garretts' Grand Tour of Europe in 1873–74 that Mary's father immersed his daughter, firsthand, into his world of railroading, giving her practical experience in accounting, correspondence, finances, and, perhaps most important, the day-to-day business of running the B&O. Within just a few weeks of departing Baltimore, Mary took over much of her ailing father's business activity. Writing from London's Buckingham Palace Hotel, across from the royal residence, on August 23, 1873, Mary apologized in a letter to her Aunt Lizzie (her father's sister, Elizabeth Barbara) for not corresponding more promptly. "Acting as Papa's secretary leaves me very little time for my own letters," she explained.[80]

Putting an ocean between himself and the B&O did not remove Mary's father from his troubles—or from B&O business. Just days after setting foot in London, after being dispatched on his curative Grand Tour on doctor's orders, Garrett immediately met with bankers to secure a profitable interest rate for a sizable block of B&O bonds, a timely move just three weeks before the economic depression at home sent the stock market plummeting. Robert regularly kept his father apprised of the country's worsening financial depression. "All the railroads are discharging hands and manufacturers all over the country are either running on short time or have stopped altogether," he wrote ominously in October 1973, as he and Mary Frick vacationed in Newport. "In Rhode Island, it is estimated that 100,000 operatives have been thrown out of employment."[81] As if the B&O wasn't enough to worry about, Harry sent regular dispatches updating his father about the latest financial worries of Robert Garrett and Sons.

In her usual fashion, practiced diligently over the years in her personal ledgers, Mary kept meticulous lists of the family's travels and her letters and gifts sent to friends and family back home. Their leisurely trip took the Garretts from London, Zurich, and Cologne to Heidelberg and Brussels, Paris and Prague. They took slow, relaxing gondola rides down the Grand Canal in Venice, watched the whales off the coast of England, rested in the curative spas of Baden-Baden, and trekked to the timeless archeological ruins of Pompeii and Herculaneum. They received "special orders" to visit Queen Victoria's private chambers at Windsor Castle. "It was magnificent," Mary enthusiastically wrote, though she did not indicate if the family met the monarch. While in London, they drove by George Peabody's estate. The financier-philanthropist had died four years earlier. "I stopped to take a look at it," Mary wrote. "It is very fine & is placed near the Old Lady of Threadneedle St . . . near the Royal Exchange." In Zurich, the Duke of Buckingham came to call; "a most agreeable visit," Mary concluded.[82]

Early in the trip, Mary's father consulted a physician in London about his deteriorating health. He was disoriented and in a fragile mental state. Garrett dictated a letter to his sister, Elizabeth Barbara, that Mary wrote for him. He revealed the great mental and physical toll the railroad was taking on him: "I am improving slowly," he wrote, "but I find that almost absolute mental rest is essential. I suppose my brain has been so hard worked for so long a period that its disturbance can only be remedied by much repose." The physician's orders were stern. "Whilst he [the physician] said I might get entirely well, he said this could only result by taking at least a year of entire relaxation with the cessation of thought upon subjects that have for so long occupied me." The physician assured Garrett that "he had had a number of similar cases in London resulting from the same cases of overtaxed brains and that this had been the only course wh. [which] produced permanently good results."[83]

Even with his daughter's valuable assistance, Garrett hardly got the "complete cessation of thought" prescribed by the physician. The Garretts tried to keep their itinerary private, but to no avail. The business of the B&O and its international web of finance hounded Mary's father relentlessly wherever the family traveled. An endless stream of letters, business appointments, and obligatory social rounds awaited them at each stop. Despite his frail health, Garrett never missed an opportunity to promote Baltimore. "He made them [his trips abroad] of much value to his native city by consultations with steam ship owners and capitalists, to whom he has presented the great advantages of Baltimore as a commercial center," an observer noted.[84]

Cables, communications, and contracts—"heavy mails and correspondence," as Garrett described in a letter to his sister—poured in each day, with Mary reviewing each one and presenting the information it contained to her father.[85] She drafted telegrams and helped him compose letters. With every telegram, every contract, and each piece of correspondence, Mary was learning the details of railroading and the inner workings of the B&O. Probably more than any young woman of her era, she was immersed in the masculine world of railroad management. It was an unconventional education, an apprenticeship that could not have been equaled at Miss Kummer's School for Girls or any other school in the country. John Work Garrett, in turn, began to trust his daughter's solid common sense and business judgment. He depended on her.

Mary also fielded visitors. Junius Morgan, now head of Peabody's company, was one of the few to get through Mary's barricade. He was a frequent visitor but one who more often than not brought bad news about the deepening financial crisis affecting the B&O back home. "Papa is not getting much rest," Mary fretted in her letters to her brothers and aunt throughout their trip.[86] By the time they reached Nice in February 1874, Garrett's health still had not improved. He wrote incoherent, often rambling letters to his mother and sister.

John Work Garrett's prolonged absence from Baltimore made him homesick for the beloved city he left behind. "All is very different in Europe," he wrote to his sister, "but to me, nowhere do I find surroundings more delightful than those of home." Apparently, Garrett's illness did not prevent him from appreciating the local scenery in Paris. "Papa was highly amused by the beautifully dressed and extremely stylish girls, who are the salesgirls," Mary quipped.[87]

As their trip progressed, Mary managed to slip out as often as she could to enjoy the sights, often wandering through historic areas on her own. She kept a detailed journal describing her wondrous discoveries. Her health was robust, and she adored everything she saw. Her letters convey the enthusiasm of an awestruck nineteen-year-old whose life was unfolding day by day before her. She especially admired the architecture of the ancient European capitals. In Brussels, she returned time and time again to look at the Hotel de Ville, "a very fine specimen of the Gothic."[88]

In Europe, Mary embarked upon her lifelong passions for archaeology and classical statuary, interests inherited from her father. Writing to Aunt Lizzie in April 1874, Mary marveled over the sights in Pompeii and Herculaneum. "Do you remember a piece of statuary / Marble / in that Museum, Psyche? I think it is one of the loveliest things we have seen." She gushed over the excess of gorgeous ancient artifacts that the family bought, one after another, for their personal collection. "We are all guilty," she wrote home. Throughout their trip, Mary's father lavished jewelry on his wife and daughter. From Paris, sapphire and diamond rings; from Rome, gold and filigree combs and gold earrings with intaglios.[89]

In Paris, Mary and her parents met up with Robert and his wife, Mary Frick. Robert wrote home to Aunt Lizzie: "There are quite a number of Baltimore people here. They all seem to like the place very much."[90] Harry and Alice could not join the family in Europe. They had just welcomed their second son, Horatio Whitridge Garrett, in 1873. Their first son, John Work Garrett II, had been born in 1872.[91] Mary was anxious to see the newest addition to the family, hoping soon "to take a peep at my new nephew."[92]

In February 1874, Mary sent a special letter of congratulations home to her grandmother Elizabeth Garrett, who was celebrating the fiftieth anniversary of one of her special charities. In 1824, while a young wife married to an up-and-coming merchant and living on Fayette Street, Elizabeth had helped to found the Society for the Relief of the Indigent Sick. In its half century of ministering to Baltimore's needy, the charity had "succored over 20,000 of the sick and poor, regardless of creed or color." Fifty years later, she was one of two surviving founders. A fête was held in Baltimore to honor the long-lasting charity and its equally long-lived founders.[93]

Mary's letters to her family during the family's 1873–74 trip reveal much more than the lavish, leisurely Grand Tour itinerary of a wealthy American family. This was the first time Mary was away from many of her family members for any length of time. The trip provided one of the earliest opportunities for her to express herself, outwardly, in writing. Mary wrote beautifully, with excellent script, precise grammar, and expressive descriptions. At an early age, she already had honed her habit of personal frugality, often writing crossways and in the margins on stationery in order to save space. Her daily correspondence, letters to and from her aunts, grandmother, and brothers, reveal Mary's warm, loving relationship with her family. The letters, while written in the typical respectful, embellished nineteenth-century style, disclose a family comfortably at ease with each other—friendly, companionable, warm, and very caring about each other's lives.

One piece of correspondence, however, was not as congenial or eagerly received as family news. On the first day of 1874, B&O interim president John King telegraphed Mary's father, notifying him of an engineers' strike in Pittsburgh. It was a troubling sign that did not bode well for Garrett's scheduled return to Baltimore later that fall. As predicted, simmering labor unrest greeted Mary's father upon the family's return from Europe in October 1874. Any health improvements Garrett might have obtained from his eighteen-month trip abroad were instantly obliterated. He returned from the trip to face, as the *Baltimore American* noted, "the gravest crisis of his life."[94] The economic depression of 1873 had not abated. It had worsened. Competing railroads continued their rate feuds to desperately hold on to as much freight and passenger business as possible. Garrett and other industrialists slashed workers' meager wages even more. Wage earners across the country—railroad workers, miners, and factory workers—suffered dreadfully. There was little relief in sight. Even Baltimore's renowned philanthropists could do little to ameliorate the impoverished living conditions of starving workers and their families.

On the B&O, the average annual pay of a fireman was $421, and the wages of a brakeman were $493. Railroad work was especially perilous and terrifying and often fatal. The equipment often was unsafe, unreliable, and aging. In the 1870s, there were no laws protecting industrial workers or ensuring their safety. Workers and their families suffered the abysmal effects of poverty. Suicide and depression were common. "In two instances, it is said, brakemen after the loss of rest and under the pressure of the depression of lost wages, etc., have purposely thrown themselves under the wheels," one Baltimore newspaper reported in the summer of 1877. "Nearly all the men talked with said at one time or another when melancholy, they meditated about stepping over the bumpers and meeting instant death."[95]

Workers' pent-up anger simmered, and in the summer of 1877, it finally exploded. With little to lose and knowing their company's president would more than likely bring in strikebreakers, on July 16, 1877, B&O workers at Baltimore's Camden Junction walked off the job, setting up blockades to prevent freight trains from moving. B&O agents opened fire on them. Within a week, the labor violence spilled over to the streets of Baltimore. It did not take long for Mobtown to again be mobbed, this time with fifteen thousand angry rioters.

The strikers turned their anger from their company to the man who ran it. They hunted him down, heading to the Garrett mansion on Mount Vernon Place, where they did not find their reviled president. The strike spread like wildfire up and down the B&O lines to West Virginia. Garrett brought the full force of the federal government against the rioting workers. Federal troops soon quelled the Baltimore riot, but the damage was done. Contagious strike fever soon spread to other labor hotspots in Pittsburgh, Chicago, Buffalo, and St. Louis.

Garrett stood steadfast. "We have the power. We have the public sentiment with us. We have the interests of the whole people in accord with us against a few," Garrett exhorted of the strike less than two weeks after it started. The violent strike proved to be a misstep for the nascent organized labor movement, as strikers earned the wrath of many labor leaders. Garrett offered amnesty, assuring that all who stood up "against the tyrannical influences of the demagogues . . . will win position and entitle himself . . . to the confidence of the Company."[96]

The timing for Garrett could not have been worse. His mother, Elizabeth, who had been in declining health for some time, died at age eighty-six on July 17, the day after the strike started. Garrett, in New York at the time, quickly rushed home. His mother died moments before he walked through the door. Mary and her Aunt Lizzie were at Elizabeth's side.

Within weeks, the workers' strike subsided. They had lost their battle. More than a hundred workers, from Baltimore to St. Louis, died in the violence. Workers went back to their impoverished living conditions and difficult, dangerous work on the railroad. As a concession, Garrett established the Workers Relief Fund, which became a model in the industry by paying medical bills and providing temporary monetary relief to workers' families.

But the Garretts did not return to their previous pre-strike routine. Their lives grandly improved. Garrett once again had proven himself to be the man in charge. His workers had been cowed and his railroad saved. Baltimore could rest assured of its commercial competitiveness.

At no time did Baltimore show its gratitude to the railroad tycoon more so than on June 1, 1881. John Work Garrett, Rachel, and Mary had just returned from what had become their frequent months-long stay in Europe. As their ship edged closer into Baltimore Harbor, the guns at Fort McHenry fired a salute to welcome home the city's royal family. Harry and Robert greeted the family at Locust Point, the booming transportation complex John Work Garrett had built after the war to breathe life back into moribund Baltimore. The reunited family clamored aboard a private rail car for the short trip around the harbor to Camden Station, where four years earlier the labor strike had erupted. This time, the scene was far different. Flags waved, committees welcomed, and thousands of grateful Baltimoreans cheered as John Work Garrett, the man of the hour, imperiously waved to the

throng. The mayor conveyed the city's gratitude that its rescuer had safely returned from his trip abroad.[97]

John Work Garrett was a man of his word. As he had promised more than two
decades earlier when he took over the floundering B&O, he continued to extend
the railroad and to assure Baltimore's prosperity. As important, he secured his
own future prosperity and expanded his own empire. The Railroad King ruled his
kingdom.

—◦◦◦—

CHAPTER 3

EXPANSION AND RESTRICTION

THE LIFE OF A NOBLEMAN

The Garrett domain began to extend well beyond railroads, politics, and commerce. In the postwar years, Mary's father purchased some of the most lavish and historic properties in Baltimore and the state. In 1871, following the lead of his friend Johns Hopkins, John Work Garrett purchased Montebello, a historic country estate in the bucolic, spacious area northeast of Baltimore. Here, the city's wealthy had built luxurious summer retreats since the days following the Revolutionary War, with manor names straight from the landed gentry's finest real-estate register: Coldstream, Huntingdon, and Chestnut Hill. The vast country estates were a world away from grimy downtown Baltimore and provided grand living for Baltimore's postwar captains of industry.

Three decades earlier, in 1836, Hopkins had purchased the old Clifton house and the surrounding 166 acres. By the 1850s, Hopkins was one of Baltimore's wealthiest merchants and, as an early investor in the B&O, became one of its largest stockholders, holding an estimated fifteen thousand to seventeen thousand shares. His fortune nearly equaled John Work Garrett's. Hopkins also was influential in Baltimore's banking industry. He was president of the Merchants' Bank and served on the boards of the First Nation's Bank, the Mechanics Bank, the Central Bank, the National Union Bank, the Citizens and Farmers Bank, and the Farmers' and Planters' Bank. [1] Over the years, Hopkins tripled the size of Clifton to five hundred acres. He commissioned the dean of Baltimore's architects, John R. Niernsee, to transform the modest, one-story house into a splendid, expansive, three-story Italianate mansion.

Approaching the grounds of Clifton from the main road, the visitor first passed through a "Roman gateway," signaling the passage into a mythic dimension, one far removed from endless economic depressions and the pestilence of Baltimore's harbor. Entering the impressive 173- × 73-foot mansion from a porte cochere, visitors disembarked from their coaches and stepped inside onto a marble floor in the foyer. A twenty-three-foot walnut staircase wound to the rooms above. The second-floor library, the most well-known of the mansion's rooms, featured a ceiling painted with portraits of Shakespeare's characters and pastoral scenes of Clifton. From the mansion's three-story "prospect's tower," Baltimore's affluent merchant could watch his ships sail in. In 1852, the *Baltimore Sun* noted that the tower afforded "magnificent and extensive views of the entire city and surrounding country and Patapsco and Gunpowder rivers, and the broad expansive Chesapeake whitened by the sail of increasing commerce."[2]

Hopkins hired William Waddell, a renowned Scottish gardener, to landscape sixty acres of the estate with ornamental plants, walkways, bridges, and fountains evocative of a fairy-tale land. Over one hundred statues dotted the finely manicured landscape. Waddell filled the gardens with exotic and rare botanic specimens that Hopkins's ships brought from around the globe. Clifton soon earned the title of one of "Baltimore's most opulent showplaces." It was a relaxing retreat for a busy merchant, as the *Maryland Farmer* noted in 1872, one that offered "[a]n air of quiet repose, of independent stillness with a sort of hush of security that so pervades this lovely spot that the very birds and squirrels seem domestic, as if they felt they had a protector, with none to make them afraid."[3]

But while guests might have enjoyed quiet repose on the tranquil grounds of Clifton during the day, the nights livened up considerably. Hopkins, the refined, gentlemanly Quaker bachelor, was renowned for merriment and all-night dances held in the expansive ballroom that ran the length of the mansion. The Prince of Wales, who became King Edward VII, was among the many visitors to enjoy Hopkins's hospitality. Not surprisingly, Hopkins himself described Clifton as "a heaven on earth."[4]

Adjacent to Hopkins's Clifton estate lay Montebello, another, far larger, heaven on earth. Built by Revolutionary War hero Samuel Smith, it was near the country estates of Baltimore's most notable families. Enoch Pratt's Tivoli, the Abell family's Woodbourne, and Edward Patterson's Homestead were close by. The Smith mansion, considered one of the most beautiful estates in Maryland, featured, among other amenities, a fireplace of the finest Italian marble and an oval dining room.[5] For Mary's father, owning a prime property such as Montebello represented the long journey the Garretts had taken since the 1790s, when

Mary MacMechen Garrett struggled on her humble farm in West Middletown, Pennsylvania, to eke out a living with her fatherless children.

After the deaths of Samuel Smith and his widow, the mansion passed into the hands of the Mount Vernon Place Tiffany family until John Work Garrett bought the property in 1871. Garrett expanded the estate, buying adjacent land parcels. The new and enlarged Montebello eventually counted not one but two mansions and required separate geographical descriptions: Lower Montebello, which included the historic Smith mansion, and Upper Montebello, with a mansion built by Archibald Stirling. Montebello eventually stretched over fourteen hundred acres and included the old Herteles brickyard, with its fifteen buildings and kilns.

It was, as many noted at the time, simply the enormity of Montebello that most overwhelmed. The sprawling estate encompassed 2.1 square miles. Standing at one corner of the estate, an observer could walk 1.5 miles east and 1.5 miles north to gain full appreciation of the expanse of the Garretts' weekend retreat. Montebello dwarfed New York's Central Park, which had opened to the public in 1853 and, in contrast to Montebello's 1,400 acres, counted a mere 843 acres.[6] Montebello gained fame as one of the country's largest estates, reminiscent of the expansive antebellum plantations of generations earlier.

Baltimoreans soon dubbed Montebello and its surrounding area "Garrett's Woods." Although Harry and Alice briefly lived in Lower Montebello early in their marriage, the once-grand Smith mansion was seldom used and in time fell into disrepair. Garrett focused on renovating the newer Stirling mansion in Upper Montebello. Unlike Hopkins's graceful Italianate style at Clifton, Garrett chose rural and rustic. Under the direction of the original architect, Edmund Lind, Garrett transformed the mansion from an elegant, stucco-walled structure into a more countrified clapboard house with a wide, wrap-around veranda, bay windows, and porch brackets for hanging vines.[7]

But rural hardly meant uncivilized. Every convenience that Mary and her family enjoyed at their Mount Vernon Place mansion or their trips abroad was replicated, if not greatly augmented, a few miles north of West Monument Street at Montebello. Montebello soon equaled, if not surpassed, Clifton in extravagance. Alderney and Devon cattle and Southdown sheep languidly roamed its spacious pastures. A year after the Garretts purchased the estate, in 1872, a writer from the *Maryland Farmer* described his visit to John Work Garrett's "elegant suburban retreat." There he found a grand work-in-progress, with abundant flowers flowing out from the terrace, "rare plants in the conservatory," and the "grapery in perfect order . . . [with] fine specimens of European grapes." The writer was at a loss to adequately describe "all that we saw." But he assured his readers there was no better way for the wealthy to live. "Can moneyed men apply a portion of their large capital to a better, more rational, more humanizing purpose than adorning their homesteads with beautiful flowers and trees and useful birds and fruits?"[8]

John Work Garrett's plan for Montebello eventually encompassed far more than flowers and rare plants. He was never far removed from his Scots-Irish farming ancestry. Finally, on a large scale, he could unabashedly indulge his passion for husbandry, first honed years earlier at the family estate at Landsdowne, which he still owned. He studied his avocation whenever he could. On the family's 1873–74 trip to Europe, three years after purchasing Montebello, Mary wrote to her Aunt Lizzie, describing how she and her parents "had stopped at Prince Albert's dairy and went over the model farm. As you can readily imagine, Papa was exceedingly interested and we looked at all the calves, bulls, etc." Mary was not quite so enthusiastic as her father about traipsing around the royal farm inspecting the livestock. She deserted the tour "at the pig sty." Her father was "delighted by not finding any calves—or pigs for that matter—better than the Alderneys of Montebello," Mary wrote. While on their eighteen-month trip, Mary's father pined for Montebello, "the woods, the meadows, the horses & colts, the [unreadable], the sheep and the garden & the flowers are to be found elsewhere & I long to enjoy these beauties in preference to the very interesting & interesting objects wh [which] I am now seeing for the first time," he lamented while resting in Zurich in September 1873.[9]

Garrett's pride and joy were Montebello's old stone "Arabian stables" with his "150 internationally famous thoroughbreds." He presented one named Damascus to King Umberto I of Italy. For many years, Garrett published annual catalogues of his inventory of horses available for sale. The "Catalogue of Trotting Stock," from the "Estate of John Work Garrett," often ran thirty-six to forty pages in length, with the detailed lineage of each thoroughbred. Maryland Volunteer, Garrett's favorite stallion and sire to most of the stock, was listed as a "Dark rich bay Horse, with black points, 16 hands 2 inches high; foaled in 1875."[10]

On their 1873–74 European trip, the family was invited to visit Queen Victoria's stables. Mary's father found the Queen's horses paled in comparison to his own at Montebello. "I have not yet seen any thoroughbreds equal to our own beauties, although I have seen the Queen's best at her celebrated farms and at Hampton Court," he boasted in a letter to his mother from the Buckingham Palace Hotel in August 1873.[11] Garrett also built a racetrack at Montebello to run his fine horses. In 1873, he enlarged the existing lake on the property to make it more suitable for boating.

With the Upper Montebello mansion expanded and renovated, the family entertained constantly with "liberal and unostentatious hospitality," according to the *Baltimore Sun*.[12] The guest list included international VIPs. Former Army General George McClellan, a longtime Garrett friend despite his fall from military grace during the war; English scientist Thomas Huxley, grandfather of Aldous; and philosopher Herbert Spencer were just some of the many visitors who passed through the gates of Montebello. Editors, bankers, members of Parliament and Congress, and railroad presidents all enjoyed the amenities of the Garretts' extravagant estate.

Andrew Carnegie visited Montebello and found it much to his liking. The steel magnate knew a thing or two about grand country living. He owned a twenty-thousand-acre estate, Skibo, in his native Scotland. Writing about Montebello in his autobiography, Carnegie noted that John Work Garrett "was one of the few Americans who lived then in the grand style of a country gentleman, with many hundreds of acres of beautiful land, park-like drives, a stud of Thoroughbred horses, with cattle, sheep, and dogs and a home that realized what one had read of the country life of a nobleman in England."[13]

Montebello provided more than pastoral acreage for cattle and sheep. During the violent railroad strike of 1877, the vast estate offered safe refuge for the family. The B&O strikers, not finding their president at his Mount Vernon Place home, stormed north to Montebello, shaking their fists in fury. "Men bent on assassination laid in wait for Garrett at both his townhouse and his country residence at Montebello," a commentator wrote. Years later, Mary recalled how fate had saved her father's life. While the family took cover at Montebello, one of the rioters fired a gun into the mansion. The bullet, intended for John Work Garrett, had instead lodged into a book in the family library.[14] The mob eventually subsided and drifted away.

Mary enjoyed the outdoor life that Montebello offered in such abundance. Through her adolescent years, rigorous outdoor exercise helped to strengthen her once injured leg. She loved to hike through Montebello's woods, wander down the estate's many paths, read in the gardens, and sail on the lake. She became an accomplished, fearless equestrian, as a friend observed, choosing the finest thoroughbreds from her father's stables to gallop through the hills of Montebello.[15]

Aside from providing an idyllic weekend retreat for his family and a place to breed his prized thoroughbreds, Garrett, never passing up a prospective investment, had other interests in the northeast region of Baltimore. By the time Garrett bought Montebello, the surrounding area had been under development for two decades as one of Baltimore's first northern suburbs. In the early 1850s, Robert Gorsuch Jr. and Edward B. Jackson began to stake off streets and to sell residential lots. The new development was first advertised in the 1853–54 *Matchett's City Directory*.[16]

But there was, perhaps, another far more important motivation for Garrett's purchase of Montebello. It was here, in northeast Baltimore, that Johns Hopkins more than likely wanted to locate his new university. Garrett later insisted that Hopkins had "designed that the buildings of the university should be constructed upon his vast Clifton estate, where each building would enhance beyond its cost." According to Garrett, Hopkins envisioned that situating the new university on the Clifton estate would provide expansive space for the university and help to develop the northeast corridor of Baltimore, making it a prosperous growth area for the city. Hopkins had instructed his trustees about "the grading of the surface to its proper drainage, to the laying of the grounds, and to the careful and the deliberate choice of a plan for the erection and arrangement of the building."[17] The 1876 *Atlas of Baltimore* shows Clifton as the site of the proposed Johns Hopkins University.

Locating the new university campus at Clifton would, Garrett later stated, attract students and relatives to live in the area: "Thus squares of beautiful houses would in time be erected, with parks and ornamental grounds adding to the healthfulness and charms of the surroundings."[18] And it was no accident that Montebello was right next door. Hopkins and Garrett's combined holdings in the northeastern region totaled nearly two thousand acres of land and would afford the new university and a future community more than ample space. It would also afford John Work Garrett, vast landowner, more than ample profits should the region develop more fully as a result of the new university.

Mary's father set his sites on other areas of development beyond northeast Baltimore. Soon after his election as B&O president in 1858, he looked to the pastoral, scenic vistas in the mountains of Western Maryland as the perfect spot to cater to the nation's growing tourism business. The Garretts had vacationed there for years, and Garrett had acquired more than five thousand prime acres of land in the area that eventually would bear his name. The B&O's earliest lines ran through Oakland, a booming little mountain town incorporated in 1861. The town's famed Glades Hotel opened in 1859 and attracted notables from around the country to take in the cool mountain air. "Buffalo Bill" Cody stayed there. Jefferson Davis lived in the hotel during its first summer before taking his place as the ill-fated Confederate president in 1861. After the war, former Union General Lew Wallace penned parts of *Ben Hur* while enjoying the hotel's amenities.[19] Timber and coal barons from around the country also flocked to Western Maryland. They benefited from the mountains' curative effects while, no doubt, calculating the infinite profits that lay underground in vast mineral and coal deposits.

Unfortunately for Mary's father and for the country, the Civil War disrupted his early dream to develop the region. Instead of luring tourists to enjoy their bountiful pleasures, the picturesque western territories of Maryland became a thoroughfare to and from some of the bloodiest battles of the war.

Seven years after the war's conclusion, Garrett finally got his wish. In July 1872, he broke ground on a new hotel in Deer Park, not far from Oakland, where he had built a church in his brother's memory in 1868. A year later, on July 4, 1873, just days before departing on his eighteen-month trip to Europe to restore his health, Garrett opened the splendid new hotel to rave reviews. The four-story, two-hundred-room hotel's glass-domed natatorium enclosed two swimming pools, one for men and one for women. The four-hundred-acre resort proved to be a veritable playground for billiards, bowling, archery, and baseball and featured both Turkish and Russian baths. The beautifully appointed ladies' parlor gained fame near and far. Newspapers boasted that the new hotel, with its sparkling, restorative spring waters, was "the most enjoyable summer resort of the Alleghenies." To assure its exclusivity, the hotel's guests were "strictly of the highest order."[20]

Not by happenstance did the B&O greatly profit from its tourism venture. The resort beckoned to restless city dwellers eager to escape disease-ridden urban summers. Enthusiastic visitors came from both sides of the mountains, not only from the East Coast, but from the Midwest as well, via the B&O's lines to Cincinnati and beyond. Soon, twelve B&O trains stopped at Deer Park each day, six going east, six going west. The trip from Cincinnati took eleven hours, from Baltimore, eight hours.[21]

Spurred by the success of the Deer Park Hotel, in 1876, Mary's father opened the three-story Oakland Hotel near the B&O station. The ballroom could accommodate hundreds of revelers, and visitors could walk to nearby Washington Springs, rumored to have been favored by the first president during a surveying trip in 1784. Like its counterpart at Deer Park, the Oakland Hotel soon attracted notables from around the country. In 1883, Alexander Graham Bell visited the hotel, where he directed the installation of the first telephone service in Western Maryland between the two resort hotels.[22]

Garrett's resorts in Western Maryland entertained American royalty for half a century. Each summer, the well-to-do decamped for several weeks to frolic at the grand Deer Park and Oakland hotels. To accommodate the top-end tourists, under Garrett's direction the B&O built a family compound of "cottages"— eighteen- to twenty-five-room getaways near the Deer Park Hotel for the Garretts and their friends to enjoy. The cottages were christened simply "#1–5." For Rachel,

Mary, and himself, Garrett built a nineteen-room cottage with five bedrooms, which Mary and Rachel decorated with abandon. Mary was thrilled with their new mountain home. "The rooms are all much larger than I supposed from your description," she excitedly wrote to her mother. Nearby, Harry, Alice, and the boys enjoyed their twenty-five-room cottage, famed for its beautiful stairway and paneling.[23] Mary Frick Garrett's father, William Frick, built one of the most glorious of the Deer Park cottages.

John Work Garrett and his sons' personal real-estate domain eventually included three mansions on Mount Vernon Place, fourteen-hundred-acre Montebello with two grand homes, summer retreats at Uplands and Lansdowne in Baltimore County, Tiverton in Newport, and cottages in Deer Park in Garrett County. But there remained one more prime property that John Work Garrett coveted. In 1878, he purchased Evergreen, the last and finest jewel in his real-estate crown.[24] He gave the manor home, one of Baltimore's most exquisite, to Harry, Alice, and their three young sons.

Evergreen sat majestically high atop a hill on fifty acres on Charles Street in the rolling terrain of north Baltimore. Even from a distance, through the trees from the road below, the two-and-a-half-story, twelve-room mansion—which would be expanded many times in the years ahead—commanded attention, with its four stately Corinthian columns, huge ornate moldings, and crowning cupola. Twelve sturdy stone steps led up to the formidable front door. The grand Italianate mansion had been built twenty years earlier by Stephen Broadbent, who had the foresight to include the most up-to-date amenities imagined at the time: indoor plumbing and central heating. Each room featured a hand-carved mantelpiece. Down a slight hill, toward the back of the house, the two-story carriage house with its own cupola housed the horses and finely embellished broughams used to transport the family in style about town.

Within a decade of the end of the Civil War, the Garrett imprimatur enveloped Baltimore and much of Maryland—in commerce, in culture, and in the state's most visible signs of Gilded Age elegance and extravagance. Mary's brothers had taken their positions as Baltimore's new generation of merchant princes. Like their grandfather Robert Garrett and their father before them, they had every outward sign of status, prestige, and accomplishment. Each had married well, had risen to the top of the "family" businesses of the B&O and Robert Garrett and Sons, and now reigned over some of Maryland's most extravagant estates. Mary's brothers had been given every opportunity to succeed.

But what about Mary? She, too, had served her "apprenticeship" in the family firm as "Papa's secretary" at her father's side for a decade. She, too, had learned the ins and outs of railroading—possibly more so than her brothers—and of the family business, Robert Garrett and Sons. What would this bright, inquisitive young woman do with her life? How would she leave her mark on the world as her father and grandfather had done?

As Mary would soon discover, the father who had brought her into his business world, whose influence and wealth had brought her enviable advantages and opportunities, could just as easily tighten the reins. John Work Garrett's province stretched not only into every nook and cranny of Baltimore and the B&O but into every aspect of his daughter's life as well.

A SILENT REVOLUTION

"Women have leaped from their spheres," commentator Maria Weston Chapman boasted of women's advancement in the years following the Civil War.[25] With its million-plus death and casualty rate, the war had depleted a whole generation of men, turning society upside down. Not surprisingly, for Mary's generation, long-held social restrictions began to erode in the war's tumultuous wake. In the last quarter of the century, women by the thousands forged ahead, reinventing themselves, creating new roles in the workplace and community, and defying old expectations for marriage and motherhood. No matter what creative path they chose for their personal or professional lives, many women had one common goal: to resist the repressive social conventions of the day.

Mary, however, did not easily leap from her sphere. Like many of her young, leisure-class contemporaries, she tried to chart her path in a new world that offered exciting options hardly imagined by her mother's generation. Unfortunately, with each new plan, she came up against a surprising roadblock, someone who was not nearly as enthusiastic about the new social order as she was. For the first time, Mary stood toe to toe with her uncompromising, domineering father. The once comfortable, close relationship that had been nurtured during her childhood and training as "Papa's secretary" showed signs of strain. Her father, who had once so greatly expanded her world through travel, companionship, and introduction to wealthy and renowned individuals from Europe to the Far East, now began to limit her options one by one.

John Work Garrett was not alone. In the rapidly changing, postwar landscape, few Americans agreed on exactly where women should "leap." One issue became strikingly clear in the war's aftermath: women's financial independence or, more specifically, their financial vulnerability. Without husbands or fathers to fall back on, women often faced grave uncertainty and peril. The topic of independence, particularly economic security, once thought to be only the plight of "decayed gentlewomen," moved from hushed parlor conversations and stormed to the forefront of women's issues. From religious pulpits, medical journals, newspapers, and popular magazines flew a volley of opinions, often polarized, about exactly where women belonged and how they could achieve economic security while maintaining social propriety.

The "woman question" became a lightning rod of dissension and endless debate. The *New York Evangelist*, the publication of the American Bible Tract Society, whose readers included well-to-do Protestant women across the country, praised women's advancement and efforts at economic self-reliance. "Fifty years have witnessed a silent revolution of unprecedented importance in woman's work, lot and outlook," the editors noted. "The truly cultivated woman respects labor and takes pride in her ability to engage in some useful, creative occupation." A feeling of independence "is the best protection a person can have in this world." Not so, stormed other social critics, with one echoing concerns shared by many Americans. He lambasted women, the "least valuable of created beings," for competing with men in the workplace, thereby lowering men's wages and threatening the core of American society. Worse, woman's work ruined her health, making her "unfit to be the helper and companion of man."[26]

Undaunted by such polarized diatribes, "New Women" flocked to women's colleges such as Vassar, Smith, and Wellesley. In 1870, eleven thousand women attended college nationwide; within a decade that number doubled.[27] Women took office jobs in the postwar industrial boom, and their proportion in the workforce increased from 15 percent in 1870 to more than 20 percent three decades later.[28] Expanding beyond the traditional role of teaching, they entered new professions, becoming librarians, nurses, journalists, lawyers, and social workers. Some created entirely new professions for themselves. Elisabeth Marbury, from a well-to-do New York family, became a theatrical agent. Socialite Elsie De Wolf developed a career in interior design. In the next decade, Jane Addams and Ellen Gates Starr would found Chicago's Hull House, helping immigrants to adapt to their new homeland. In Baltimore, Henrietta Szold would do the same. New York arts patron Candace Wheeler unleashed her entrepreneurial drive and forged a commercial partnership with designer Louis Comfort Tiffany. As Wheeler noted of women's newfound visibility in the public sphere: "Women of all classes had always been dependent upon the wage earning capacity of men . . . but the time was ripe for a change."[29]

Mary, too, was ready for a change. By her early twenties, she had matured into an attractive but still socially shy young woman. Her sensitive nature, developed in adolescence, carried into adulthood. The "fullness" of which she had once written gave way to a slim, strong figure. Photographs show her to be a serious, pensive young woman, often wearing the spectacles Robert and Harry had ridiculed years before. Although she would soon tend to favor unadorned fashions, she obligingly wore the requisite bustles and embellished silk and taffeta dresses with puffed leg-of-mutton sleeves required by the fashion magazines of the day. She often pulled her dark brown hair back sternly into a chignon at the nape of her neck. Her father's strong will and fortitude, so apparent in his photographs, reflected in Mary's face as well.

In 1877, Mary's schoolmate from Miss Kummer's, Bessie King, introduced Mary and Julia Rogers to her cousin Martha Carey Thomas and Mary "Mamie" Mackall Gwinn. Carey was three years younger than Mary, Julia, and Bessie, and Mamie was the youngest of the group, four years younger than Carey. Mamie's grandfather had served as a U.S. senator and ambassador and her father was Maryland's attorney general. She lived a few doors away from the Garretts on Mount Vernon Place. From a respected Quaker family, Carey's father was a favored Baltimore physician and her mother was an avid reformer and activist. Mary immediately liked her new acquaintances, soon calling Carey "Minnie"—a childhood name that Carey would soon outgrow but one Mary always preferred. Like Mary, Carey had suffered a serious childhood injury at the age of seven, when she had been severely burned in a kitchen accident, leaving her permanently scarred over much of her body.

The five women had much in common. Their fathers, except Julia's, who had died, were prominent Baltimore leaders and trustees of the fledgling university just taking shape in downtown Baltimore and named after its benefactor, Johns Hopkins. But they shared a greater bond than well-known family names. All bright and inquisitive, they shared a love of reading and a sense of adventure. Most important, they felt a profound need to put the pressing issue of the day, the "woman question," to the test.

Mary, Julia, and Bessie's original reading group, formed years earlier at Miss Kummer's, soon expanded to include Carey and Mamie. The five young women christened themselves the "Friday Night," named for their biweekly gatherings in each other's parlors. From a vantage point of a half century later, in 1938, Mamie Gwinn recalled how the group originated as a "small club of the like-minded, to convene at one another's houses fortnightly and to read to one another bookish papers."[30] They inaugurated their group by commissioning a photograph of themselves. Though they looked sedate and sophisticated in their group photo, their meetings proved otherwise.

Intense female friendships were particularly important to young women of the nineteenth century and helped adolescent girls to make the awkward transition to adulthood. Such relationships helped to bolster women against a male-dominated world, allowing women to freely express themselves to each other in a culture that demanded conformity and conventionality. Middle- and upper-class women usually spent most of their lives with other women—in their clubs or tending each other through pregnancies, childbirth, and childrearing—in homosocial or homoemotional relationships.[31] They often wrote chatty, hyperbolic, introspective, and intensely romantic letters to each other, professing love and pledging undying devotion.

At last, Mary had found lively friends, surrogate sisters, with whom she could play and laugh, not schoolmates who would tease her and bring her to tears. The group eased her out of some of her shyness and incited a streak of rebelliousness in her. Mary loved the Friday Night, calling it her "intellectual machine."[32] Their fathers' stewardship of the new Johns Hopkins University, which had just opened in 1876, fired up the young women's lively imaginations and sense of activism. The Friday Night, through readings and late-night talks, articulated their hopes and fears and explored the mysterious world of sexual relationships, marriage, and women's place in the world. They wrote a collective novel—never published—with each of the five budding authors penning a chapter or two in small notebooks. In heated discussions, they debated the tug between women's independence, the confinement of marriage, and the need for women to be better educated.

Religion was one topic seldom discussed. Robert Garrett's Presbyterian "peculiarities," first experienced in West Middletown seventy-five years earlier, were of no interest to his granddaughter in the more secular postwar years. In late adolescence, Mary dabbled a bit in religious inquiry, occasionally noting biblical passages in her journal. The interest was short-lived. In her adult life, Mary rarely wrote of attending church or being under the sway of religion. Mamie later observed that Carey and Mary "had by far (I should suppose) [the] least natural theism, least religious instinct . . . Religion was not talked of in the meetings of the Club; its members had in that respect no influence on one another, though lack of christian [sic] faith was pretty generally understood." When Mamie's mother complained that the Friday Night had turned her daughter away from religion, Mary stood up to her, asserting that "more and more people hold such modern views."[33]

Religion aside, the five young women were beginning to learn the rules of the Gilded Age social order. As Mamie later wrote, they learned "that in an altered world, a gentlewoman's culture, unsupported by [college] degrees, would not in case of need assure her independence." They pondered English feminist Mary Wollstonecraft's 1782 *A Vindication of the Rights of Women*, with its revolutionary idea of equality of the sexes and emphasis on rigorous female education. Stimulated by such fiery writings and debates, Mary began formulating her own answers to the "woman question." She criticized the prominent critic and social reformer John Ruskin, who asserted women's true place of power was in the home. "Ruskin says that a woman's knowledge on higher subjects should be elementary just so she may be able to help her husband, but to leave him to climb the scaly hill of knowledge. No! Knowledge is power and I for one am going to do my best to gain it," she concluded of stifling Victorian expectations and marital arrangements.[34]

Courtship and marriage were very much on Mary's mind. She had many examples of upper-class Victorian marriages all around her, notably her brothers and their wives, who represented very conventional images of Gilded Age domesticity and conformity. As married women, Mary's sisters-in-law provided acceptable models of Victorian female expectations. Their marriages offered a social status that Mary, as an unmarried woman, did not have. Now firmly ensconced in Baltimore's elite social circles, they held court in their sumptuous Baltimore homes, Robert and Mary Frick on Mount Vernon Place and Harry, Alice, and their three sons on the sprawling grounds of Evergreen. Each vacationed at the other's summer getaways at Uplands in Baltimore County, Tiverton in Newport, and Garrett County. Robert moved on from the Valley Railroad in 1875 and officially entered the inner circle of B&O management, ascending to third vice president. Harry was making his mark as head of Robert Garrett and Sons' banking division, which continued its seamless financial relationship with the B&O.

Mary pondered how marital arrangements such as those of her brothers and sisters-in-law would affect her own life and ambitions. Although only three years younger than her two sisters-in-law, she held different aspirations. She did not, however, want for suitors. As the daughter of an influential and well-connected family, she would have been considered very eligible in the marriage market. She thought a great deal about marriage, particularly during the time when "a man who would become a brilliant success" enchanted her. "For a long time," Mary later wrote, "he wanted to marry me." It is unclear who the mysterious love interest—or interests—might have been, for Mary wrote few details about either. During the late 1870s and 1880s, she frequently corresponded with "Mr. Marsh" and "Dr. Murray," jotting their names in her correspondence journal. Carey at one point felt that Mary was in love with Dr. Murray and later suggested that Mary consider marrying "Prof. Marsh."[35]

The Friday Night helped Mary to demystify some of the secrecy and fear of veiled Victorian marriage and sexuality. Like most well-to-do women, the young women were sheltered from and unknowledgeable about the opposite sex. Their friendships with each other offered comfort and familiarity, while men's needs and desires still proved to be unfathomable, even fearful. Their sexuality was just budding. Their female relationships, while apparently not physical or sexual at that point, were far more understandable than heterosexual interactions. As Mamie later observed of their inquisitive relationships: "We were sure we didn't like men better."[36]

One afternoon, Julia, Mary, and Carey discovered medical books, possibly a medical standard such as *What Women Should Know*, on the shelves of Dr. Thomas's library. The young women enthusiastically dove into the books, which were graphic and pathological in their medical descriptions of intercourse, venereal disease, and the indelicate topics of male anatomy and sex, subjects they knew little about. Mary, who just a few years before had been shielded by her mother from "the laws of health" and menstruation, was now shockingly confronted with the realities of sexual relations and what many women considered to be "conjugal responsibilities."[37]

The Friday Night added yet another dimension to Mary's life: intense and always shifting dynamics among the five women that not only established valuable female friendships but also sowed the seeds for jealousies and deceits that would escalate with time. Early on, Carey became infatuated with Mary—more precisely, with Mary's grand and opulent lifestyle, so different from her own modest Quaker upbringing. She was dazzled by the Garretts' everyday lives, filled with magnificent city mansions and expansive country estates, glamorous friends, couture fashions, liveried broughams, and servants to do their every bidding. Meeting up with the Garretts on an 1880 trip to Europe, Carey wrote, "Mr. Garrett has the most magnificent courier, Pietro, who waits on him and runs Mary's errands." She composed a sonnet to Mary and began unrequited advances, insisting on a special relationship. Although valuing their friendship, Mary wanted to keep it "sensible."[38]

Within two years of the group's formation, the Friday Night's emotional relationships became entangled in intrigues. Besides Mary's "sensibility," Carey faced another impediment in her developing affection for Mary: Julia. For nearly a decade, since their days at Miss Kummer's, Mary and Julia had shared all aspects of their lives, including, to Carey's chagrin, her imploring letters to Mary. Julia found Carey's overtures to Mary insulting—and upsetting. She accused Carey of encouraging a "special friendship" with Mary.[39] Mary, too, was not yet ready to sacrifice her favored relationship with Julia for Carey, who, in 1879, would set sail with Mamie to begin what would become nearly four years of graduate study in Europe. Undaunted, Carey persisted in a long-distance campaign to drive a wedge between Mary and Julia, an effort that would prove successful within a few years.

Now in their mid-twenties, late for the Victorian marriage market, the Friday Night discussed the impossibility of marriage for ambitious New Women like themselves. Young women increasingly questioned marriage and were not eager to settle for an unsuitable, stifling arrangement. Carey, who boasted that several men had fallen in love with her and that she had returned passion toward at least one, wrote: "There seems no solution of the question of marriage, for it is difficult to conceive [of] a woman who really feels her separate life work to give it up when she marries a man, and yet I think—a fact which I used to ignore—that it is and must be a giving up." Mamie later wrote that "we were the marrying brand, and didn't want to marry, and were rather smug about it."[40]

Mary felt the same. She was unconvinced marriage was the right course for her. Bessie tried to persuade her otherwise, but Mary would have none of it. "I have never seen a more thorough and complete and really unconscious surrender of principles," Mary wrote, enraged, to Carey.[41] For Mary, marriage would have been a compromise to the independence she craved. It would have meant moving from the domination of one powerful man, her father, to another.

She tried to sort it out in her mind, often walking through the gardens of Montebello to collect her thoughts. She wrote her ideas about marriage in a note she entitled "Social Questions." She turned to the great philosophers. She especially admired Aristotle, who espoused a marriage based on friendship, in which the partners complement each other sexually and emotionally. She considered what it would be like to spend a lifetime with the same person. She wrote unenthusiastically, "Marriage implies not only sexual relations, but also living together." The institution of marriage, she apathetically acknowledged, "is nothing else than a more or less durable connection between male and female after the birth of the offspring."[42] Her use of the word "durable" reveals not only a great lack of romantic passion for marriage but a sense of merely tolerating yet another unpleasant social obligation.

Perhaps it was the "the birth of offspring" that most concerned her. Throughout her life, Mary suffered from debilitating menstrual periods and related gynecological problems. The explicit drawings of sexual relations and anatomy depicted in Dr. Thomas's books might have alarmed her, as she wondered how she could physically withstand the rigors of repeated pregnancies or, perhaps, fatal childbirth, not uncommon in the Victorian era. It is also probable that Mary did not want to marry and relinquish the Garrett name. During her father's reign of the B&O, there were few family names that could top her own.

But for Mary, the problem of marriage was not confined to choosing among suitors lined up at her front door or fearing marital intimacy. Looking back on that time several years later, Mary insisted the problem had been her father, who emphatically forbade her to marry. Mary recalled that her romance with the man who became a brilliant success was doomed from the start. "My father did not intend me to marry him, or anyone else." There are many reasons why Garrett might have balked at allowing his only daughter to marry. We can speculate that his motivations were selfish. Mary had, after all, proven herself to be a skilled assistant, a confidante, and a companion, someone whose business abilities and sound judgment he valued and needed. She had also proven to be a loyal nursemaid through his frequent illnesses that required constant attention and curative trips to Europe. On the family's 1873–74 trip to Europe, Garrett had noted with envy an English friend's daughter who stayed close by and "keeps house for him."[43] Or perhaps Garrett did not share his daughter's enthusiasm for the "man who would become a great success." Possibly, the suitor was not quite as brilliant as John Work Garrett would have liked and did not live up to the spousal standards Garrett set for his children.

The most intriguing conjecture about Garrett's refusal to let his daughter marry is that, very possibly, he was trying to save her from the perils of yet another restrictive and unfulfilling Gilded Age economic arrangement in marriage. In the Victorian era, wealthy Americans more often than not valued their daughters for their economic potential to merge powerful families. Married women, unless protected by carefully worded legal documents, often forfeited their fortunes to their husbands. Perhaps Garrett was not willing to sacrifice his daughter to strike such a deal or to consign her to an unhappy, economically uncertain future. Perhaps he thought of her as more than a commodity to be traded in the marriage market. It is also possible that he might not have wanted another man to usurp the prominent position he held in his daughter's life.

By 1878, twenty-four years old and disillusioned about marriage, Mary began to think of attending college and preparing for another path. She studied for her Harvard entrance exams. While not a true application process to the all-male college, the exam provided an academic benchmark for women.[44] Mary prepared for a year, but probably not very seriously. She traveled a great deal, making her annual sojourns to Europe and New England, with her studies crammed in between. Studying geometry and geography for the exam must have seemed dull in comparison to the whirlwind amusements of her trips—socializing with poet Robert Browning, artists Sir Lawrence Alma-Tadema and Edward Coley Burne-Jones, and British philosopher and biologist Herbert Spencer. And there were countless gatherings with the extended Garrett clan at Saratoga or Newport, where Mary loved to play tennis and take tea with the Garretts' wide circle of friends. The family frequently stayed at New York's Brevoort, one of their favorite hotels on Fifth Avenue near Washington Square. The hotel's stationery boasted "a quiet hotel with a restaurant of peculiar excellence."[45]

In early 1879, Mary and Julia sat for the exam. By June, the results were in, and the news was not good. Mary, who always wrote glowingly of her friends' accomplishments, noted Julia's "great success." Her own exam, she wrote, was a "wretched failure." Julia's exam scores were impressive; she had scored 74 percent on physical geography, 80 percent on English composition, 83 percent on physics, and 77 percent on mathematics. Mary was not quite as fortunate. Her mediocre, uninspired education a decade before was apparent. "Yes, I have failed about as badly as possible," she wrote to Carey. She had scored much lower than Julia, with 65 percent in English composition, 36 percent in physics, 42 percent in mathematics 1, and 31 percent in mathematics 2.[46] She had failed in each category.

Mary became hysterical, Mamie later recalled. She was shocked at her abysmal failure, writing to Carey, "I was so sure that the knowledge that was so easy for me as a child would be easy now." She thought her inability to concentrate on her studies was physical. She had visited a doctor "for an examination about that trouble I had behind the uterus, which I'm afraid is not very much better." She finally came to terms with her scholastic shortcomings. "I am forced to the conclusion I am not cut out for the student life, either mentally or physically."[47]

It would not have made much difference even if she had passed the exam. Once again, Mary met the familiar impediment: her father. He again put his foot down, forbidding her to continue her studies. "I begged my father that I should be allowed to go to college," Mary later recalled.[48] While her brothers had received the best education at Princeton, Mary was prevented from following in their footsteps.

She tried another tactic: to study abroad. She felt certain, given her familiarity with travel to Europe and her family's wide network of acquaintances there, that her father would acquiesce on this matter. She was wrong. "Papa would gladly, if not more so, see me buried as have me go and I do not think there is the faintest chance of ever getting his consent," she wrote to Carey four months after receiving the grim news about her exam results. Bessie faced a similar obstacle with her own father, and Mary wrote that Bessie would "never go without his consent."

Mary had also asked her father a few years earlier to allow her to study abroad "with [a] teacher who had just opened a school there." That teacher was Sarah Kummer, headmistress of the girls' school on Mount Vernon Place that Mary had most likely attended in her adolescence. "Mademoiselle" had moved on to Paris, where she opened a school to provide instruction in French for American women. Again, Mary's father "positively refused to allow [me] to go to Paris." He finally allowed her to take "special classes," although Mary did not indicate the details.[49]

In an era when women's economic independence drew public debate and private anguish, Mary, in her mid-twenties, was still completely financially dependent on her father. He tightly controlled her expenditures. For spending beyond her allowance, she had to ask him to pay for purchases, even the most minor trinkets, often prevailing upon her mother to intercede on her behalf to pay for her "investments," as she called them. She submitted receipts for a wide range of such investments. Three French paintings, for $20,000, or fabric for new dresses: "44 yards @ .40 = $17.60 and other imported fabrics totaling $43.45."[50]

Despite her anger over her father's control, Mary remained intensely loyal to him and her family. Her inextricable bond with her father and the inherent satisfaction the status her family wealth and name conferred had a powerful hold over her. While angry with the restrictions her father placed on her, she wanted—craved—above all to please him. His approval and praise made her feel "crowned with laurel," a friend noted.[51]

Mary watched as one by one the Friday Night left Baltimore to follow their dreams. Her old friends were finding their way in the wider world. Julia studied at Newnham College at Cambridge and tried her hand at writing, submitting articles to magazines, although none was ever published. Still, she began to hone her skills as a writer, expanding her intellectual interests well beyond Baltimore. Julia's letters to Mary reflect her growing maturity and questioning, as Mary did, the probability—or improbability—of marriage. Carey, accompanied by Mamie, was already on her way to earning her doctorate from the University of Zurich. While Carey wrote effusive letters about her doctoral studies abroad—"I have never been so happy"—Mary, on the other hand, had never been so miserable.[52] She yearned to find a central commitment in life as her friends had discovered for their own lives.

By the age of twenty-five, with marriage and college forbidden to her, and earning her own living not even a remote possibility for the daughter of a renowned and fabulously wealthy railroad tycoon, Mary followed a not uncommon path for many thwarted, restricted, unfulfilled Gilded Age women: mental collapse or *neurasthenia*, as it was commonly called by the Victorians. Depression, withdrawal, and complaints of chronic illness were accepted for Victorian upper-class women forced into idleness and isolation who had little else to occupy their lives. Such emotional and physical vulnerability helped to bolster the popular belief of women's fragility. In this regard, Mary lived up to society's expectations. The once enthusiastic, healthy young woman, who had loved to hike and climb, to camp outdoors, to play tennis and race through the hills of Montebello on her father's thoroughbreds, spun into a downward cycle of neurasthenia, hypochondria, and depression that would last for the next several years.

The precise cause of Mary's illness is unclear, although it more than likely stemmed from a combination of physical ailments, gynecological and orthopedic, as well as psychological problems as a result of her perceived failures and frustrations. It is also likely that she was influenced by her father's example. Starting with the Garretts' 1873–74 eighteen-month trip to Europe, during which John Work Garrett convalesced from his physical and emotional breakdown, and continuing through the next decade until his death, Mary watched as her father lapsed several times into debilitating health-related problems. After her father's breakdown in 1873–74, he recovered sufficiently to return to Baltimore to face labor unrest and the 1877 strike. In 1880, Garrett again decamped to Europe to rest from his latest illness. He was able to report to his doctor from Bellagio, Italy, that he was improving: "My health has been better here, my pulse is now eighty, my appetite and digestion good, and I sleep well."[53] In the next years, the Garretts made several more curative trips to Europe. In her twenties, Mary began the same pattern of repeated physical and mental lapses displayed by her father.

Mary and her father were not the only Garretts to frequently fall ill. Mary's Aunt Lizzie, John Work Garrett's sister, also suffered from many mysterious maladies, often describing her symptoms: "My bowels were disturbed 30 times and 20 the following day," she wrote describing a probable attack by a digestive bug. A few years later, she suffered a mental collapse, which greatly concerned Mary. "Please tell me the cause of Aunt Lizzie's depression," Mary anxiously wrote to her mother while visiting Cold Spring Harbor.[54]

Mary's health spiraled down. She visited famed British neurologist Dr. J. Hughling Jackson. It is unclear why Mary visited a neurologist or who recommended him, but it is possible that her father, with his medical contacts throughout Europe, suggested Jackson. Following the proscribed advice at the time for women plagued with neurasthenia, Jackson instructed Mary "to give up all ideas of doing it [studying], lead a simple, regular life, ride, walk, dance, play tennis, etc . . . in fact, amuse myself in every possible way, *to avoid intellectual society, join friendships with ordinary, commonplace people*, drink weak tea . . . use no alcohol, above all, again and again, *do not work* . . . and do this forever."[55] She was now restricted by even more prohibitions than those her father had placed against her.

Thus, Mary forged a career of sorts: traveling, letter writing, and worrying about her health. She traveled ceaselessly, busying herself with constant moves. The logistics of her trips to Europe, the Far East, and New York, from Mount Vernon Place to Montebello to Deer Park, consumed her time and energies. She fretted about missed trains and delayed voyages, bad weather and disappointing accommodations. She occupied her time thinking of her health and her doctors and taking the cure at one famed spa after another. Her letters, once kind and complimentary almost to a fault, began to take on an uncharacteristic tone of bitterness and anger. She complained of a "pitiful little note" she had received from Lizzie Whitridge, Alice Garrett's sister. She "had yet another baby," Mary snipped.[56]

Her days became utterly mundane. Up at seven thirty; Greek lessons from eight thirty to ten; ten to two, reading and napping; four thirty, horseback riding.[57] She wrote letters, sometimes a half dozen a day, chronicling each one in her logbook. Her daily favorites now expanded to include Gen. and Mrs. George McClellan; Alice Gilman, daughter of the president of the new Johns Hopkins University; and her possible suitors, Dr. Murray and Prof. Marsh.

By 1880, Mary was obsessing more than ever about her health. Her letters during the late 1870s and early 1880s reveal a litany of concerns. "Do you think I am becoming a perfect monomaniac?" she implored Carey. She wrote of daily headaches. Visiting doctors became the primary focus of her travels. Vacationing in St. Moritz, she slipped and fell while hiking on a glacier, exacerbating her childhood ankle injury. She consulted a doctor. "After a careful, painful examination," she wrote to Carey, "he said that the skin which had been attached to the bone (at the place where the scar is, if you remember) ever since it healed when I was a baby, was detached when I hurt it in my fall." She began walking with crutches. She had to wear a "Big Boot," most likely an awkward, uncomfortable cast. She gained weight. Her once slim figure succumbed to the plumpness she had always fought. "My appetite is large and my dresses are tight."[58] She once again was physically impaired, as she had been as a child.

Her father was forced to intervene. Regretting that "Miss Garrett's progress to recovery continues to be so slow," John Work Garrett wrote to her doctors, arranging for them to accompany and transport her in Europe to complete her trip. Carey was critical of the Garretts' control over their daughter. "It is dreadful to think that a woman is such a slave that she is not even allowed to hurt herself without her owners becoming enraged."[59] Carey, on the other hand, was far removed from what she felt was the "enslavement" of her friend and on a much different trajectory, enjoying unprecedented success and unfettered independence from her parents while studying for her doctorate in Europe. Carey's accomplishments only served to reinforce to Mary her own lack of focus. Most distressing, it underscored Mary's complete financial vulnerability and uncertain future.

IDEALS OF WOMANHOOD

Despite her illnesses, setbacks, and thwarted dreams, not all was lost for Mary during her twenties. Unwittingly, this became a pivotal time in her life. These years provided Mary with her own "silent revolution." She began to make choices for her life and to think of her future direction, although the exact direction was as yet undefined. She was experiencing what American psychoanalyst Erik Erikson would later describe in the twentieth century as a "moratorium"—preparing for the yet-undefined life's task that lay ahead.[60] Mary knew she would not marry and have children. She would not progress through the conventional stages of a woman's life. Instead, she looked for other models to follow, traits to emulate.

Thrilled years before by her father's exciting world of business and incited by the pursuits of Friday Night and other women around her, Mary began to imagine possibilities beyond the traditional feminine sphere. It was during the seemingly dismal years of her twenties that her notions of womanhood took shape. She began to write enthusiastically of accomplished women and the traits that most impressed her: their demeanor, their achievements, their sacrifices for success. She carefully studied the choices successful women made to transform their lives. Women physicians, particularly her own physician Mary Putnam Jacobi, inspired her. Jacobi became a dominant force in shaping Mary's identity, self-philosophy, and later, her philanthropies.

Born in 1842, within three decades Jacobi achieved fame as one of the country's finest physicians and medical researchers. Like many women physicians of the time, she had graduated from the prominent Female Medical College of Pennsylvania. In 1864 she settled in New York, where she opened a practice in obstetrics and gynecology. The young physician, from the famed publishing family of G. P. Putnam's Sons, organized the Association for the Advancement of the Medical Education of Women in 1872 and lectured at the medical college of the New York Infirmary for Indigent Women and Children. She continued her medical studies and writing in Paris, where she moonlighted as a journalist and fiction writer.[61] She honed her writing skills, which later helped her to carefully craft medical descriptions and speeches and articles for her suffrage activities.

In 1873, Mary Putnam married Dr. Abraham Jacobi, a radical who had been banished from Europe after the 1848 revolutions that swept the continent. He went on to gain fame as the "Father of American Pediatrics." They had three children, but Mary Putnam Jacobi never lost sight of her feminist goals. She became an outspoken advocate for coeducation for women medical students, arguing that female medical colleges, such as the one she attended, could not provide the same high standards of study and training as men's medical schools that were affiliated with established universities and large hospitals.

Jacobi worked tirelessly to refute long-held stereotypes of women's physical fragility and inferiority, arguing that there was no scientific justification to exclude women from the professions. Her 1876 essay "The Question of Rest for Women during Menstruation" brilliantly refuted E. H. Clarke's widely held 1873 argument, *Sex in Education; or, A Fair Chance for the Girls*, about the limitations of women's physical activity. The trailblazing rebuttal won the prestigious Boylston Prize at Harvard University.[62]

Always fearful of her own medical conditions and in dread of contact with male physicians, Mary sought out the advice of Jacobi when she was studying for her Harvard entrance exam. From their first meeting in June 1878, Mary was impressed by the renowned physician. "She is a little woman, very neatly dressed, not in the least pretty, but with a kind, sensible face, wearing spectacles . . . [and] with a very businesslike manner," Mary wrote to Carey. Jacobi assured Mary that she had no "internal trouble." The physician tried to boost Mary's confidence, assuring her she "need not fear studying now or being afraid of the future . . . and she would feel better in a year." Jacobi prescribed "lots of iron, in the form of mineral waters, if I could get them, a quart of milk a day, meat, and some other things to [aid] digestion." Mary admired Jacobi's singular dedication to her profession. "She is uncompromising—she never would have gotten where she is in these days if she hadn't been." Mary noted the devotion of the doctor to her young child, "but she also loves her work."[63]

Another woman greatly impressed Mary, this time on the opposite side of the country. Mary traveled with her parents on a leisurely trip by private railcar to the Pacific Coast, passing through sixteen states along the way. In California, they met the governor, José Antonio Romualdo Pacheco Jr., "the only native governor they've had here," Mary commented. But it was not the governor who most impressed her. Rather, it was a woman who accompanied the governor and his wife on the visit, a Mrs. Burton. This humble woman, who had come so far in life, inspired Mary. She had married at the age of thirteen and learned to speak English. "She is a brilliant woman, I believe. She dramatized Don Quixote and is writing a play."[64]

Another, less animate, woman helped to shape Mary's notions of womanhood. In 1878 while touring the Louvre in Paris, Mary contemplated the Venus de Milo. "Isn't the Venus of Milo the grandest woman you know in art?" she rhetorically asked Carey in an 1878 letter. "She is so strong, and free and grand—utterly free of self-consciousness. She is so calm in her face."[65]

Mary similarly found inspiration from her literary favorites. While vacationing with her family in Western Maryland, Mary wrote that they had just finished reading aloud Jane Austen's *Emma*. Considered to be one of Austen's most charming, but imperfect, protagonists, Emma is young, rich, and not in any hurry to get married. She has "lived nearly twenty-one years in a world with very little to distress or vex her," the narrator explains in the opening sentence. The novel is a light, but insightful, look at love, misunderstandings, and ultimate submission to expectations. Not far beneath the surface lies Austen's recurring theme that women must acquiesce to society's demands to marry, for it is only through marriage that they attain power and economic security. Mary was not so easily convinced of such a fate, expressing hope for more free agency in her own life. "There is a great deal of kindness and goodness in so many of [Austen's] characters, but there is never the slightest desire in any one of them to rise above the dull commonplace of their lives," Mary wrote in July 1879.[66]

Mary carefully catalogued those ideals of womanhood she wanted to emulate: accomplishment, seriousness of purpose, self-reliance, and confidence. At the age of twenty-eight, Mary finally was able to put those valuable traits to use. She began to break free from her father's dominance and enjoy some measure of adult independence. She and Julia often traveled to New York, and Mary frequently went alone as well. Mary adored the glamorous, sophisticated city, so different from Baltimore. In 1882, she rented a place of her own, an apartment in one of New York's many residence hotels in the fashionable area of 39 West 33rd Street between Fifth and Broadway, across the street from where the Empire State Building would rise a half century later. She stayed there off and on, for a few weeks at a time, often traveling back to stay at Montebello or Mount Vernon Place or to launch off on another trip abroad. But she always dreaded returning to Baltimore "without a friend left in it."[67]

Away from her parents, who were now busy traveling around the country on B&O business to St. Louis, Jacksonville, Chicago, and Cincinnati, Mary began to regain some of her confidence lost during the previous years. New York, especially New York on her own, opened a world of exciting possibilities and new friendships that would last a lifetime. Mary's New York circle of friends included men and women, predominantly the movers and shakers in the arts and, specifi-

cally, the Decorative Arts movement, then sweeping across the country like wildfire. She developed a close relationship with Julia Brasher de Forest, and her
brothers: Lockwood, who for years had been engaged by the Garretts to design
their mansions' interiors, and Robert, a successful New York railroad attorney.
The de Forests hailed from an established, patrician New York Huguenot family
dating back 250 years to "New Amsterdam." Their maternal grandfather had been
president of the New York Stock Exchange, and Robert's father-in-law, John Taylor Johnston, was president of the Central Railroad of New Jersey and the first
president of the Metropolitan Museum of Art.

Mary also befriended Julia de Forest's cousin Louise "Lou" Wakeman Knox,
who in 1886 would marry widower Louis Comfort Tiffany. Lou's father, the Reverend James Hall Mason Knox, was on the board of John Work Garrett's alma
mater, Lafayette College, and served as the college's president from 1883–90.
Mary was enthralled by the sophistication and glamour, not to mention interior
decorating *savoir faire*, of her New York friends. "Lou has one of the prettiest sitting rooms I ever saw," Mary reported to her mother.[68] In New York, Julia de Forest, Lou Knox, and Mary lived close to each other and shared a common love of
art—Julia would later author a book of art history—and, as importantly, an interest in advancing women in medicine. Lou and Julia served on the board of managers [directors] of the New York Infirmary for Indigent Women and Children,
started by one of the most prominent physicians of the day, Dr. Elizabeth Blackwell. Mary often visited the infirmary, talking to the patients and observing firsthand the work of the female physicians.[69] The seeds of interest in women physicians, first planted by Dr. Jacobi, were fervently growing in Mary's mind.

Under the tutelage of the extended de Forest and Tiffany clans, Mary, too, fell
under the spell of the Decorative Arts movement, which captivated elite women
with its emphasis on bringing beauty, handcrafted art, and aesthetics to eager
fashion-conscious Gilded Age Americans. For Mary and her mother, the Decorative Arts movement arrived just in the nick of time. They had three enormous
homes to keep up to date with the required Gilded Age accoutrements. In the
early 1880s, they began decorating the family's new nineteen-room Deer Park cottage. Mary enthusiastically wrote to her mother of the wondrous decorating possibilities she saw in New York: "lovely chairs, table covers that would look lovely
in our country home."[70]

Despite the thrill of independence, Mary kept the family ties strong, writing
daily to her parents, usually her mother, and reporting optimistically and enthusiastically on her day-to-day activities. Always close to her mother, Mary fretted
when Rachel did not quickly respond. "I looked for your letter today and it did

not arrive. Please write more often," she begged. She also wanted updates on the B&O. "Please send railroad news!" In New York, Mary frequently saw Professor Marsh, who followed the Garrett family activities with interest, commenting in February 1882 that he had read in the papers of Mary's brother Robert's latest gala.[71]

All around her in New York lay the magic of the theater, which Mary devoured and attended at every chance. She saw *Oedipus*, performed in Greek, a language she had studied and understood. "It was one of the greatest pleasures I've had in a long time and would not have given up my language for a great deal," she wrote to her mother. She went to parties and museums and theater benefits—one in particular that she especially enjoyed featured black musicians, and another was put on to support "a poor artist's family" and starred actress Lucy Ingersoll.[72]

Mary often escaped to a favorite refuge in Orange, New Jersey, to stay with her father's longtime friends Gen. and Mrs. George B. McClellan. After being summarily dismissed by Lincoln after the bloody debacle of Antietam, McClellan retreated to New Jersey to await further military orders from the president. They never came. After a failed 1864 presidential bid against his former commander-in-chief, Lincoln, McClellan's political future began to brighten in New Jersey. He was elected governor in 1877 and served one term, leaving office in 1881. Mary greatly enjoyed the McClellans' company, often accompanying them to the theater and parties in New York.

Despite her small leap to the freedom of New York adventures, Mary's lack of economic independence and her uncertain financial future haunted her. By now, her brothers had every visible sign of successful adulthood: respected positions in their professions and the community, magnificent mansions, and socially brilliant wives. Mary had no such benchmarks to recognize her passage into adulthood.

She began to have long, imploring discussions with her father, pouring out her fears for her future. She had but one request: "That I should be left independent of my brothers' control— that if I had but a thousand dollars a year I would be on *my own.*"[73] A thousand dollars a year, about twice the annual wages of a female federal office worker or triple that of a female factory operative, would not have been much for a young woman accustomed to boundless world travel and luxurious homes on Mount Vernon Place, Montebello, and Deer Park. Yet, to be out from under the dominance of her brothers and their wives, with whom she had an increasingly displeasing relationship, was all she asked. She craved a bigger, more complete taste of freedom. She wanted to be on her own, on her own terms, to be self-reliant like the women and feminist ideals she had come to admire.

Her father seemed unconcerned about her plight, not answering her anguished pleas. "He kept right on talking" during her desperate appeals, she later remembered.[74] Mary and her father had come to loggerheads. She had cause to be concerned. In the uncertain economy of the Gilded Age, even the wealthiest family could be displaced overnight into poverty. In Mary's mind, without an education or an income to call her own, the fates could easily consign her to a life of genteel, impoverished spinsterhood. Or worse, financial and social subservience to her brothers and their wives.

But, more than likely, by the early 1880s, John Work Garrett was not at all concerned about his daughter's financial independence. He was far more interested in the governance and financial independence of a groundbreaking university in downtown Baltimore. He had been an integral force from its inception fifteen years earlier.

CHAPTER 4

AFTER GARRETT

WHERE ARE THE MEDICAL CLASSES?

When Johns Hopkins concluded his cordial meeting with George Peabody in the Garrett home shortly after the Civil War, Hopkins's concerns about how to distribute his $8 million fortune were greatly eased. Following Peabody's advice, Hopkins signed a will and, employing the same model used in the creation of the Peabody Institute, appointed a board of trustees to carry out his wishes. Soon after, on August 24, 1867, at Hopkins's request, the trustees gathered to form a corporation known as the Johns Hopkins University for "the promotion of education in the State of Maryland."[1] The founding trustees included Mary's father, as well as Carey's, Mamie's, and Bessie's fathers and eight other prominent Baltimore leaders.

Hopkins died six years later, on Christmas Eve, 1873, at the age of seventy-eight at his townhouse at 81 West Saratoga Street. He left all but $1 million of his $8 million estate to the new institution that would bear his name. His bequest of $7 million, comprised primarily of B&O and bank stock as well as valuable real estate, was the largest philanthropic gift ever given in the United States at the time. Earlier that year, Commodore Cornelius Vanderbilt had endowed a university in Nashville in his name for $1 million.

Hopkins gave his trusted friends considerable latitude in carrying out his will, providing only few instructions and designating that his bequest be divided equally between the establishment of a university and a hospital, two separate legal entities. Charles S. Peirce, one of the great intellectuals and philosophers of the day, commented on the flawlessness of Hopkins's will, that it was "a certain testament, happily free from all definite ideas."[2] Hopkins did, however, make one important financial stipulation: that the trustees not sell the fifteen thousand shares of B&O stock that comprised most of his estate and that only the stock dividend, not the principal, be used for construction and operational costs. He wanted not only to create a sound endowment for the university, but also to ensure the stability of the stock from political influence or a sell-off. Hopkins had helped to lead the B&O for decades and had fought to keep the railroad in private hands during the embattled 1858 election of Mary's father to the presidency. Like Garrett, Hopkins had complete faith in the future profitability of the railroad—and its reliable cash dividend.

Medical care for the indigent and needy had been of particular concern to the benevolent Quaker. In a letter dated March 10, 1873, nine months before his death, Hopkins emphasized the urgency that the trustees move quickly with the establishment of the hospital. "I cannot impress this injunction too strongly upon you," he wrote. "It is my desire that you should complete this portion of your labor during the current year and be in readiness to commence the building of the hospital in the spring of 1874." He also was concerned with medical education— or the deplorable lack of it—in the United States at the time. "You will bear constantly in mind," he instructed the trustees, "that it is my wish and purpose that the institution should ultimately form a part of the Medical School of that university for which I have made ample provision in my will."[3]

Within two months of Hopkins's death, the trustees began in earnest with their charge to create an outstanding university and a modern hospital that would reflect the far-reaching vision of the benefactor, one of Baltimore's great leaders. The majority of the trustees were college educated, yet knew little about creating a new university from the ground up. Rather than replicating prevailing educational models found at the country's four hundred other colleges and universities, the trustees wanted to create a new prototype of higher education. They investigated and interviewed, writing to preeminent college presidents to guide them. The right three stepped forward: Charles Eliot of Harvard, James Angell of the University of Michigan, and Andrew White of Cornell, considered to be "heroes of American university development."[4]

The trustees were active participants, not passive bystanders, in shaping the new university. They delved into the literature of the day to learn about European and American educational systems. They ordered twenty-two books, ranging from *Higher Schools and Universities in Germany* and *The History of Harvard University* to *Education: Intellectual, Moral, and Physical* and Horace Mann's *Lectures and Annual Reports on Education*. Two of the twenty-two books dealt with a controversial issue of the day, coeducation: E. H. Clarke's popular and controversial *Sex in Education* and J. Orten's *The Liberal Education of Women.*[5]

The trustees were divided on the scope of the new university, with some arguing to think big, on a national level, to attract students and faculty from far beyond Baltimore's borders. John Work Garrett and a few others cast dissenting views, favoring instead to make the university of practical, vocational benefit to the immediate community of Baltimore. Voting him down on what he thought was an important concept that he insisted Johns Hopkins had endorsed, this would not be the last time his fellow trustees angered Mary's father.

On some issues many trustees agreed. The nation did not need more elite liberal arts colleges, such as Harvard, Yale, or Princeton. Nor was there a pressing need for more public higher education. The Morrill Act of 1862, often called the Land Grant College Act, designated thirty thousand acres in each state for public colleges, "Democracy's Colleges" as President Lincoln had called them, that focused primarily on technical training in agricultural and mechanical arts.

This was a propitious time for the development of a new kind of university, a time when higher education was accelerating in the years after the Civil War. The increasing middle class hungered for better education. The Hopkins trustees started from scratch to create an entirely new brand of American higher education. Although most of the trustees were devoutly religious men, they wanted a secular university. In the late nineteenth century, the nation teetered on the ideological cusp of change, with much heated debate over the secularization of education, of pulling away from prevailing, traditional religious doctrine and moving toward more scientific scholarship.

What was needed, President Angell recommended, "was a great graduate university."[6] The emerging age of scientific discovery and bacteriology of the late nineteenth century inspired an entirely different kind of research-based higher education in the United States to rival the best European graduate universities. The time was at hand to bridge the research of the library and laboratory to the classroom and everyday lives.

The trustees agreed on yet another point. The most forward-thinking educator for the job of president was Daniel Coit Gilman, who then presided over the University of California. Gilman had acquired not only outstanding academic credentials but also firsthand knowledge of the European model of higher education that stressed graduate-level original research and scholarship, which the trustees hoped to adopt for the new university in Baltimore. Unencumbered by traditional notions of American higher education or religious dictates that defined other colleges, Gilman assembled some of the best minds in the humanities and sciences for the new university. Believing that an institution could excel through the accomplishments of gifted individuals, he recruited scholars with sterling research pedigrees. He spent a year traveling through Europe and the United States, inviting academic luminaries such as Henry Rowland in physics, Basil Gildersleeve in Greek, and Ira Remsen in chemistry, among others, to join the faculty. Gilman emphasized research in order to expand students' knowledge and craft excellent faculty. "The best teachers are usually those who are free, competent, and willing to make original researches in the library and the laboratory," he stated.[7]

On October 3, 1876, the pioneering model of higher education opened its doors. Earlier, on September 12, Thomas Huxley, eminent scientist and grandfather of Aldous, the future author of *Brave New World*, presented the dedication speech. In a move that shocked the nation and firmly established Hopkins as a secular institution, Huxley, a leading proponent of Darwinism, did not offer the usual opening prayer. Instead, the ceremony was conducted "without priestly ceremonies."[8]

The first university building was equally unpretentious. "Men were more important than buildings," the advisors emphasized.[9] The university opened in humble quarters on Howard Street, just north of Centre Street. Since the university did not yet have a library, its central location in downtown Baltimore allowed students to use the well-stocked libraries at the Peabody Institute and the Maryland Historical Society. The University of Maryland's medical school, already in its seventh decade, was located just a few blocks away from the new university.

Medical education was very much on Gilman's mind. In his inaugural speech, the president emphasized one point of particular concern to the university benefactor: the poor quality of medical education that then existed in the United States. Gilman vowed that the Johns Hopkins University would soon fulfill its benefactor's wishes to open a medical school and set an improved, higher level of medical training and care. "We need not fear that the day is distant . . . which will see endowments for medical science as munificent as those now provided for any branch of learning, in schools as good as those now provided in other lands," Gilman stated during his speech. He assured that the medical school would soon open. "It will doubtless not be long after the opening of the university, before the opening of the hospital; and this interval may be spent in forming plans for the department of medicine." Gilman envisioned a seamless ideological integration between the university and the hospital, in what would soon be called the "bench to bedside" mode of applying groundbreaking scientific research from the laboratory to improved patient care in the hospital wards. "It is impossible to have a hospital without its becoming a place for medical education," he noted.[10]

The new university on Howard Street soon acquired a reputation for producing serious scholarship—and equally serious young scholars. "Sober Johns Hopkins. It is a university of manly young men. Dudes are seldom found there," the *New York World* proclaimed. "Johns Hopkins University is a steady-going place, containing few dudes and no students who lead the sumptuous lives that characterize the Harvard men. The classes are made up largely of manly fellows who mean business and who have little time to devote to college frivolity."[11]

Mary was enthused by the university, but emphatically thought it should not be restricted only to "manly fellows who mean business." During her twenties, when she was floundering and desperately trying to convince her father to allow her to attend college, she looked hopefully at the new university as the answer. A month before the university opened in 1876, at age twenty-two, she decided she wanted to take classes. This was, after all, a university created by a longtime Garrett family friend, Johns Hopkins, whom she knew well. Why should she be excluded from taking classes at his university? Hopkins was a Quaker, and Quakers believed in equality of the sexes. He had not stipulated that women could not be students. In 1876, Mary had approached Gilman with the idea. She thought Bessie King and Julia Rogers might also be interested in attending the new university. She wrote to Julia that she had asked Gilman, "If I can find two other girls who are in earnest & if we are willing to give 3 hours a day to it [could you] arrange with some of the young chemists and physicists to give us the requisite training to begin the elementary course in Biology?"[12] Gilman flatly denied her request. Carey, too, applied to take courses and was similarly dismissed.

The problem of coeducation had nagged at trustees from the start, with one member of the board citing women's conundrum: "How are women to get the highest education provided [when] the avenues of education are closed to them?" Eliot asserted the answer lay in separate education exemplified by the new women's colleges. Eliot was especially firm on this issue, pronouncing that coeducation was a "thoroughly wrong idea which is rapidly disappearing." He cited several reasons for his adamant stance. Students might fall in love, which could produce socially unequal marriages. Academic rigors might bring on physical ailments that would destroy a woman's chance of marriage. Women simply could not keep up intellectually with male students. And, finally, there was no point to educating women, since a woman's future was so different from a man's.[13]

Angell, who presided over a public university that admitted women, commented indifferently that "the young men have, so far as I know, borne themselves with the greatest courtesy and prudence toward the ladies . . . The girls go to and from the College undisturbed." Gilman, while president of the University of California, had admitted women to all departments of the university. He noted the intellectual aptitude of the female students: "Among the regular students the proportion of ladies who have been good scholars has been greater than that of young men."[14]

Unmoved by Angell's ambivalent concern for commingling or Gilman's earlier approval of coeducation, and perhaps considering Baltimore's postwar conservative sympathies, the Hopkins trustees designated that the new university be all male. Gilman steadfastly resolved that at Hopkins, at least, young women should "not be exposed to the rougher influences which I am sorry to confess are still to be found in colleges and universities where young men resort."[15] The trustees agreed. Perhaps sensing an avalanche of female applications well beyond their own daughters, the trustees enacted a policy on November 5, 1877, that allowed women to take special classes, but not to matriculate to a degree. The trustees and Gilman stood firm. There would be no official place for women at the Johns Hopkins University. At least not yet.

Coeducation was hardly the trustees' biggest problem. Even before the doors opened, the university, with its rich endowment, faced a string of financial difficulties. With almost all of its endowment tied up in B&O common stocks that Johns Hopkins had directed the trustees never to sell, the university began a wild financial ride on the B&O roller coaster. In 1876, there were hints of trouble with the B&O and within two years the railroad paid out its dividend, not in much-needed cash, but in stocks. The trustees were forced to pull back on plans for university expansion. They took an unorthodox step to raise needed cash: they sold the dividend stocks. They still held on to the original stocks of the bequest, as mandated by the benefactor.

For the second time, John Work Garrett was outraged at his fellow trustees' actions. Furious, he stormed into a board meeting on October 6, 1879, and harangued the trustees for neglecting Johns Hopkins's directive to hold on to the stocks. Perhaps he felt himself to be Hopkins's personal, posthumous advocate. Or, more likely, he was nervous about the fifteen thousand shares of B&O stock held by the university. The trustees had opened the door on a future, potentially disastrous course of action should they someday vote to liquidate additional stocks — in direct contradiction to Hopkins's advice to "not dispose of said capital stock, but to keep said stock as an investment."[16] Such a sell-off would have serious consequence for the B&O. The stock value could plummet or principal ownership of the railroad could shift out of Baltimore and Garrett control.

Garrett reiterated the benefactor's belief that stock dividends were the best course for the university, citing Hopkins's last will and testament as a "special request" and adding that he had advised Hopkins on such a plan, "in having these very instructions given to you in the interests of the University."[17] With that, he pronounced that the B&O would pay a 4 percent dividend the next day and that the university's income would double in the coming years from the B&O stocks. The first promise held true. The second proved a disastrous prediction.

Garrett's fury with the trustees was fully reciprocated. His arrogance, his insulting tirade—he had accused the treasurer of the board, Francis White, of being "singularly ignorant" about the B&O—outraged the trustees.[18] Garrett's outburst strained the board's relationship with the railroad president, producing an untenable and unfortunate position, given the university's complete financial dependence on the B&O. Garrett's omnipotent control over the B&O—and much of Maryland—stirred both resentment and fear among the trustees.

There was yet another matter that angered Garrett about his fellow trustees: Clifton. Garrett asserted that Hopkins had designated Clifton as his choice for the location of his university, which probably had been Garrett's motivation for buying nearly fourteen hundred acres of land right next door at Montebello. Garrett had pressed for the Clifton location from the start, even encouraging the hiring of a botanist to the faculty in 1879 to improve Hopkins's beloved Clifton. In spring 1882, as the university needed to expand its science laboratories, Garrett continued his persistent campaign to move the university to the more expansive area of Clifton and near to his own adjacent fourteen-hundred-acre holdings in the region. The issue was so volatile that, for the first time, the trustees requested that their votes be tallied in the minutes.[19]

"Then began a fight which is memorable in the annals of [Baltimore]," the New York Times later reported of the showdown. "Mr. Garrett fought with the earnestness and vigor of his intense nature." Garrett, along with three other trustees, was voted down. Not accustomed to being outdone, in 1882, Garrett, along with Johns Hopkins's cousin Lewis Hopkins, resigned in rage from the board. The issue would continue to gall him until the day he died. "Garrett never flagged, and to the end of his life, he continued to reproach privately and publicly the action which he declared treason to the wishes of his friend," the New York Times explained.[20]

A letter Garrett received may have stirred his invective to the board and his subsequent resignation. Earlier that year, businessman F. B. Mayer wrote to him, lamenting the "destination of Clifton."[21] The once-magnificent country estate, the "heaven on earth" with its Roman gateway and exquisite gardens that Hopkins had so loved, had fallen into disrepair and decay in the years after his death. The beautiful Italianate villa, where the nineteenth century's rich and famous danced away the hours, was now dilapidated. The estate where Johns Hopkins had—possibly—envisioned locating his university, remained isolated, abandoned, and forgotten in the area northeast of Baltimore next to Garrett's Montebello.

Mayer laid out a plan to resurrect what he felt was Hopkins's original plan to locate the university at Clifton. Mayer suggested a radical idea to restructure the existing commercial roadways in Baltimore, to unite the languishing northeast region, where Garrett's enjoyable, but unprofitable, Montebello lay undeveloped, to the vibrant downtown entrepôt and harbor. Mayer proposed creating a "natural radiating system" that would connect downtown Baltimore to the proposed Clifton campus. Montebello, as well, would be connected to "the B&O Central office, the Post office, Battle and Washington Monuments, Peabody Institute, Greenmount, the University, the waterworks"—all the major areas of Baltimore. A grand promenade would run through the center, "three hundred feet wide with six rows of trees could be made to rival the Champs Elysées of Paris." Clifton would become the center of it all, a new Jardin des Plantes of Baltimore.[22]

Mayer's intriguing, irresistible idea to realign Baltimore's commercial highways to northeast Baltimore, to finally put Clifton—and Montebello—to good commercial use, simmered in John Work Garrett's mind. His resentment continued over his failed bid to locate the university at Clifton. A few months after receiving Mayer's letter, Garrett took the opportunity—a very public opportunity—to continue his battle with the Hopkins board of trustees. The occasion was the thirtieth anniversary celebration of the founding of Baltimore's YMCA, in which Garrett and Johns Hopkins had played a critical role. On January 30, 1883, Garrett delivered a stinging excoriation of the trustees and the progress of the university. His speech shocked the audience. The next morning, the *Baltimore Sun* featured the event—and the verbatim speech—on the front page: "Mr. Garrett Speaks Out," the headline read, "A Pointed Speech Last Night Criticizing the Johns Hopkins Trust."[23]

On that evening, Garrett presided over the large banquet, held in the YMCA hall on North Charles Street. Joining him on the dais were many of Baltimore's most distinguished citizens, including several Hopkins trustees and President Gilman. After starting with "congregational singing," scripture reading, and prayers, Garrett stood to deliver his speech. He proudly enumerated the many successes of the YMCA since its founding: 505,000 visitors to the building; 2,000 men who had "availed themselves of the advantages of the gymnasium; 3,000 who had attended classes in German, phonology, elocution, and music; 2,394 association meetings" held over the three decades. Garrett reminisced how he had convinced Johns Hopkins to contribute to the construction of the YMCA building.

Hopkins had confided to Garrett that his annual income was more than $450,000. Certainly, Garrett had insisted, he could contribute $10,000 to the building fund "and be made relatively happy by the reflections connected with the facts and this act of beneficence."[24] With Garrett's similar contribution of $10,000, the building was constructed.

Garrett continued on with his speech, recalling warmly how, years earlier, he had brought his two great friends, "these two remarkable men," George Peabody and Johns Hopkins together in his home on Mount Vernon Place to discuss "the subject of the disposition of [Hopkins's] estate." After the successful meeting, Garrett said, Hopkins "informed me on the following day that he had determined to commence making his will—that will which, full of wisdom, humanity and earnest determination for great usefulness, must bear rich fruits for all time."

Suddenly, his speech turned angry and accusatory. What had happened to Hopkins's vision for his institutions in the decade since his death? The university that Hopkins planned had indeed opened in 1876, Garrett conceded, but not where the benefactor had intended in the bucolic and spacious area of Clifton. Instead, the trustees chose a "noisy, thickly populated section of the city" on North Howard Street. Johns Hopkins, Garrett assured the audience, wanted the university to be located at Clifton, not in downtown Baltimore. The trustees had spent "an enormous sum in the City of Baltimore and not at Clifton Park," Garrett admonished.[25]

And what about Hopkins's dream for a modern hospital? Garrett railed. The benefactor had left half his estate, $3.5 million, for a hospital. "The grounds and the buildings for the hospital have already cost more than $1,200,000 and more than nine years have elapsed since the death of the founder and not one patient, not one of the indigent sick of Baltimore has yet received any benefit from this vast expenditure."

Most egregious, Garrett stormed, was the trustees' failure to create Hopkins's dream of a great medical school. "Where are the medical classes that should now be engaged in preparing physicians with the highest culture and the best advantages to be derived from clinical instruction at the hospital, as designed by the founder?" Garrett asked, accusingly. Hopkins, Garrett reminded the audience, had left very clear instructions about the formation of a medical school as part of the university.

Garrett ended his long speech—probably much to the relief of many members of the audience—by adding that the trustees should "at once establish medical and other additional schools and arrange for the commencement of the beneficent work of the hospital in a single year." He added that, "I hope, in no distant day, my friends, to see hundreds of students of the university connected with all branches of culture, representatives of the great professions, and especially of medical science."[26]

Garrett's public condemnation of the progress of the opening of the hospital and medical school at the time of his speech in January 1883 was correct—to a point. Plans were well underway by that time. The trustees had commissioned John Shaw Billings, a brilliant Civil War surgeon, author, medical librarian, and visionary on hospital construction, to advise on the design of the hospital and its academic facilities. Architect John Niernsee, who had designed many of the splendid buildings of Mount Vernon Place, was chosen to bring Billings's innovative ideas to life. The Boston firm of Cabot and Chandler completed the design. Construction on the hospital had begun in a timely manner in 1877 on the thirteen-acre site that Hopkins himself had carefully selected. He had paid $150,000 for the city's debt-ridden Insane Asylum on the site on Loudenschlager's Hill in East Baltimore. The new hospital buildings slowly rose from the ground, as the trustees, bound by the terms of Hopkins's will, used only income, not principal, from the always-teetering B&O endowment income to finance construction.

By the time Garrett delivered his speech in January 1883, an embryonic medical school already was taking shape at the university, with faculty teaching a core curriculum of medical courses in anatomy, physiology, and pathology. Gilman had traveled to Europe specifically to investigate the relationship of hospitals and medical schools. In May 1876, the trustees had purchased a parcel of land near the hospital for the site of the medical school. Over the next years, Gilman enlisted some of the era's most renowned physicians, all skilled medical researchers and instructors, including pathologist William Welch, surgeon William Halsted, and gynecologist Howard Kelly. Canadian physician William Osler, unsurpassed in the English method of instruction, which Gilman and Billings thought best for medical education, was appointed as the first professor of medicine and physician-in-chief.

But progress was slow, and John Work Garrett was not a patient man. The problem for the trustees was not a lack of vision for the medical school and hospital. The problem was a lack of money, or more specifically, a lack of income from the B&O stocks. The construction of the hospital and the development of the medical school inched forward as much as the dwindling B&O dividend allowed. But soon, another far more grievous heartbreak consumed him.

In October 1883, Mary and her parents returned from what had become over the past decade their annual trip to Europe to bolster John Work Garrett's health. The trip had been "largely for the benefit of his health and while he was there he was several times unwell," the *Baltimore American* reported. Three days after their return from Europe, on October 11, Rachel set out from Montebello in her carriage with her driver for a trip into town. Within moments, tragedy struck. The horses, "which were in high spirits from not having been driven as much as usual during the absence of Mr. John Work Garrett in Europe," suddenly became frightened and galloped down the road. The carriage overturned. Rachel was thrown "with terrible force from her seat, and in falling from the carriage, struck her head upon the road, causing a concussion of the brain."[27] Onlookers rushed her, unconscious, back to Montebello. Mary and her father were quickly summoned. The family physician, Dr. Alan P. Smith, grimly told the family there was little hope of recovery.

Mary's father moved his office—secretaries, telegraph operators, and attachés—to Montebello. He never left his wife's bedside. Five weeks after the accident, at eight in the morning on November 15, sixty-year-old Rachel died, surrounded by her family. She had never regained consciousness.

Grief-stricken, the family carried on. Rachel had been the glue that kept the family together. She had enjoyed a warm relationship with her own family, particularly her sister, Florence, who lived in the Georgetown area of Washington, D.C. "You are always flitting about," her sister often teased Rachel about her many travels. Rachel had nursed her husband back from a dozen lapses of health, and had been his protector and confidante. She provided the gentle hand that guided the family through the turbulent years of the Civil War, and afterward, her sons' successful marriage matches. Her daughters-in-law greatly admired her, writing to the matriarch frequently and warmly, always addressing her formally as "Mrs. Garrett." "She was a lady of most amiable disposition and was ever noted for liberal and unostentatious charity," the *Baltimore American* concluded.[28]

Mary did not write of her mother's death. During this time, she developed a habit that she would carry in the years ahead of not writing in the midst of family tragedy.

John Work Garrett was completely inconsolable. His mental and physical health acutely declined. It was said that he had two loves: one was the railroad and the other was his wife.[29] And now, one great love was gone. The death of his beloved wife of thirty-seven years sounded the death knell for John Work Garrett—and forever changed his daughter's life.

DEATH OF THE RAILROAD KING

For months, Mary and her father moved incessantly, traveling from Montebello to Deer Park to Mount Vernon Place and back to Montebello to start all over again. Mary, ever attendant at her father's side, made the arrangements for private railcars to transport them around Maryland and up and down the East Coast. John Work Garrett's opulent estates could do little to soothe his aching heart or cure his many ailments. The once imposing, powerful man was restless, aimless, and dying.

The family spent a cheerless Christmas 1883 at Montebello without Rachel. The memory of her tragic, untimely death just a month earlier weighed heavily. Mary cabled Mr. Andrews, her father's assistant, to order "a saddle of venison and some pheasants or partridges from the mountains to be brought to Montebello for Christmas day." By March, Mary encouraged her grief-stricken father to take the cure at the spa at Lakewood in southern New Jersey. The fashionable winter resort offered polo, golf, and other activities Mary hoped would divert her father's attention from his heartache. In the blustery dampness of a New Jersey winter, Mary wrote that "Papa and I have settled in and I'm afraid I'm going to find it dreary."[30] Dr. Mary Putnam Jacobi; Dr. Alan Smith, the family's personal physician who had attended Rachel in her final days; and Julia Rogers accompanied them. By early June, the unhappy ensemble moved on to yet another New Jersey resort, Elberon. Showing signs of strain from constantly caring for her ailing father, Mary wrote to Carey that she continued "to take care of Papa and arrange for his comfort." Her father, while "a sweet tempered patient," demanded all her time and devotion.[31]

Taking care of her father was not her only concern. She began to supervise the houses on Mount Vernon Place, Montebello, and Deer Park. "So many things have to be thought of, and it takes a good deal of time to give orders on paper," she wrote. Mary focused on the "smallest of details" that required her attention— the digging of a well at 101 West Monument, the care of her father's thoroughbreds at Montebello, the interior decorating at the Deer Park cottage, or the needs of his business correspondence. She was much comforted by Julia Rogers, "who makes my duties as light as possible," she wrote to Carey.[32] They passed their time reading aloud. They counted *Middlemarch* and *Vanity Fair* among their favorites during the long, demanding months.

Mary's kind ministering was of little help. John Work Garrett simply gave up. The man who had ruled Maryland with an iron hand for a quarter of a century, whose abilities, influence, and personality had been larger than life, soon lost interest in all around him. He began to fade away from the dual blows of heartbreak and years of "nervous exhaustion from long and continued application of the business of the company," the *Baltimore Sun* explained.[33]

He showed little concern for the spacious, two-story art gallery that he had just started to build onto the back of 101 West Monument Street to house his vast collection of statuary, artifacts, and paintings. He had recently ordered seventeen full-sized pieces from a sculptor in Rome. They meant nothing to him now. He was invited by Joseph Drexel, chairman of the American Committee of the Statue of Liberty, to attend a special reception commemorating the laying of the pedestal for the great monument in New York harbor on August 5, 1884.[34] That, too, was of little importance to him. Even attending his college reunion at Lafayette College that year did not appeal to him.

Most profoundly, Garrett lost interest in his beloved B&O. Exhausted and defeated by illness, he "separated himself almost entirely from the active cares of the business to which for many previous years he had so closely and indefatigably devoted himself," the Baltimore American wrote. He turned over all of his business to his sons. Robert was appointed interim president of the railroad. Mary's father, possibly unsure of his son's capabilities, warned him to look over his shoulder in the perilous railroad business: "Do nothing to be published. Do nothing," he warned Robert about an important matter in January 1884. "Beware of your Chicago friends—some of them are great tricksters."[35]

He showed little concern for the new Mount Clare Passenger Car Shop, built on the site of the cornerstone of the B&O, where the country's first major railroad had started fifty-six years earlier. In 1883, Garrett approved the construction of a larger building to replace one that had burned down in January of that year. Often called the Rotunda, the enormous, twenty-two-sided, 245-foot-wide building featured a 123-foot-tall central cupola. It gained fame as the largest passenger car shop in the world, as well as the world's largest circular building at the time. It should have been the symbolic crowning achievement of the B&O and its long-reigning king, but he no longer cared. Nor was the ailing president interested in the magnificent, newly completed B&O Central Headquarters Building on Charles Street in downtown Baltimore. By then, he was too ill to pay much attention.

Longtime friends and business associates noticed his marked decline, frequently writing to inquire about his health. Mary always wrote the same response: "The President is about the same to-day," signing her messages "Miss Garrett."[36] The end seemed to come surprisingly quickly, despite years of chronic bad health and unabated despair after Rachel's death. In late June of 1884, Mary and her father decamped to the cool mountain air of Deer Park. Another family physician, Dr. Nathan Gortor, accompanied them. Garrett languished through the summer. On August 8, he signed a new, and final, last will and testament.

A friend noted that Garrett "appeared in measurably good health when I last conversed with him on the 5th of September, but his change became sudden."[37] Within days, Garrett's chronic ailments turned acute, as his kidneys began to rapidly fail. Word soon reached Baltimore that his condition was worsening by the day. Reporters began their death vigil outside the front door of the cottage, reporting moment-by-moment accounts of his final hours.

Robert, on business in New York, was summoned immediately to Deer Park. Harry, Alice, and Mary Frick—and, of course, Mary—already were there. Their forceful and often fearsome father lay unconscious "in a pleasant room on the second floor facing north." Doctors and nurses bustled about. "Miss Garrett was with him constantly," the papers assured anxious readers. The family posted hourly bulletins, each more foreboding than the one before it. The once indomitable Railroad King was "dying in inches." Outside, surrounding the Deer Park cottage compound that John Work Garrett had recently completed, the autumn-tinged mountains were tranquil. Mary wrote on September 21, "The woods still keep their fall fashion and are most beautiful."[38]

As the family kept the deathbed vigil marking the end of the great man's life, Mary must have wondered about her future. How would she survive? What would be her source of income? Where would she live? Would her life simply shift from her father's control to her brothers'? She knew, as her father faded away, that her own path was not nearly as well charted as her brothers' and their wives'. Robert had been primed for more than a decade to succeed his father at the helm of the B&O. Harry's success at Robert Garrett and Sons was guaranteed. Mary Frick and Alice reigned as Baltimore's grande dames. At that moment, as she watched her father's life ebb, her own life was rudderless.

John Work Garrett "passed peacefully away" at 5:25 on Friday morning, September 26, with all members of his family at his side, the *Baltimore American* announced in a special edition. The news of his death flashed over the wires, making headlines across the country the next day. Mary's father was sixty-four years old. His twenty-six-year reign as B&O president was over. The cause of death was listed as renal failure, but all who knew him understood that he died of a broken heart from his wife's tragic death ten months earlier. "When she died," the *New York Tribune* reported of Rachel's death, "his heart broke."[39]

It was only fitting that Mary's father should die amid the gentle Allegheny Mountains in the Maryland county that had been named in his honor twelve years earlier. A friend noted that "there is something strikingly beautiful in the thought that this eminently busy man should have breathed his last on top of the huge mountain solitudes of the Alleghenies, far away from the strifes, the jealousies, the rivalries and the turmoils of men."[40]

John Work Garrett and his father had helped to tame the once formidable mountains. It was here, twenty-five miles to the north of Deer Park, that the first generation of the Garrett dynasty, in the early decades of the nineteenth century, began to shape and connect the far reaches of the new nation, first as successful merchants trading along the National Road and later forging the nation's first major railroad, the Baltimore and Ohio, across half the continent. Not far away, at the critical mountainous juncture of Maryland, Pennsylvania, and West Virginia, John Work Garrett had collaborated with President Abraham Lincoln against Robert E. Lee and Thomas "Stonewall" Jackson's constant Confederate bombardment. Despite all odds, Mary's father had kept the B&O running during the turbulent years of the Civil War and helped to put Baltimore back on the map in the war's terrible aftermath. He had built up a struggling railroad that allowed Baltimore to keep up with its fearsome competitors, the Erie, the New York Central, and the Pennsylvania. He was, as the *Pittsburg Dispatch* wrote upon his death, "unrivaled among the railroad kings."[41]

There was an outpouring of grief for the railroad president, whom many credited with keeping Baltimore financially afloat during the Civil War and the following decades. The tributes poured in. "No citizen was more intimately connected with the business interest of this community and no one has done more to further its prosperity," the *Baltimore Sun* insisted. The Baltimore City Council passed a wordy resolution commemorating his life. Similarly, the B&O board of directors stated that its late president "had but one purpose, the giving to Baltimore the unequalled advantages of its geographical position." The *Railroad Gazette* emphasized, "No man in Baltimore has been so closely or extensively identified with the progress of the city as has Mr. John Work Garrett."[42]

For nearly three decades, Garrett had transformed the B&O, once a penniless line and political football, to a national railroad system that stretched from Baltimore to the Great Lakes and the Mississippi River with connections to rail lines out to the Pacific. He had fulfilled the B&O founders' hopes and dreams for the untested, humble, horse-drawn line in 1828. And he had transformed war-torn Baltimore to the world entrepôt he had envisioned. He was "the first to conceive and execute the grand terminal facilities that have given our port its great advantage and which other Atlantic ports have been compelled to initiate," the *Baltimore Sun* wrote in a special edition, "Tributes for Mr. Garrett." During Garrett's tenure, the stock increased from $57 to near $200. The lines extended from 514 miles at the outbreak of the Civil War to 2,250 at the time of his death. The gross revenues of the B&O increased in his twenty-six years from $4.5 million to $20 million, and the number of employees jumped from five thousand "officers and men" to twenty thousand. He tripled the number of cars and locomotives. Only a month before his death, the B&O had logged its largest monthly revenue in its fifty-six-year history.[43] He had, by whatever means necessary, kept the B&O and Baltimore running.

The family planned "a quiet and unostentatious funeral."[44] It did not quite turn out that way. Maryland had never seen anything like it. Garrett's funeral was the largest ever held in the state. Not since June 1881, when thousands of cheering Baltimoreans had lined the harbor for the Garretts' return from Europe, did Baltimore pay such tribute to the man who had pulled the flailing city back to its feet after the war.

On September 28, the morning of the funeral, eight hundred family and friends gathered at Montebello at nine o'clock for the service. Many mourners had gathered there in Rachel's final days just ten months earlier. Garrett's rose-covered coffin was placed in the main parlor, which faced Montebello's pastoral lake where Garrett had often sailed with his guests. At the foot of the coffin stood a locomotive engine fashioned from flowers. Observers noted of Garrett's remains, "He had little changed. He had lately let his beard grow, and his face was a little thinner." The service was simple, with a few words delivered by the family's longtime pastor, the Reverend Jonathan Leyburn, followed by the family's favorite hymns. Outside, Montebello's lush lawn was "thronged with people with covered heads as the remains were brought out." Thousands of mourners "solidly packed" the funeral route between Montebello and Green Mount Cemetery. More than "one thousand B&O employees stood on either side of Green Mount Avenue as the cortège neared the cemetery," the *Baltimore American* stated. Those living closer to town gathered at the B&O's newly completed Central Headquarters Building, "the last and most beautiful of his work for the company," the *Baltimore Sun* reported.[45]

As church bells tolled along the way, more than two hundred stately, elegant carriages, carrying railroad presidents from around the country, somberly made their way to the cemetery. Many of the men had been Garrett's adversaries for decades. From the New York Central, the Lake Erie and Western, the Pennsylvania, the Pittsburgh and Western, all the men Garrett had fought and conspired with for years were there to pay their respects. Politicians—governors, ex-governors, congressmen, former presidents, and senators—along with other distinguished Maryland citizens joined the procession. When they reached the cemetery, ten thousand people crowded in for the burial service. John Work Garrett was buried next to his beloved wife on a scenic knoll not far from the cemetery's Gothic chapel. Just a few feet away lay the gravesite of his great friend Johns Hopkins, who had died eleven years earlier.

Three months later, at Christmas, Mary was finally able to again correspond with friends. She penned a note of thanks to Carey for her steadfastness through the ordeal of her parents' deaths: "I wish I could tell you what a comfort it is for me that your love for me is unchanged. I hope if we live to be old, we may be able to look back on a long series of years of friendship."[46]

John Work Garrett's daughter had lost her beloved inspiration and exemplar, her warden and guardian, unquestionably the most important force in her life. Her father had expanded and constricted her world, given her opportunities, yet denied her greatest aspiration—to leap from her sphere. But, as she was to soon discover, John Work Garrett's greatest impact on his daughter was yet to come.

THE PHILANTHROPIC ERA FOR WOMEN

"I was much surprised," Mary later wrote about her reaction to learning the details of her father's last will and testament. The young woman, who just months before her father's death had pleaded with him for a modest thousand-dollar yearly allowance, found that at the age of thirty she had inherited one of the largest fortunes of the day. In an era in which the *New York Tribune* estimated that there were 4,047 millionaires in the United States, Mary, in her own name, now solidly ranked as one of them.[47] Over the next decades, she would hold status as one of the wealthiest women of the Gilded Age.

No sooner had John Work Garrett died than Baltimore newspapers immediately began the public debate on the extent of his estate. Based on the known amount of Garrett's publicly held stock and value of his real estate holdings, as well as the assets of Robert Garrett and Sons, the *Baltimore American* estimated that his estate was valued between $5 million and $30 million. When his will was made public a week after his death, it was discovered that the actual amount fell closer to the middle, at $16,815,592.97.[48]

It is not known exactly when Mary first learned about the terms of her father's will. John Work Garrett signed his will on August 8, eight weeks before his death, while he and Mary were at Deer Park. There are no records indicating that he shared the contents with her at that time, and she did not write of any such revelation in her letters. More than likely she learned of it only after her father's death. Understandably, she was more than "much surprised."

Garrett made extraordinary provisions—"princely generosity"—in his will, as the *Baltimore American* noted.[49] Mary fared especially well. Her father had appointed her, with Harry and Robert, as one of the executors of his estate, the sprawling, tangled, almost incomprehensible web of cash, securities, properties, and railroad investments that comprised his seemingly endless holdings. He divided his assets equitably among the three siblings, giving Mary one-third of his cash and investments. John Work Garrett, the father who wished that his daughter "had been born a boy," had, in death, firmly and finally placed his daughter on equal footing with her brothers to manage the Garrett empire.

Garrett bequeathed to Mary the mansion at 101 West Monument Street, the Montebello estate and all its surrounding property, the Deer Park cottage, and all the contents in each—"furniture, plates, pictures and other household effects." Mary also inherited her father's beloved thoroughbreds and elegant stone "Arabian stables" at Montebello. With each provision, Garrett reiterated an important, absolutely essential, legal phrase required to keep Mary's inheritance in her hands. He stated that everything she inherited was to be "free from the control of any Husband she may have."[50] The father Mary claimed had insisted she never marry no longer controlled her fate after his death. But he could ensure that, should she marry, her large inheritance would stay intact and in her control.

Mary's inherited real estate holdings totaled more than twenty-five hundred acres of valuable land in Western Maryland, northeast Baltimore, Mount Vernon Place, and lucrative residential and commercial rental properties scattered throughout Baltimore.[51] In addition to being very, very rich, she was now one of the most prominent female landowners in the country.

To his sister, Elizabeth Barbara, fifty-seven years old and unmarried, Garrett left the townhouse at 12 East Mount Vernon Place where he, Rachel, and their family had moved in the early years of the Civil War. He gave Robert official ownership of the house at 11 West Mount Vernon Place, and he gave Harry ownership of Evergreen. He also provided for his youngest son, the invalid Henry, designating a minimum of three thousand dollars annually "or such amount as may be necessary for his maintenance, care, and comfort."[52]

Baltimoreans were less concerned about the disposition of Garrett's real estate to his family than they were about the future of the city's lifeline, the B&O, and what Garrett had in mind for his majority shares of B&O stocks. The fortunes of Baltimore and the Johns Hopkins University were as much connected to the B&O as were those of the Garretts. Baltimore newspapers immediately raised the issue of the impact the distribution of Garrett's estate would have on the city's economy. "In the event of the death of a man whose property consists largely of the securities of corporations in which are interested numbers of other persons," the *Baltimore American* wrote the day after Garrett's death, "there is always a general desire for information as to the disposition that will probably be made of the estate."[53] Such interrogation, the paper assured, was "not only quite natural, but proper and not indelicate, as would be the case under other circumstances."

Baltimore justifiably was nervous, and the *Baltimore American* had every right to ask such "indelicate" questions. The assets of the Garretts and the fiscal well-being of the city the family had helped to shape for two generations were inextricably intertwined in an intimate, seamless relationship.

At the time of Garrett's death, there were 147,925.66 shares of B&O common stock. Of that amount, the three Garrett heirs—Mary, Robert, and Harry—were collectively the largest stockholders, with 40,000 shares. The number of shares held by the Johns Hopkins University had risen over the decade since Hopkins's death from 15,000 to 17,500 shares, the city of Baltimore held 32,500, and other Baltimore stockholders an aggregate 16,500 shares. This concentration in Baltimore accounted for 106,500 of the nearly 148,000 B&O shares, 72 percent of the stock. Baltimore's mayor affirmed the urgency of maintaining control by Baltimore stockholders. The city's share of stock, he noted, was "of great value to the city for the abundant income derived from the investment . . . it is essential to the lasting prosperity of the city that this large share in the ownership of the great railroad should be retained."[54]

Were the largest stockholders, such as the Garrett heirs or the university trustees, to suddenly sell a significant amount, the control and the future routes of the B&O might shift away from Baltimore, cutting off much of the city's livelihood. In his 1879 tirade against the trustees, Garrett had warned against such a course of action for the university. There were enough examples of cities that had lost their commercial primacy when their railroad route was diverted. Cincinnati, which had reigned supreme before the Civil War as the "Queen City" or, as fittingly, "Porkopolis" for its thriving slaughterhouse industry, lost ground when "important men had been caught sleeping at their posts," and major railroad expansion was rerouted north to Chicago.[55]

Garrett had assured anxious businessmen that the balance of B&O power would not be jeopardized after his death. He "had so provided and arranged in his will that there would be no such change in the existing status of his holdings of various securities," the *Baltimore American* speculated.[56]

Garrett *had* so "provided and arranged"—and done much more. His will reflected the critical and highly integrated business relationship between the Garretts, the university, the B&O, and Baltimore. Garrett made a final, astonishing gesture. The provisions of his last will and testament were as generous to his beloved Baltimore and the B&O as to his family. Much as Johns Hopkins had directed his trustees not to sell the B&O stocks, his protégé employed the same strategy. Garrett stipulated unambiguously in his will that his trustees—Mary, Robert, and Harry—hold "Thirty Thousand (30,000) shares of the Common Stock of the Baltimore and Ohio Railroad Company for twenty (20) years after the date of my death." That date stretched into the next century, to 1904. "I feel confident that these three large proprietors [his heirs, the Johns Hopkins Trust, and the City of Baltimore], cooperating with others alike interested in the welfare and growth of Baltimore, will control the management of the Road in the interests of that City." Garrett had emphasized his plan as being "beneficial to the City of Baltimore and to the State of Maryland, as well as to the many other States and communities which have been brought by the Baltimore and Ohio Railroad into close business relations with the City of Baltimore."[57]

The thirty thousand shares, valued at more than $6 million, represented three-fourths of Garrett's B&O common stocks. Only after 1904 could the shares be liquidated. During the twenty-year holding period, the three siblings would hold their own shares, ten thousand each, in trust and receive the dividends. At the time of Garrett's death, B&O common shares were valued at approximately $200 each and paid a 10 percent dividend. This meant that in addition to their other inheritance, each of the three siblings could hope to earn $200,000 annually from the dividends. The remainder of John Work Garrett's estate, comprised of other investments and valuable real estate, was distributed to the three siblings and the other designees in Garrett's will. To his very end, Garrett, like Hopkins, put his complete faith in the stock of the railroad his family had helped to build for half a century. "He was a firm believer in the intrinsic value of the stock, to-day and permanently," Lewis Hopkins noted at Garrett's death.[58]

As the *Baltimore Sun* succinctly explained, "John W. Garrett meant that the control of the Baltimore & Ohio should be kept within the Garrett family."[59] Garrett hoped to stabilize and ensure the future prosperity of the company, at least posthumously, and to prevent a sell-off of the stock. With Garrett's mandate to retain thirty thousand shares, Johns Hopkins's will restricting the sale of the university's 17,500 shares, and other Baltimore-held shares, the majority of the stock shares were guaranteed to stay in Baltimore and, by inference, within Garrett control.

Perhaps Garrett also hoped to hold together his family in their capacity as stewards of his estate. However, as time would tell, John Work Garrett, the once-domineering father, could not control the future stability of the relationships among his children or predict the financial well-being of the railroad that his family had been involved in since its earliest years. Through the extensive inheritance he provided for his daughter, John Work Garrett finally had given Mary the free-dom to achieve what she wanted, to pursue her own path, with no strings—or brothers—attached. She no longer had to fear being dependent on her brothers and their wives. Her father had understood the importance of equally including her in the family wealth. She was now an independent woman of great means, free and clear of anyone's control. In death, Mary's father at last had liberated his daughter, allowing her to leap from the restricted boundaries he had once placed around her. Her inheritance finally allowed her to escape the malaise and un-certainty of her tumultuous twenties.

She later recalled that how, during that difficult span of her life, when all options had seemed closed, she resented her father's seeming "antagonisms and prejudices against women." Yet now, after his death, after their disagreements and disharmony, his earlier transgressions and restrictions against her were instantly absolved and forgiven. With the distribution of his extravagant estate and her ele-vated role as co-executor, she fully understood the societal pressures that had pre-vented him from encouraging a more public role for her in the B&O while he was alive. She also fully understood the extent of his admiration for her. "He thought to give me, a woman, an equal value in the management of his estate, with full ex-pectation that I would use that power," Mary later surmised. She believed he eventually would have seen the error of his ways in excluding her from an official position in the family business. "If my father had lived a while longer, he would have realized, I am sure, the impossibility of my being able to accomplish any-thing if I were always an outsider and he would have provided against it."[60]

Knowing her father's love of wealth and power, her appointment as equal ben-eficiary and co-executor of the estate was the ultimate validation of her worth as a woman. "He regarded the possession of money as power and trust," she wrote. His trust for her had been made explicit. Her father's posthumous message was clear and her understanding of it unambiguous: "If a woman is competent to in-herit, she is competent to have a share in life's activities." She later remembered that instant when she first learned of her father's will as being the pivotal point of her life. From that day forward, she vowed to "use her father's trust and money to live a life worthy of him and to help women."[61]

Within two months of John Work Garrett's death, on November 20, 1884, the B&O board of trustees elected Robert, then first vice president, to the presidency of the formidable railroad empire. Robert had been filling in for his ailing father for several years. Although the B&O was still headed by a Garrett, Robert's elec-tion marked the beginning of the "after Garrett" phase of the B&O. To all famil-iar with the great line, this meant that no longer would the B&O be led by a strong, uncompromising, seasoned president. Robert was thirty-eight, the same age his father had been when elected B&O president in 1858. Although unready and perhaps terrified of his burdensome new status, Robert became, as the *Baltimore Sun* noted, "the youngest of the railroad magnates and capitalists in the United States."[62]

Already, he began to show signs of the emotional instability and weakness that would trouble him for the remainder of his life and mar his presidency. He made uncertain executive decisions. Most critically, he had failed from his first weeks in office to show state politicians who ran the show, as his father so adroitly had done, the most important move in assuring the B&O's dominance in the state. John Work Garrett's children and all of Baltimore began to adjust to the "after Garrett" period of their lives. For Mary, as co-executor, managing her father's estate became a full-time occupation in itself—and a not very pleasant one. The execution of her father's financial empire was a responsibility that had tremendous consequences far beyond just the immediate family. It meant proceeding with scrutiny and the utmost diplomacy. The knowledge of the B&O and the business skills she had acquired over the years as "Papa's secretary" would prove invaluable as she slowly tried to untangle and distribute the complicated estate.

Harry headed Robert Garrett and Sons, still a successful business after sixty-five years. The family firm managed the bulk of John Work Garrett's estate, a closely guarded arrangement that excluded Mary from seeing for herself how the estate was being handled and what was being charged against her accounts. Shortly after her father's death, Mary began to press for access to the firm's accounting books. With each new request, she was roundly rebuffed, always with the same excuse, "that the affairs of the B. & O. R.R. were in a disastrous situation and her brother Robert's mental condition made it impossible to bring up financial questions of this kind."[63] The situation would become increasingly problematic and disastrous for family relationships over the next two decades.

It did not take long for Mary to understand the drawbacks of her unexpected celebrity as a railroad heiress. Along with the usual requests for charitable contributions came letters from strangers around the country asking for employment or handouts. "I saw a statement in the paper recently that you were the richest woman in America," one such letter writer, an unemployed minister, explained, "and my wife said 'write to Miss Garrett and ask her to help us. You knew her father and he heard you preach in Dr. Leyburn's church.'" A request came from Oakland, Maryland, asking for employment on the B&O. "I am writing to you today as a perfect stranger to see if you would use your influence with the B&ORR to get me a job as a cross-tie inspector." Another correspondent, from Washington, D.C., wrote in beautifully embellished cursive writing, "I ask of you a little help and oh, please do not think me fraud and that what I say is false." The letter continued, "I know of your great power and extreme wealth and I think if anyone could be kind to me 'tis Miss Garrett." The writer added, "You would not miss the money." Mary relied on Amzi B. Crane, her father's, Robert's, and now her own, assistant, for help sorting through the barrage of letters. She grew tired of the endless stream of letters asking for money, writing impatiently to Crane of "a crank whose letters are becoming too frequent."[64]

In the wake of the death of their powerful, controlling, father, the new generation of Garretts, Mary and her brothers, began to carve out their own separate identities. The first visible step was to establish their own very distinct domains and personalities. Mary soon took ownership of 101 West Monument Street, the house her grandparents Robert and Elizabeth had proudly built in 1856 to announce their move up in Baltimore society. For two generations, the ancestral Mount Vernon Place mansion had symbolized the family's stature. By moving into the grand mansion, Mary pronounced her new position as a wealthy independent woman.

Over the next years, Mary completely refurbished the mansion—several times over. She hired the New York architectural firm of McKim, Meade and White, where Stanford White, the most celebrated of the Gilded Age architects, reigned. Mary essentially gutted the house and started anew, deciding first to banish the gloomy red brick exterior in favor of a "delicate cream tint." In 1886, the *American Architect and Building News* described the renovated mansion: "The house is one of the older structures in the city and is of charming Italianate design . . . The basement, and all door and window enrichments, and other exterior details, are of white marble. The interior is sumptuously fitted up . . . the dining room is said to have cost $30,000 and is entirely in dark oak, richly carved."[65]

Despite the costly renovations and the luxurious lifestyle her inheritance provided, Mary soon developed a reputation uncommon among Gilded Age heiresses. Always publicity-shy, her name increasingly made the headlines, more often than not for her involvement with provocative and interesting causes. "For years, Miss Garrett has devoted herself to literary pursuits, to the utter neglect of those amusements and frivolities commonly indulged in by others of her age, sex, and position," the *New York Times* explained to its celebrity-obsessed readers.[66] She also continued her keen interest in the B&O and its management, now under the tenuous presidency of her brother Robert.

Mary began to carry on her father's work, to sustain his memory and to continue his legacy in a far different way than her brothers were doing at the B&O

and Robert Garrett and Sons. In the last year of his life, Mary's father had begun adding a two-story art gallery and conservatory to the back of the mansion at an estimated cost of $100,000. It remained unfinished at the time of his death. New York architect Henry Rutgers Marshall supervised and directed the ongoing construction. "In all the work, only the finest and costliest materials are to be used," the *Baltimore American* described the quintessential Gilded Age extravagance. "A broad stairway and spacious vestibule are of Italian statuary marble, with columns and decorations of the finest bronze cast from the design of the masters. The picture gallery will be a magnificent room, rich also in marble and bronze, and the light from above into the gallery and conservatory is admitted through vaulted ceilings and glass of which is to be set in elaborate frames of solid beaten brass. A magnificent mosaic floor, from Italian design, is being laid, which will be one of the most noteworthy examples of this art in the country."[67]

Mary's father had insisted on providing a public entrance to the gallery from Cathedral Street. Like his friend George Peabody, whose popular cultural institution on the other side of Mount Vernon Place opened its doors to the public, Mary's father had ambitions to eventually make his private collection available to a wide audience. For years, he had bought artwork with this idea in mind. "It was Mr. Garrett's intention, and in fact his chief desire, that not only should the gallery be one of which the city might be proud, but one that the people might enjoy and be personally benefited by," the *Baltimore Sun* stated the day after Garrett's death. Mary finished the job her father had started. "The picture gallery [is] wainscoted in dark oak, carved and inlaid with Italian designs in satinwood," the *American Architect and Building News* reported upon its completion. "The glazed gallery leading to it from the library is in polished Sienna marble, with a domed ceiling, having a frieze and cornice of polished brass."[68]

The art gallery and conservatory were but the latest of John Work Garrett's artistic flourishes to the mansion. In 1881, he had commissioned famed designer Lockwood de Forest, whom Mary had befriended in New York, to fashion what would become one of Baltimore's most extraordinary and imaginative creations: the "East Indian Room." In the Gilded Age, when Americans were captivated by all things Oriental, the East Indian Room or the "Teakwood Room," as it was often called, thrilled those visitors to 101 West Monument who were fortunate enough to see it firsthand. Only a select handful of the rich and famous around the country could boast such an exotic de Forest treasure. "Here one finds the most elaborate teak-wood carvings," a visitor wrote.[69] The intricate, prized carvings and frescoes that covered the room were done by the "natives of Ahmedabad" and complemented Garrett's extensive collection of ancient Greek and

Roman statuary and paintings purchased on the family's many trips abroad. Mary's renovation of the art gallery would continue for years as she fine-tuned it to perfection.

She also put her mark on her newly inherited three-story, nineteen-room Deer Park cottage, one of the five built in the B&O compound by her father in 1881. She redecorated it yet again, just a few years after she and her mother had completely overhauled it with the newest decorative arts embellishments. She re-upholstered, redecorated, and refurbished to her heart's content. For the "large, first-floor sitting room," she bought lady's chairs and a rosewood frame sofa, upholstered in *cretonne*, a colorfully printed unglazed cotton fabric popular at the time. For the wide veranda that wrapped around three sides of the cottage, she bought fifteen rockers, and for the smaller, enclosed sitting room, matching wicker chairs and sofas. For the large, second-story bedroom on the north side of the house, the one in which her father had died, she bought new bureaus, towel racks, an armoire, and a bed with a "hair mattress." As always, she kept precise lists of every piece of furniture, and its exact location in the cottage, along with swatches of fabric to describe each upholstered piece.[70]

A few doors away from Mary's Monument Street home, at 11 Mount Vernon Place, Robert and Mary Frick were similarly occupied. Their marriage produced no children, allowing Mary Frick to devote all of her time to her uncontested role as Baltimore's reigning social arbiter. In 1884, Robert and Mary Frick purchased 9 Mount Vernon Place, next door to the mansion that John Work Garrett had bought for them as a wedding present in 1872. They, too, commissioned the firm of McKim, Meade and White to transform their Baltimore townhouse into one that would rival the grandest of the grand manor homes of the Astors and the Vanderbilts of New York. "It will be the most elaborate and costly house in the city," a commentator noted at the time. And exotic—the mansion eventually housed an enclosed aviary, with rare tropical birds, plants, and a resident monkey. Indeed, Robert and Mary Frick's home on Mount Vernon Place became the largest, most expensive residence ever built in Baltimore. The renovation eventually cost $1 million—in today's currency, well over $15 million.[71] To associate with Robert and Mary Frick meant that one had arrived at the top of the social ladder. "A nod from her [Mary Frick Garrett] in church or at the opera" meant everything.[72] An invitation to their Mount Vernon Place mansion was the most coveted in Baltimore. Mary Frick entertained in royal style. She hosted tea each afternoon at five in the ladies' drawing room. Guests ate from golden dishes and sipped wine from golden Venetian goblets. At one memorable dinner, ninety terrapins—Maryland's unique culinary delight—were used in the soup course alone.

Railroad president Robert held his own. Known as a *bon vivant* about town, his wardrobe was so flamboyant as to attract notice in the press. "Mr. Garrett figured as the best-dressed man in the city," the *Baltimore American* exclaimed. "He always wore a flower in his buttonhole, the violet being his favorite. A florist procured a peculiar violet from the West, which he grafted with a dark rich blue violet in his hothouse, and after careful nursing, he produced for the fashionable world a new violet which he called the 'Robert Garrett.'" The *Chicago Tribune* reported that Robert owned 140 pairs of finely tailored pants.[73]

Robert beautified Baltimore as well as himself and his home. On Mount Vernon Place, he installed a fountain and commissioned a bronze reproduction of a statue of George Peabody, sitting in a reposed position overlooking the beautiful park.

When not enjoying their newly refurbished home on Mount Vernon during Baltimore's social season, which ran from November to Easter, Robert and Mary Frick removed each spring to Uplands in Baltimore County. In 1885, E. Francis Baldwin, the B&O's architect, renovated the country estate. They stayed through June at their house in the county, with its large conservatory and panoramic view of the scenic Maryland countryside. Their moves from one residence to another were punctuated by trips abroad or to New York or Newport, and stops at the family compound at Deer Park.[74]

Transporting household equipment from one home to another often proved to be a logistical nightmare for railroad stationmasters up and down the East Coast. Wealthy Victorians did not travel lightly and the Garretts were no exception. Hundreds of telegrams, spelling out precise travel arrangements, preceded each move. Accompanying Robert and Mary Frick were not only their favorite bed linens and food, but also draperies, selected paintings and statuary, and other prized decorations. On one such move, the private B&O car holding the Garretts' personal possessions was too big to pass through a tunnel. On an 1889 trip between residences, the general agent of the B&O telegraphed ahead concerning the extent of the Garretts' shipment: "Mrs. Garrett will have 8 horses to ship, also 2 Victorias, 1 coup and buggy, also a dog cart and vis-à-vis. Horses will be transferred on arrival at Jersey City to Fall River Boat. There will be about 100 packages consisting of trunks and boxes and 4 wagons."[75]

A few miles north up Charles Street at Evergreen, it was not the lady of the house but, rather, Harry who was overseeing the daunting renovation of the mansion. Alice was otherwise occupied with rearing their three sons. Having had five full-term pregnancies in six years, she was often in frail health. Their fifty servants helped to tend to the mansion. Harry expanded the house in two directions. The

first major renovation, completed in 1885 under the direction of Baltimore architect Charles L. Carson, included a porte cochere and a north wing that housed a
state-of-the-art gymnasium. Like many Americans of the day, Harry and Alice
were interested in the new ideas about the benefits of health and exercise and encouraged physical activity and team sports for their three sons. They commissioned Dr. Dudley Allen Sargent of Massachusetts, the "father of gymnastics," to
design a modern, up-to-the-minute gymnasium. The wing also held schoolrooms
for the boys' home tutors, a billiards room featuring a mantel of Sienna marble,
an oak and mahogany marquetry floor, and a bowling alley. An octagonal dining
room was added to the new east wing of the house and showcased amenities typical of the era: an ornate ceiling and sideboards, wainscoting, and heavy, massive
furniture. The adjacent conservatory wafted pleasant floral fragrances to conceal
unwelcome food odors.

Most engaging, though, was Evergreen's noticeable nod to the Gilded Age:
the Gold Bathroom. It was not simply *a* gold bathroom, it was *the* Gold Bathroom, and it dazzled Evergreen guests with its gilded wooden shutters, tank, and
twenty-four-carat commode. One observer wrote that the "bathroom is so bright
and shiny that King Midas would be jealous." It cost $2,360 and gained notoriety
across the country as symbolic of the excesses of the Gilded Age. Not to be up-
staged by her sister-in-law, Mary soon installed her own headline-grabbing bathroom. "Miss Garrett of Baltimore has a bath in her home lined with Mexican
onyx that cost $6,000," the *Chicago Daily Tribune* pronounced.[76]

Harry and his family also enjoyed their yacht, the *Gleam*, reputed to be "one
of the swiftest boats on the Chesapeake."[77] The family traveled in their private
B&O railroad car, the *Maryland*.

Wealthy Gilded Age Americans had other responsibilities besides living well.
Along with their preoccupations with sumptuous homes, constant moves, endless
acquisitions, and glittering social circles, they enthusiastically lived up to the in-
tractable responsibilities of *noblesse oblige*, the age-old obligation of the wealthy
to extend benevolence and charity to the needy. As Mary immersed herself in her
father's estate and grappled with the terms of his will, she became aware of another aspect of her father's finances aside from the business of the B&O: his philanthropies. If Mary did not know it already—and more than likely she did—her
father's death in 1884 revealed the indelible mark of philanthropy the Garretts had
made on Baltimore.

Aside from his support of the YMCA, Mary's father also gave generously to the
Peabody Institute, notably casts of Greek and Roman statues and friezes. He financed cultural lectures and exhibitions throughout the city, supported the Bal-

timore Zoo by helping in the acquisition of exotic animals such as camels and sea lions, and improved parks throughout the city. During the city's frequent small-pox epidemics, Garrett regularly contributed "subscriptions for the sufferers."[78] He also sent regular contributions to his alma mater, Lafayette College in Pennsylvania, to Robert E. Lee's former domain, Washington and Lee College in Lexington, Virginia, and donated land for a school in Oakland, Maryland.

As she began to grasp the enormity of her inheritance, Mary began her own foray into voluntarism and philanthropy. She became a part of what commentator Annie Nathan Meyer in 1891 described as the "philanthropic era for women."[79] Like her mother and grandmother before her, Mary also found that philanthropy opened many doors of opportunity.

In the postwar era, women across the country caused a seismic cultural shift beyond reinventing their roles in the workplace and the professions. They built on and strengthened generations of voluntarism and fundraising expertise, forging new social programs in their communities and creating a strong national network of voluntary organizations. From coast to coast, women became interconnected through their voluntary organizations, sharing ideas and building a strong women's culture. "It is the most important sociological phenomenon of the century," author Charlotte Perkins Gilman noted of the late-century surge. "The whole country is budding into women's clubs."[80]

In the antebellum years, women had focused their voluntarism primarily on their communities, in churches and in local charities such as libraries, poorhouses, and orphanages. The Civil War decade proved to be a watershed for change. Thousands of women were politicized through their work with the U.S. Sanitary Commission, as they rushed to build a national network to aid soldiers and their families. The Woman's Christian Temperance Union, with the indefatigable Frances Willard at the helm, transformed women's often-ridiculed anti-alcohol campaign into the first nationwide postwar women's group—and a very formidable one. WCTU galvanized thousands of women from coast to coast. Joining in their common crusade to abolish alcoholism, middle-class women marched arm in arm down the main streets of America, smashing saloon windows and becoming a force to be reckoned with, all the while broadening their scope to include a range of municipal and domestic reforms.

Emboldened by their early successes, women of all backgrounds accelerated their activism, creating national coalitions to communicate their shared interests in countless efforts: promoting the arts, working toward women's suffrage, improving their communities, and helping women in their struggle with financial security, among myriad issues. Usually segregated by racial and socioeconomic divides, like-minded women from Boston to San Francisco began to connect and communicate their shared concerns. Better travel and publications and, not least, the invention of the telephone in the mid-1870s, helped women across the country quickly mobilize and effectively agitate for their causes.

Always frugal about personal accounts, Mary did not contribute to each charitable request that came her way. Amzi Crane sorted through the bundles of solicitations that arrived regularly, and Mary carefully judged the merits of the organizations. "I have just received a report of the Society for the Suppression of Vice, which I send to you in the same mail," Crane wrote to her. She enthusiastically supported many Baltimore causes: the Maryland Prisoner Aid Society, the Northeastern Day Nursery, the Baltimore Orphan Asylum, the Society for the Prevention of Cruelty to Animals, and the Shelter for the Aged Colored People.[81]

Mary focused on her goal to "help women." In 1886, she and Bessie joined the board of the Baltimore Woman's Industrial Exchange on North Charles Street, near Mary's home on Mount Vernon Place. The Baltimore Exchange, like many others in the nationwide movement, evolved from the interest in using the decorative arts to help "decayed gentlewomen" discreetly earn money through the sale of home-produced merchandise. Started in 1880 by Mrs. J. Harmon Brown, the Baltimore Woman's Industrial Exchange's "Lady Managers" included the city's most notable female Quaker activists. Carey's family, the extended King-Carey-Thomas clan, provided the foundation for the Baltimore Exchange. Mary Whitall Thomas, Carey's mother, was among the founders. Also active on the Baltimore Exchange board were Elizabeth Hopkins, cousin of Johns Hopkins; Anne Tyson Kirk, daughter of one of the founders of Swarthmore College; and Sophia Orem, whose successful merchant husband enabled Baltimore to create Druid Hill Park next to his estate, Auchentoroly. Like many exchanges, the Baltimore Exchange gained fame from its elegant Ladies' Tearoom, where well-to-do shoppers lunched daily, and by selling finely embroidered goods and Gilded Age favorites such as knee warmers, hand-painted china, and "bachelor comforts"—little sewing kits for the unattached man. Mary's sisters-in-law, Mary Frick and Alice, enthusiastically supported the Baltimore Exchange through their frequent purchases of "slips and negligees" sewn by the needy but talented consignors.[82]

Baltimore's Woman's Industrial Exchange left a great impression on reformer Jane Addams. She had spent two years in Baltimore in the 1880s as she, like Mary, tried to find a calling for her life. Wanting to escape her privileged, protected life to do something useful for the needy, while in Baltimore she examined various kinds of charities, including the Woman's Industrial Exchange, where she often lunched in the popular tearoom and learned about the anonymous "ladies in reduced circumstances" who consigned their carefully crafted merchandise. At the exchange, she studied ideas of charitable self-help that eventually found their way to Chicago's Hull House.[83]

By the closing decades of the century, women expanded their activism in other creative directions, particularly in education. In 1848, Elizabeth Cady Stanton had issued the call to arms: "When woman, instead of being taxed to endow colleges where she is forbidden to enter—instead of forming sewing societies to educate 'poor, but pious' young men, shall first educate herself, when she shall be just to herself before she is generous to others; improving the talents God has given her; and leaving her neighbor to do the same for himself, we shall not hear so much about this boasted superiority."[84]

In droves, women answered the great suffrage leader's clarion call. Women began to focus on their own educational needs, from kindergartens to colleges. They set out to debunk long-held notions of women's physical fragility and intellectual limitations and to expand female expectations beyond wifedom and motherhood.

For too long restricted by such stereotypes, it would not take Mary long to join the crusade to fulfill her self-directed mandate "to help women," particularly in education. Earlier, Mary had spent hopeful years as a young student with Miss Kummer, who, much to Mary's disappointment, "did not believe in college."[85] Now, with her large inheritance, Mary could unleash her frustrations and anger at being held back. She could make sure that other young women did not face the same obstacles.

———·αʌ*·———

THE PRACTICAL HEAD
OF THE GARRETT FAMILY

TO RISE ABOVE THE DULL COMMONPLACE OF THEIR LIVES

"Dear Girls," Mary began with her familiar salutation to Carey and Mamie in a letter from Montebello on August 1, 1885.[1] The summer had been unbearably hot in Baltimore, with temperatures of well over 100 degrees for days on end. Mary had escaped to the cooler air of the New Jersey countryside for a few weeks to visit with the McClellans in Orange. She had now returned to Baltimore and more serious matters. She needed to put the finishing touches on an advertisement to be placed in the newspapers announcing a brave new educational experiment the Friday Night had envisioned. For some time, the five women had been discussing how to transform their ambitious ideas about women's place in society—the vexing "woman question"—from mere discussion to reality. In the summer of 1885, their plan finally came together.

Despite their ever-shifting personal dynamics, the five women remained committed to each other and their shared feminist goals. By 1885, Mary, Julia, and Bessie had known each other for eighteen years. As a group, the Friday Night had been meeting and communicating from near and far for nearly a decade. Carey and Mamie returned from Europe, where Carey had graduated *summa cum laude* in 1882 with her doctorate from the University of Zurich. She was immensely proud of her achievement, writing to Mary that "because no other woman has a German degree I care more for it."[2]

The advertisement Mary wrote and rewrote on that August morning described a new girls' school the Friday Night proposed to open the following month:

The Bryn Mawr School for Girls' first year opens on September 21—193 North
Eutaw Street near Monument. Circulars at Cushing & Bailey's and Murphy's—
No extras. The prescribed course will be so arranged as to include the highest
requirements for entrance made by any college—drawing and elocution obligatory. Miss Eleanor Andrews, the Secretary of the School, will be at the schoolhouse from 9 to 2 on or after the 25th of August to receive applications and answer inquiries.[3]

In her usual meticulous attention to detail, Mary agonized over each word. Of particular concern was one point she and the others knew would attract attention—
and not particularly positive attention: college preparation. While preparing young
women for college would be the primary objective of their new girls' school, they
also knew this was the issue that would draw the most criticism. Mary wondered if
"the point about preparation for college needs more presentation than all else put
together." The reason, Mary wrote, was "the prejudice of the community."[4]

Mary's concern was justified. The school's proposed philosophy of female education and college preparation flew in the face of all conventional wisdom at the
time. While female education was slowly breaking through many of its moribund
chains of tradition, rigorous education, especially that thought demanding
enough to prepare a young woman for college—or even worse in the eyes of many
Americans, a career—still remained highly controversial. But there were glim-
mers of hope. Beginning in 1821, Emma Willard started a national grassroots
movement among women to improve female education. Willard founded the
Troy Female Seminary in New York. Hoping to elevate women's education to
more rigorous academic standards, Willard testified to the New York Legislature
in 1819 that education for women had for too long been dictated by "the taste of
men, whatever it may happen to be, and has been made into a standard for the
formation of the female character."[5]

Farther north, in Mount Holyoke, Massachusetts, Mary Lyon, inspired by
all-male Amherst College, in 1837 raised nearly $30,000 from women in New
England to create Mount Holyoke Seminary. Reportedly, when activist Lucy
Stone heard of Lyon's plan to start a rigorous academic school for girls, Stone, at
that very moment, was "at a sewing circle, where she was stitching a shirt to raise
money for a male theologian's education." Stone later recalled, "Those who had
sewed and spent time, strength and money to help educate young men, dropped
the needle and toil and said, 'Let these men with broader shoulders and stronger
arms earn their own education, while we use our scantier opportunities to edu-

cate ourselves.'"[6] Later in the century, Mount Holyoke evolved into the first of the famed "Seven Sisters" women's colleges.

The Friday Night hoped to keep the momentum going. They set an unprecedented condition for the new Bryn Mawr School. The curriculum would be challenging enough that students would be expected to pass Bryn Mawr College's rigorous entrance examination, similar to Harvard's entrance exam, in order to graduate. This requirement must have been of particular importance to Mary, since she had scored so poorly on the Harvard exam six years earlier, a failure she attributed to her weak academic preparation at Miss Kummer's.

For Mary, who had just inherited a massive fortune and was directed by her father's will to co-manage his $17 million estate, the notion of women's abilities equaling men's more than likely held special resonance. She had been bolstered by her father's confidence that she would use her inheritance to the fullest, "to use that power" he had given her. The Friday Night wanted to reverse traditional ways of thinking about education that stressed female frailty and subservience as opposed to male strength and fortitude. Antebellum educational reformers such as Mary Lyon and Emma Willard had astutely integrated their argument for women's education into prevailing notions of separate spheres. Building on notions of the eighteenth-century "Republican Mother"—whose primary duty was to instill values of democracy, virtue, and piety in her children—and inherent differences in the nature of men and women, they argued persuasively that society would benefit from well-educated mothers and helpmeets. While this successful rationale had opened the doors for women's education in the early part of the century, the argument had grown stale for a newer generation of women hoping for opportunities beyond marriage and motherhood.

The challenge Mary and her colleagues faced was to dispel ideas about women's limitations and to replace them with ideas about women's possibilities. Bringing about such seismic cultural change would not be easy. They devised a brilliant counter-strategy. They would build their argument on women's *similarities* to men, not their *differences*. They knew it would be an uphill battle. Many Americans still were under the sway of influential authors such as Dr. E. H. Clarke, a Harvard medical professor and member of the university's Board of Overseers. In his widely publicized 1873 *Sex in Education*, which Mary Putnam Jacobi had fiercely rebutted and which had influenced the Hopkins trustees in their creation of the university, Clarke stressed that without a doubt overly rigorous education resulted in irregular female development, "monstrous brains and puny bodies; abnormally active cerebration and abnormally weak digestion, flowing thought and constipated bowels."[7]

Could the Friday Night disprove such prominent critics as Professor Clarke? They envisioned a curriculum that would be on par with the most demanding courses of the best boys' preparatory schools. Gone would be outdated finishing-school classes, such as Mary had noted of Miss Kummer's emphasis on "cultivation, not college." Banished would be odes to "The Wonderful Water Lily" or admonishments on "The Advantage of Resisting Temptation," such as had prevailed when Mary attended Miss Kummer's right after the war. At the new Bryn Mawr School, students would study classical languages, mathematics, and science, subjects then restricted to males and thought far too rigorous for the fragile female mind. An early catalogue emphasized that the school would "provide for girls the same advantages that had for some time existed in the best secondary schools for boys."[8] As important, the school would emphasize physical education to discredit prevailing stereotypes of female frailty.

Since another objective of the new school in Baltimore was to provide a pool of well-educated students for the Quaker women's college near Philadelphia, Bryn Mawr, preparing to open in fall 1885, the school would be similarly named, although it would not be located on a picturesque "high hill," the source of the Quaker college's Welsh name. Instead, the Bryn Mawr School would be located in downtown Baltimore, in an old three-story schoolhouse next to a Quaker meetinghouse on North Eutaw Street. Next door sat that bastion of maleness, the Johns Hopkins University, now entering its second decade.

Not only would the new school provide ably trained candidates for Bryn Mawr College, but it would also, the founders hoped, serve as a prototype for higher standards of female college preparation nationwide. The founders hoped the new model of education would be replicated across the country, as Mary wrote in the planning stages, to "prove the possibility of the existence of such schools and so be indirectly the means of creation of similar ones in other places."[9]

Each member of the Friday Night, particularly Mary and Carey, brought unique skills to their daring project. Carey, with her new doctorate and unbridled enthusiasm, already was thinking of innovative and pioneering ways to elevate women's education. The previous year, in 1884, she had been appointed dean of Bryn Mawr College. Clearly influenced by the rigorous standards of European higher education that she had experienced, Carey hoped to bring the same high academic principles to the new college she was helping to shape. Although lacking the firsthand academic experience of Carey, Mary, too, had good reason to start an exacting college preparatory school for girls. It was she who had been denied higher education, failed miserably at her Harvard entrance exam, and simmered in anger for years over her uninspiring academic preparation at Miss Kum-

mer's. Since then, she had had to resort to self-education for her own enlightenment. She had watched as her brothers, simply by virtue of their gender, had been
educated at Princeton and handed prestigious and demanding corporate positions. It was she who had been advised by Dr. Jackson in 1880 to forgo strenuous
activity and intellectual pursuits, to "avoid intellectual society and to join friendship with ordinary, commonplace people."[10] In shaping the ideas for the new
school, Mary called as much upon her own mediocre female education as Carey
drew upon her exhilarating, superior education.

Mary also drew from the qualities of womanhood she had catalogued in the
previous years. She hoped to see future generations of women enjoy the intellectual and physical stimulation she had been denied and to develop the qualities
she found to be important in womanhood: independence, intellectual aptitude,
physical fortitude, and confidence. She wanted to see women "rise above the dull
commonplace of their lives," as she had noted of the characters in Austen's *Emma*,
and to gain the professional stature that she admired in Dr. Mary Putnam Jacobi
and others who had influenced her.

Carey and Mary's backgrounds and goals were a perfect, complementary
match. They became the driving force behind the school. Carey reviewed the applications for teachers, all of whom she required have a college education. Daniel
Coit Gilman, an advisor to the new school, frowned upon such a requirement.
Carey expressed her exasperation with what she felt were Gilman's outdated notions of womanhood. She wrote to the Friday Night that Gilman felt the whole
idea of women's higher education was futile, that "women were so different from
men that they had not the same need of education as men and for them a college
education was oftener a liability than an asset."[11]

While Gilman's position as a university president offered prestige to the fledgling girls' school, his role as an advisor often proved problematic. On most issues,
he represented the very kind of authoritarian father figure and old-fashioned ideas
the young women hoped to rebel against. Unmoved by his advice, the founders
recruited eight new faculty to teach subjects ranging from mathematics and science to languages and elocution. All had college degrees.

Luckily for the founders, they did not have to follow Gilman's—or anyone's—
advice. They could create the institution of their dreams, thanks to Mary, who,
flush with her abundant new inheritance, financed the whole venture. While the
academic standards of the new school were appealing to some applicants, Mary
and the Garrett name were also attractions. Her status as one of the country's
wealthiest heiresses added a much-needed dash of celebrity and prestige that
would guarantee widespread press coverage.

To manage the new school, the founders hired Eleanor A. Andrews, mentioned in the advertisements, as secretary, a title that would later be changed to headmistress. Mary became treasurer. As her father had managed the B&O, Mary, too, supervised every detail of the Friday Night's educational enterprise. As the opening date of the new school neared, Mary suggested that the founders make Montebello their "headquarters." Mary often called upon Amzi Crane for assistance in running the school. Aside from helping Mary to untangle her father's complicated estate and manage her own increasingly complex financial matters, he also helped to keep the new school on track. He tended to a range of matters, from the mundane, making sure the flowers were watered and the rooms painted, to the more serious, such as fielding requests for employment at the new school. Of one applicant, Crane wrote, "She is of good reputation and has some means in her own rights. Her husband was for many years manager of the hosiery department at Hodges."[12]

The founders gave equal attention to students' qualifications. The new students hailed primarily from nearby neighborhoods in Baltimore, although Mary noted of one applicant that "she is Parisian and one of her endorsers says her knowledge is most superior." Clara Brown, the granddaughter of former Mayor George Brown, who had helped to quell the April 19th riots in the days preceding the Civil War, became the youngest student at the school. She was affectionately nicknamed "Baby Brown."[13]

The founders carefully scrutinized each potential student, looking for academic aptitude. Mary, always the pragmatic businesswoman, took the additional step to check the families' standing in the community and to assure that candidates could pay the tuition. She asked Crane to do background investigations on the applicants' families. While considering students in the first years of the school, Mary wrote to Crane that "before they are definitely entered, I should like to be sure that their [families'] business reputation is acceptable."[14]

The founders also fretted about the faculty. While on a trip to Oxford, England, Mary looked for new teachers for the school and warned her cofounders to be careful about applicants' "respectability and moral character as we might find we had introduced a wolf into our fold."[15] Possible improprieties could doom the new school.

After a month of advertising in newspapers up and down the eastern seaboard and placing circulars throughout Baltimore, the new Bryn Mawr School for Girls opened on September 21, 1885, ten days before its higher-education counterpart, Bryn Mawr College, opened its doors. There was little fanfare, only scant notices in the newspapers. The first class counted a "handful of students," who each paid

$150 tuition. It was a modest beginning to a bold educational experiment. But despite its unpretentious inauguration, the new school apparently did manage to attract the freethinking, inquisitive students the founders had in mind. At least, the students were unconventional enough to actually stage a student protest against unfair restrictions forbidding them to go to the ice cream store for their daily treat. After Miss Andrews refused to let the girls leave school for their lunchtime indulgence one afternoon, the disheartened students in unison banged their desktops. Miss Andrews did not succumb to their classroom collusion, and soon order was returned to the little school on North Eutaw Street.[16]

The founders, renamed "the Committee," ran the school by a majority vote to make decisions about academic and fiscal matters. Increasingly, the responsibilities of managing the school began to strain the five friends' relationships, a strain that would become more marked in the years ahead and would eventually split the group. Miss Andrews often was caught in the middle of the Committee's disputes and hastily summoned to Mary's house for impromptu discussions about the latest crisis, real or perceived.

Within a year of the school's founding, the Committee began to align against each other, often firing off letters questioning each other's decisions and loyalties. In May 1886, Mary wrote to Carey that Bessie had taken an action that Mary did not agree with. Enraged, Mary feared her wishes were being overruled. In red ink—highly unusual—she angrily wrote to Carey, "there is a majority against us!" Mary and Mamie began to quarrel, not over school administration, but over their rivalry for Carey's affection and attention. Mary, once cool to Carey's awkward advances and professions of affection, now warmed to Carey's magnetism and intensity. After her years with Carey in Europe, Mamie could see her relationship with Carey—and with Mary, of whom she had once been "very fond"—changing.[17] Julia, too, knew that her longtime, intimate bond with Mary was fraying over Mary's growing interest in Carey.

In 1886, the founders faced a crisis, one far more serious than their own shifting personal dynamics. Carey was adamant about not allowing Jewish students to attend the school. Mary, perhaps understanding the public ramifications of accusations of anti-Semitism in a city with an influential Jewish population, insisted the school accept Jewish students. Carey balked, writing an angry note to Mary criticizing her judgment: "Cannot your action be withdrawn: we should not risk all that we care for in the success of the school for such a thing about which I think at least I should have been allowed to give my reasons . . . I wish them at all hazards. It is so important."[18] The debate over allowing Jewish students soon spilled over into the press. The *Jewish Exponent* accused the school of anti-Semitism.

Carey eventually relented, assuring the school would admit all academically qualified students. The bitter disagreement over the issue of admitting Jewish students
caused a rift between Carey and Mary, one that did not heal for several months.
Carey, who often miscalculated Mary's tenacity, too often assumed an imperious
tone with Mary in their business matters. She later apologized to Mary for her
terseness in mishandling the volatile issue, explaining that she "had been very
tired in June and therefore not kind."[19]

A year after the school opened, Mary enjoyed an important and welcome diversion from the growing pains of the new school. In spring 1886, she received exciting news. The president of the United States, forty-nine-year-old Grover Cleveland, a longtime acquaintance of John Work Garrett's, and his twenty-one-year-old
bride, Frances Folsom, decided to spend their honeymoon in Deer Park in one of
the cottages near to her own. The honeymooners stayed in what was known as Cottage #2, as six B&O guards stood watch outside. The couple took daily, undisturbed
strolls and enjoyed "the magnificent views of the surrounding areas." The next year,
a future president, Gen. Benjamin Harrison, and his wife, Caroline, made the first
of several trips to Deer Park. The mountain resort started by John Work Garrett in
the aftermath of the war soon earned the title "the Spa of Presidents."[20] In the years
ahead, Mary would come to know the two first ladies well.

The joy of the presidential bridal trip to Deer Park and the initial success of the
Friday Night's educational experiment quickly ebbed for Mary. She soon faced
back-to-back tragedies and, as devastating, escalating family legal battles that
would last into the next century.

ROBERT AND HARRY

By 1886, Robert, too, faced the burden of keeping an organization financially
afloat. But his problem was not a fledgling girls' school on North Eutaw Street.
His dilemma was the B&O.

Although Robert's ascendancy to the presidency of the B&O had been all but
assured in the fall of 1884 following his father's death, the future solvency of the
railroad was not. Within months of taking office, Robert found himself faced with
mounting railroad debt and untenable political forces. While John Work Garrett
had been able to quell the chaos of B&O mismanagement, settle labor strikes, and
wrestle with competitors in fare wars, Robert could not pull in the reins tight
enough to bring order to the troubled line. Nor could he dominate local politicians as his father had done. He was not the astute political strategist his father had
been. Robert, and the railroad he led, floundered.

Perhaps most critically, he had to face the "creative" bookkeeping methods of his father, a legal and economic time bomb that would plague the Garretts and the B&O for years. The B&O's annual report the next year diplomatically noted of John Work Garrett's management of the accounting ledgers, "the condition of the property a year ago was much worse than was supposed at the time. Not only were the securities over valued . . . but the apparent earnings of the company were exaggerated by tricks of book-keeping."[21]

Robert tried to be the aggressive president his father had been. But railroading was perhaps not Robert's natural vocation. The *Baltimore Sun* later recalled an incident in which one day Robert stopped to talk with a group of B&O workers. "'I suppose,' said Mr. Garrett, 'that this work is sometimes irksome to you men.' The workmen replied that it was. 'Well, we all have to work,' said the road's president. 'I have to work, and to work hard sometimes, and very often I fret and chafe under it. I often wished that I had learned some trade. But in this world we all have our responsibilities to shoulder, and we have to make the best of it.'"[22]

Robert tried to make the best of it, but his presidency did not improve with time. On December 8, 1885, he arranged what would become a fatal meeting with William H. Vanderbilt, president of the New York Central Railroad and son of the omnipotent Commodore Cornelius Vanderbilt. The meeting at Vanderbilt's mansion pitted the two adversaries against each other to hammer out a contract dispute. "Here was a President of a railroad with a broken contract staring Mr. Vanderbilt in the face and burning under a sense of injustice and injury face to face with an irascible old man of portly habit [and] obstinate of disposition," the *Chicago Tribune* reported of the hour-and-a-half meeting. Suddenly, Vanderbilt "lurched forward . . . and fell prostrate, senseless and dying, stricken down by apoplexy."[23] He fell dead in Robert's arms. Rumors flew that Robert had brought on Vanderbilt's shocking death during the heated dispute, allegations that Robert vigorously denied. Robert's already fragile mental health went from bad to worse. Like his father, Robert felt the crushing weight of keeping the B&O running. The railroad was taking its terrible toll on yet another Garrett.

Following the example of his father, in the summer of 1886, Robert sailed with his wife, Mary Frick, Mary, and Julia Rogers on an extended tour of Europe to regain his health. Their travels took them to the usual therapeutic spas and glittering social resorts. In London, Mary and Julia went their own way, traveling through the bucolic English countryside to see Winchester Cathedral, while Robert and Mary Frick stayed in London. Reunited, the group next traveled to France. From the ancient twelfth-century Benedictine monastery at Mont St. Michel in France, Mary wrote to Aunt Lizzie in Baltimore: "Do you know at all what a beautiful part of the world we are in here? It is like a little old walled town on the coast of Brittany which has recently become quite a fashionable place."[24]

More than likely, Robert could not enjoy the beauty of Mont St. Michel or any other famed European vista. Like his father's, his curative trips offered little cure. B&O business awaited him at every turn. His mental and physical health was rapidly failing, and he spiraled into depression and exhaustion.

With Robert's mental health deteriorating, and Harry focused on other matters, Mary was gaining control of the Garrett name—and much more. She was now acting as proxy to her late father to fulfill his legacy and to carry out his wishes for the university and the B&O. As Robert's faculties slipped, Mary became more dominant in the family. "After the death of her father, Miss Garrett's influence over her brother, Robert Garrett, was so marked that it became a matter of current talk in Baltimore," the *Chicago Daily Tribune* noted.[25] Mary seized the vulnerability to renew her father's long-lost ambitions. In February and early March 1887, Mary met privately with Daniel Coit Gilman several times to discuss a bold proposal for the university. Three years after John Work Garrett's death, Gilman must have thought the ghost of the troublesome trustee had appeared before him. Instead, it was someone equally as persistent: Garrett's daughter.

By that point, Mary knew Gilman well—but not particularly favorably. He had rejected her admission to the university ten years earlier. He tried, unsuccessfully, to temper the Friday Night's daring plans for the Bryn Mawr School's elevated scholastic standards. But most egregious for Mary, he and the Hopkins trustees repeatedly had angered her beloved father and thwarted his plans for the university.

The plan that Mary presented to Gilman reiterated in no uncertain terms the points that had galled her father for years about the management of the university. In a not very carefully masked proposal that resurrected many of her late father's grievances with the trustees, she proposed to move the university to Clifton—which the university still owned—to make the university a technical school that would serve the community, to convert the university's Howard Street property to an industrial training public school, and to reform the Baltimore city schools to focus on industrial training. It was an item-by-item listing of every issue on which John Work Garrett had been voted down years before—plus some demands of her own. Most brazenly, Mary insisted the trustees admit women to all departments of the university. To make sure Gilman understood the seriousness of the plan, she hinted that there might be a repeat of the "public unpleasantness" of her father's 1883 tirade at the YMCA.[26]

The price of Mary's bribe: $35,000 annually. If the trustees agreed to carry out the plan, the Garrett family would erect university buildings at Clifton and rent the buildings to the university. Not only was Mary blatantly seeking to avenge her father, but she also hoped to increase the flagging value of Clifton, and by association, Montebello. She offered to forgive the rent on the buildings if the value of the property did not increase after the relocation of the university.[27]

This was Mary's first stab at what would become her trademark "coercive philanthropy" to change institutional male-dominated policy in order to advance women's status and opportunities. She did not seek to initiate a women's college. She did not want a separate but equal division of the Johns Hopkins University for women. Rather, she wanted to fully integrate women into all departments of the modern research university, and she was willing to pay the price to attain that equality.

The trustees balked. Despite Robert's new position as trustee to fill the seat left vacant by his father and his personal plea on March 7, 1887, to argue for Mary's proposal, the board "respectfully declined." The New York Times later explained, "If the trustees would consent to the removal [to Clifton], Miss Garrett would heavily endow the university."[28] But the matter was not yet settled.

Through the spring of 1887, as the railroad continued to falter under the proposed threat of a syndicate buyout that would end the Garretts' control, Robert and Mary tried another tactic: to gain control of the university's large block of B&O stocks. Robert took out an option to buy all the shares of the university's stocks at $175 a share, worth nearly $3 million. Taking the option, his prerogative as president, was an attempt not only to promote the proposal Mary had discussed with Gilman but also to conceal from the public the susceptibility of the B&O stocks. John K. Cowan, a B&O director, and Thomas M. King, B&O second vice president, supported the proposal, suggesting that the Hopkins board take advantage of the buyout offer to reinvest the money from the sale into more diversified and stable stocks. The trustees again refused to be manipulated into a financially enticing offer that would, in essence, cede their control of the university.

For a brief moment, when the university was most financially at risk, it appeared that Mary and Robert would gain control of the university's devalued B&O shares and corral a majority of B&O stocks into Garrett hands. It also appeared that Mary would finally make the university coeducational. The move would have put the Garretts in charge of the university's stocks—and the university.

Although her proposal was unsuccessful, this was not the last time Mary would offer an extraordinary financial bribe to coerce the Hopkins trustees into changing their policies. She now fully understood the university's greatest weakness: money, or specifically, the lack of it.

The B&O continued to spiral down. Many people placed the blame for the B&O's decline squarely on Robert's shoulders. Jessie K. Hines, state insurance commissioner and a member of the Maryland Democratic Party's inner sanctum, told John Cowen, B&O general counsel: "Bob Garrett is completely under your thumb. He does whatever you tell him to do, and it is well known that that is the case, for he has very little sense, and knows nothing about business, hates work, and cares for nothing except to have a good time, and his recklessness and dissipation not only here but elsewhere have become notorious."[29]

In July 1887, Robert again traveled through Europe, this time trying to secure foreign support for the failing railroad. While in London, he heard rumors that B&O directors in Baltimore were clandestinely negotiating with John Pierpont Morgan to raise more capital for the company. J.P., judged by many to be the most powerful man in the world, had succeeded his father, Junius, at George Peabody's former company, renamed J. S. Morgan in the mid-1850s. Robert knew the talks with Morgan spelled doom for his presidency. He consulted a physician, who advised him to resign. On his return from Europe in the fall of 1887, Robert met with the devastating news that confirmed his loss of control of the company. Another powerhouse, Jay Gould, one of the Garretts' longest-running commercial adversaries, was after the B&O Telegraph Company, which Robert had held on to dearly as a profit-making venture. He could not compete with Gould's Western Union. In a final, crushing defeat for Robert, Gould won.

On October 12, 1887, Robert submitted his resignation letter to the B&O board of directors. He stated simply: "It is well known to many of you that it has been for some time my fixed desire and intention to withdraw from . . . my position as President of the Baltimore & Ohio."[30] He remained a university trustee to provide the crucial link to the railroad.

For the first time in nearly three decades, a Garrett did not head the B&O. Immediately upon his resignation, Robert, Mary Frick, and Mary left by private railcar on a trip to the West. Robert's two physicians, Dr. Nathan R. Gortor and Dr. W. T. Barnard, accompanied the party. As the train pulled out of the station, several witnesses watched as Robert, disoriented from his mental collapse, shouted: "They have stolen my telegraph! Don't let Jay Gould capture Maryland before I get back!"[31]

The farther away from Baltimore—and B&O business—the train chugged, the more Robert's health improved. As if the vigor of his youthful soldiering with Robert E. Lee twenty years earlier had been suddenly restored, Robert heartily took in all the palliative pleasures of the trip. He hiked, hunted, and fished. He enthusiastically immersed himself in the culture of the Indians, arranging for a dinner with Sitting Bull. He reveled as "the beef was roasting over the camp fires, around which the Indians held a mimic war dance."[32]

Mary, too, enjoyed the trip, particularly the "Yellowstone River scenery." From her adolescent years, Mary always enjoyed meeting new people on her travels, writing about them in great detail and, presumably, benefiting from learning about lives very different from her own. While visiting the Flathead Indian Reservation in Idaho, Mary wrote long letters about the education of Indian children in the Jesuit mission schools. In a heartfelt thirteen-page letter that any travel chronicler would envy, she described how the children were taught skills in shoe-making, dressmaking, sewing, scripture, and history. "A blind man who speaks English, French and six Indian languages" also intrigued her.[33]

By the time Mary and her traveling companions, including a retinue of servants and physicians, reached the Pacific Coast, they enthusiastically agreed to extend their two-month Western trip to a trip around the world. "Our sudden decision makes us fearfully busy," Mary wrote excitedly on December 13, 1887.[34] Nine days later, they set sail on the San Pablo to Yokahama, Japan.

When they stopped along the way in Hawaii, King Kalakaua entertained the Garretts at his palace. The travelers continued on to China, Hong Kong, and Egypt, where they sailed up the Nile to Luxor to see the great pyramids. They trekked deeper into Africa and went on safari, where Robert shot lions. They went on to Constantinople, St. Petersburg, and Berlin.[35] Mary wrote excitedly of their trip, the architecture, the music, the theater, and climate. All the fascinating sights they encountered along the way captivated her, from Kobe, Japan, where she was photographed in an elaborate geisha costume, to the Nile and Germany. Well trained from her many trips abroad with her parents over the years, Mary never missed an opportunity to buy an ancient relic or well-known painting to display in her father's art gallery at her Monument Street mansion. In her letters to the Dear Girls, she always inquired about the progress of the Bryn Mawr School. Anxious about its well-being, she made every effort to keep up with the day-to-day management from the other side of the world.

By the time they reached Paris, Robert's depression was much improved, which in turn, lightened the spirits of his concerned wife and sister. But it was in the City of Light that the happy little group met with tragic news. They received word that Harry had drowned in a boating accident on the Chesapeake Bay.

Early on the morning of June 7, Harry had set sail on his sleek yacht, the Gleam, with several friends and business associates. They left Baltimore's South Street dock around eight in the morning and sailed south to Annapolis to watch "the drill of the cadets" at the United States Naval Academy. From there, they leisurely made their way back north up the Chesapeake, enjoying the summer afternoon. Around ten o'clock on the starlit night, the steamer *Joppa*, making its way from Baltimore to its moorings on the Choptank River, suddenly found itself on a direct collision course with the *Gleam*. Alert crews on both ships immediately scrambled, sounding warning whistles and frantically veering away. But it was too late. The *Joppa* crashed into the port side of Harry's yacht. While passengers on both vessels were merely shaken, Harry was thrown overboard. "Someone said there was a cry for help near our stern before we got our [rescue] boat out," Captain J. H. Wheeler of the *Joppa* later stated.[36] Other witnesses reported that they had seen Harry holding on to the *Joppa*'s anchor chain. Then he disappeared into the dark water.

News of the tragic collision quickly reached Baltimore. The next day, newspapers began their endless, detailed coverage of the accident. Baltimoreans were stunned that such a tragedy could befall the handsome, energetic, forty-year-old husband, father, and scion of one of the state's most renowned families. Crowds gathered on shore to keep vigil at Sandy Point on the Chesapeake Bay, where they could watch the search efforts. Others crowded the B&O's Locust Point in Baltimore's harbor, where it was assumed each bit of news would reach them first. The B&O's Central Building downtown was draped in black, "as it was when his father died," the *Baltimore American* reported.[37]

Much to everyone's horror, rescuers could not locate Harry's body. Divers went down to the sunken wreck to search. A large vessel, the *Britannia*, was brought in to fire its cannons into the water in the hope of bringing the body to surface by concussion. The effort only served to "shatter every pane of glass" on the ship. June 11, four days after the accident, produced another "day of anxiety" for Baltimore. That day, the pastor of the Associate Reformed Church, where the Garrett family had been faithful members since Robert Garrett Sr. had first come to Baltimore more than eighty years earlier, spoke the words on everyone's mind: "This, my friends, is a sad day for all. A day inexpressibly sad and tragic for the family that is bereft; a sad day in the history of this city, a very sad day in the history of the Associate Reformed Church."[38]

Everyone offered a theory on the location of the body—and the papers reported each one in gruesome detail. Senator Charles Ridgely Goodwin, Harry's close friend, took command of the rescue operations. He insisted the body must have lodged in the yacht. Crews worked through the night of June 11 to raise the boat. When it finally was brought up, onlookers gasped at the sight of it. "The once beautiful yacht was a complete and utter wreck," the *Baltimore American* reported. The next day, the papers ran a detailed sketch of the ruined vessel. The boat was hauled to Skinner's shipyard. Passenger ships immediately set sail across Baltimore's harbor so curious onlookers could view the crushed furniture, divans, piano, silver, and broken chinaware of the once elegant schooner. Damage was estimated at $8,000.[39]

The search dragged on. Local boat owners and companies offered their boats and tugs to help in the recovery efforts. A $1,000 reward was offered for recovery of the body. Alice, the "prostrate wife," and the boys remained in seclusion at Evergreen.

A week later, on June 13, the ordeal finally ended. "The bay gives up its dead," the *Baltimore Sun* announced. Harry's body had been spotted less than a mile from the site of the collision at 5:30 A.M. by a small boat of watermen setting sail for their day's work. The coroner found that "none of Mr. Garrett's jewelry or money were missing. He had several diamonds on his person, and his Russian pocketbook was where he had placed it."[40]

The funeral was held immediately at Evergreen. In droves, carriages— twenty-five from the B&O's Central Building and six from the Camden Station— converged at Harry's much-loved Evergreen. Solemn, silent crowds lined North Charles Street outside the house. In "one of the most touching incidents of the funeral," the *Baltimore Sun* reported, the captain and the crew of the *Gleam* stood outside Evergreen. When the procession passed by, the captain's "frame was convulsed with grief."[41]

With Harry's death, Robert Garrett and Sons, still thriving since Mary's frontier-merchant grandfather founded his modest western trading business in 1820, took on new leadership. Like at the B&O, a Garrett no longer presided over the family business.

If Robert had made any improvements in his health during his trip around the world, all was lost on that June day. The news of Harry's drowning was too much to bear. After returning from Europe, Robert "was taken to a quiet cottage at Ringwood, near Tuxedo Park, New Jersey." He stayed there "for some time."[42]

The papers wrote sympathetic accounts of Robert's breakdown. "It was thought that his trip around the world had improved his health," the *Baltimore Sun* reported, "but the shock caused by his brother's sudden death was very great." Robert and Mary Frick stayed in Ringwood for about a year, but "finding that he was injured rather than benefited, he returned to his home."[43]

Mary tried to quash the reports about Robert's mental collapse. "She says that her brother is in excellent health, though reduced in weight from his travels," the *Washington Post* explained. But the situation was far graver than a mere weight loss. Robert slowly faded, dropping out of most of his civic activities. "Robert Garrett at one time was one of the most conspicuous club men in Baltimore. He belonged to every swell club in the city," the *Baltimore American* lamented on Robert's absence from his favorites—the Maryland Club, the Baltimore Club, the Athenaeum, the University Club, and the Elkridge Club.[44] He sequestered himself in his Mount Vernon Place home and was rarely seen in public again. Despite her husband's illness and absence from social activities, Mary Frick carried on her duties as Baltimore's premier hostess.

After Harry's death, the *Chicago Daily Tribune* presented an intriguing interpretation of Robert's 1887 option to buy the Hopkins stocks and an incident about the Garretts' around-the-world trip following Robert's resignation. "When the schemes that led to the invocation of the aid of [the syndicate] culminated, Robert Garrett saw the wisdom of his sister's counsels, which he had failed to follow, and practically surrendered to her the management of his interest of the road." The *Tribune* added that on the Garretts' trip, "[Robert] was induced to give her the control of all his interests in the Baltimore & Ohio Railroad Company."[45]

While Mary certainly knew the inner workings of the B&O, it is unlikely that Robert ever gave her "control of all his interests," meaning assets, certainly not while Mary Frick was to be reckoned with. Rather than wresting control of Robert's shares of the B&O, as the *Tribune* might have implied, Mary persuaded Robert to step aside as an executor of their father's estate.

As the only able heir, Mary became the primary executor. In agreement with Mary Frick and Alice, Mary appointed two new co-executors to fill the positions left vacant by Harry's death and Robert's incapacitation: Charles F. Mayer, president of Consolidation Coal Company and a longtime family friend who had been an honorary pallbearer at Rachel's funeral, and Mary Frick's father, William Frick, insisted upon by his daughter. With the appointments of Mayer, representing Mary's and the B&O's interests, and Frick, watching carefully over his daughter's, Robert's, and Alice's shares of the Garrett estate, the opposing forces and the battle lines were drawn, assuring that John Work Garrett's once hopeful plans for his legacy would end in disunity among his heirs.

A few weeks after Harry's death, Carey wrote to Mary, asking why she did not speak more of her brother's untimely death. Mary's response was to simply state that she had been lost in thought about the tragedy, thinking remorsefully about words that had been left unspoken to her beloved brother: "I was thinking so much [more] of the things I did not say than of those I did," she wrote in July.[46]

She also had other matters on her mind. Samuel Spencer, a former assistant to her father, was elected to succeed Robert as B&O president. He was strong, forceful, and brilliant, implementing many long-overdue reforms that Robert had neglected. But he made a fatal mistake. He openly criticized John Work Garrett and set out to expose Garrett's faulty bookkeeping. Some B&O directors also suspected he was open to a syndicate takeover of the company. The press reported: "Mr. Spencer's ambitions led him into other combinations adverse to the interest of the Garretts." And that meant only one thing. He had to go. Mary worked behind the scenes to bolster the Garrett stakes and to make sure Spencer's presidency was a short one. She extended cash and credit to the troubled line in the aftermath of Robert's failed presidency and lobbied for Spencer's ouster. He was soon voted out by Garrett-sympathizing B&O directors, having served only one year and four days in office.[47]

Mary and the Garrett factions found a new president more to their liking, someone who could far better keep the family's hold on the company: Charles Mayer, the newly appointed fellow executor of her father's estate. When the dust had settled after Spencer's departure, and Mayer was firmly ensconced as president, the *Chicago Daily Tribune*—in a direct affront to Robert's mental fragility—reported that Mary "not troubled with paresis or failing mental powers . . . undertook the overthrow of Spencer and the result of her labor was the election of Charles F. Mayer . . . Once more the management of the Baltimore & Ohio will be dominated by the Garretts."[48]

The press portrayed Mary as the astute and shrewd behind-the-scenes manipulator she was becoming in order to keep Garrett friends in leadership positions in the company. "Her knowledge of the [rail]road and its management gives her a position in the councils of that corporation not possessed by any other individual," the *New York Times* noted. And devoted daughter and keeper of the family flame, "she worshipped her father and her most ardent hope is to see the great road which he built and brought to such great importance kept up to the position where he left it and perpetuated as one of the great institutions of the country," the *Chicago Daily Tribune* assured.[49]

With one brother dead and the other incapacitated, Mary finessed her role as clandestine head of the Garrett empire. Her decade of sitting by her father's side as "Papa's secretary" paid off. "Miss Garrett today, although few persons know it, controls and manages the Garrett interest in the Baltimore & Ohio Railroad and for some time has been the most potential factor in the manipulation of the interest of that great corporation," the *Chicago Daily Tribune* reported after Harry's death. The *Springfield Republican* conferred on Mary the title of "the present practical head of the Garrett family."[50]

Harry's death and Robert's mental collapse exposed the enormous flaws in

John Work Garrett's posthumous plan for the family to control thirty thousand shares of B&O stock for twenty years. Had Robert been able to reverse the financial decline of the railroad, had he been able to put the railroad back on track, Garrett's plan might have worked and proven profitable to all parties. Instead, the B&O continued to disintegrate, as did the family ties that Mary's father had hoped to maintain through the far-reaching terms of his will.

Although Mary had managed to help overthrow Spencer in favor of a more malleable president to keep control of the B&O, stewarding her father's estate proved far more formidable. If the newspapers viewed Mary as the "present practical head of the Garrett family," Mary, herself, by 1888 must have thought her role as estate trustee far more titular and frustrating. The challenge for Mary, the major obstacle that stood in the way of her diligent stewardship of her father's estate, was that Robert Garrett and Sons, headed by Charles Nitze after Harry's death, closely guarded much of the estate. Keeping a controlling stake in the B&O proved far easier than getting into Nitze's inner circle of Robert Garrett and Sons. Harry's death exacerbated the untenable situation. Harry's estate could not be settled because it, like everything else involving the Garretts, the university, the B&O, and Baltimore, was inextricably—hopelessly—intertwined with John Work Garrett's twenty-year plan to control the majority of B&O common stocks.

A year after Harry drowned, Mary began a pitched battle against her family, specifically her sisters-in-law, that, like the terms of her father's will, would stretch into the next century and increase in acrimony over time. Since her father's death four years earlier, she had suspected mismanagement of his estate and had pressed to see the books at Robert Garrett and Sons for herself. The increasing rancor with her family consumed her energies and drained her emotions. She employed a stable of attorneys up and down the East Coast, beginning with Judge William Fisher of Baltimore. B&O president and estate co-trustee Charles Mayer served as a legal advocate. She also sought the advice of her friend, New York attorney Robert de Forest.

Mary desperately needed to examine the records of Robert Garrett and Sons to determine how the estate was being managed and what had been charged against her accounts as compared to those of her brothers and their heirs. In 1885, the thirty thousand shares earmarked for the twenty-year holding plan had been distributed in trust to Mary and her brothers. This, in theory, would provide each sibling with a $200,000 annual cash dividend.

But within a few years, the distribution of the remainder of the estate became increasingly messy and blurred. By 1889, when the value of a share of B&O stock plunged to $90, less than half what it had been at the time of John Work Garrett's death, Robert Garrett and Sons settled part of the estate, at a great loss to Mary. On her behalf, Charles Mayer wrote to co-trustee William Frick, charging that, "In this one transaction Miss Garrett was cheated by Robert Garrett and Sons (to the profit of her sisters-in-law) of $906,666 and the estate of John W. Garrett of $2,720,000."[51] It was one of many acrimonious, accusatory letters that would volley between the Garrett heirs and their representatives over the next decade. Mary would never forget that she thought she had been cheated out of hundreds of thousands of dollars in a major transaction. The battle escalated to the settling of John Work Garrett's unworkable will.

Despite Mary's coups in holding on to the B&O, the instability of the company and the faltering stock dividend in the late 1880s did not bode well. She must have realized that the seemingly unlimited income the B&O had provided to her family for two generations, the income that had allowed her to live in the lap of luxury her entire life, was slowly, unmistakably coming to a painful and jolting end. By 1887, the $200,000 in income anticipated by her father's will for her shares of the stock held in trust had been replaced by a stock dividend. Like the Johns Hopkins University's, Mary's finances were slowly being derailed by the B&O.

Robert and Mary Frick and Alice and her sons probably would not have felt the B&O income loss as acutely, since both Mary Frick and Alice held wealth of their own. Mary was still a wealthy woman, even by the lofty standards of the Gilded Age. She had other sources of income, notably lucrative rental properties scattered throughout Baltimore that brought in about $85,000 annually, other more secure investments inherited from her father's estate, and income from the sale of timber on her lands in Western Maryland.

But the Gilded Age was fickle—and Mary knew this. The roller coaster economy could displace millionaires to poverty overnight. "Decayed gentlewomen" and "genteel poor" were not uncommon terms used to describe the fate of many wealthy women who, left without employment or income, faced sudden financial reversal. She had long supported charities that helped such women.

Despite such uncertainty, Mary began a pattern of philanthropic giving that in the years ahead would take her near the edge of financial ruin and cause episodes of great emotional distress. Her first major cash outlay, one that would establish the standard of her large-scale philanthropy, was to the Bryn Mawr School.

MISS GARRETT'S SCHOOL FOR GIRLS

Three years after their "experiment" opened, Mary and the other founders had every reason to believe the Bryn Mawr School would succeed. By the end of the third year, the school produced its first graduates, two young women who, as expected, matriculated to college. But the school's classrooms on Eutaw Street were dark and shabby, and the makeshift basement gymnasium, with its dirt floor and noisy furnace, hardly boasted of a grand educational experiment that purported to do no less than elevate women's status in society and advance female education. The school needed larger, more modern facilities that reflected its trailblazing educational philosophy.

In 1888, Mary purchased an odd, wedge-shaped lot at the corner of Cathedral and Preston Streets, "the heart of the best residential area of the city."[52] It was from the homes of the nearby families that the Bryn Mawr founders hoped to draw most of their students. Always the pragmatist, Mary selected a site near to the trolley lines that could transport students to and from the new school.

As a woman accustomed to owning some of Maryland's finest homes and estates, Mary knew well the powerful message expressed by a grand, stately, nononsense building. To convey the importance of Bryn Mawr School and its innovative approach to girls' education, she assembled a stellar team of architects and educators to express, in no uncertain terms, the school's important educational mission. Not only would the school's educational philosophy serve as a model, but its new building would also exemplify, in bricks and mortar, how young girls could prevail as educated and physically robust students. Designing and overseeing the new school gave free rein to Mary's imagination and unleashed her business skills.

Mary hired New York architect Henry Rutgers Marshall, who had recently completed the two-story art gallery and conservatory on her Mount Vernon Place mansion, to design the school building and the firm of William Ferguson and Bro. to construct it. Early estimates of the cost of the Bryn Mawr building ran around two hundred thousand dollars, although the final cost more than doubled that amount. Mary personally financed the entire project, as she had the school's more humble beginnings three years earlier in rented rooms on Eutaw Street.

To fit the lot Mary had purchased, Marshall designed a six-story, 90- × 76-foot Romanesque Revival building. There was nothing remotely demure or feminine about the design of the fortress-like girls' school building. It bespoke strength and sturdiness, firmness of mission. The first floor was built of solid sandstone, the second floor constructed of pressed brick, all topped off by a heavy iron roof covered with English tiles. The entrance on Cathedral Street could be reached at the top of a wide flight of stairs. Immense iron lamps stood sentinel on either side of the heavy front door, one "so heavy my nanny had to open it," a young student later recalled.[53]

Mary reported to the Dear Girls on the progress of the construction: "I have just had a three hours interview with the architect and things are really moving along very well now," she wrote in October 1889. "I think we all can feel much brighter about the prospects for an early completion." Onlookers soon grew curious about the sudden burst of construction at the corner of Cathedral and Preston. Newspapers near and far began reporting about "a building that has created a great deal of curiosity."[54] Not shy about their grand educational experiment, once construction was underway the founders hired not one, but three, clipping services—the National Press Intelligence, Burrell Press Clipping Bureau, and Henry Romaine—to keep up with the national publicity about the school. Soon, dozens of articles began to appear from Boston to Cincinnati, Altoona to Chicago about "Miss Garrett's School for Girls."

The national press began to sit up and take notice of this shy but influential philanthropist, a woman who seemed to wield such power behind the scenes. "Miss Garrett secludes herself and conceals herself so thoroughly that unless the recipients themselves disclose what they have promised to keep quiet, no one ever hears of the benefaction, though it must have taken thousands of dollars out of the lady's purse." Mary preferred it that way. Always reticent about personal celebrity, Mary reveled in the national publicity the school received. She enthusiastically kept each newspaper clipping, sending copies to Carey, now dean at Bryn Mawr College. Mary urged Carey not to lose them: "Please do not let them lie around where anyone could get hold of them—return them to me," she advised.[55]

The New York Times seemed taken aback that such an impressive building could arise so discreetly, almost mysteriously, at the direction of Mary Elizabeth Garrett. "It is generally known that Miss Mary Garrett's charity is most liberal and practical," the Times noted in a "Special Telegram," "but so carefully does she guard it from public notice that the world at large never learns of her good work unless its nature is such that secrecy is entirely impossible." The newspaper claimed that even the workmen had no idea about the nature of the building they were erecting or "the identity of the lady who visited and inspected the place." News was "leaked out that the building is intended for the Bryn Mawr School."[56]

Many commentators noted that the school will "constitute a splendid monument to the memory of the large-hearted daughter of the man who made the Baltimore and Ohio railway company what it is, and who did much for the city of his choice. The name Garrett is already revered in Baltimore. This new and splendid benefaction will make it more revered than ever." The Harrisburg Patriot noted cheerfully that Mary Garrett made "the world a brighter and better place by being in it." The *Richmond State* felt compelled to comment on Mary's personal qualifications to undertake a large construction venture on her own, opining "[t]his Baltimore lady . . . is at one in the same time perfectly feminine and perfectly business." The *Times* concurred on her abilities. "Being a thoroughly practical business woman as well as a philanthropist, she undertook the matter personally, purchased the lot and signed the building contracts."[57]

Not surprisingly, in an era when women's preparation for college and careers served as a lightning rod, the curious new building and the school's mission drew polarized comments. Many reports reflected well on the "Baltimore branch of Bryn Mawr College" and its efforts to prepare women for higher education. But not everyone was enthused. As Mary had feared, "the prejudice of the community" had to be taken into consideration. The *Kitchen Magazine* asked, "Why does not Miss Garrett or some other philanthropist invest a quarter of a million dollars in a model school of domestic economy, in which we prepare girls for housekeeping and homemaking," adding that "without thoroughly trained, competent housekeepers it is a folly to hope for well-trained, pleasant homes." A Baltimore physician criticized the plan of the new school building, advising a young female patient "to avoid the school because climbing the stairs would affect future childbearing."[58]

But Mary was not interested in creating a school to train competent housekeepers or succumbing to fears of climbing stairs. She wanted to create a school building that would be a testament to women's strengths. To accomplish this, she turned to Dr. Dudley Allen Sargent to design a showcase for women's physical stamina. Just a few years earlier, Sargent had completed the impressive gymnasium at Evergreen for Harry's three sons.

Sargent had gained fame as the country's leading proponent of physical exercise. And not just for men. He heartily endorsed its benefits for women as well. In an age still grappling with the "woman question," physical exercise represented a radical departure from conventional ideas that stressed women's physical limitations in everything but childbearing.

For Mary, who had spent most of her first ten years in leg braces and continued to suffer from a host of physical and psychosomatic illnesses, the school's emphasis on physical education and the design of an up-to-the-minute gymnasium was of ultimate importance. Always inspired by her longtime friend Dr. Mary Putnam Jacobi, Mary was ready to put Jacobi's thesis on women's stamina to the test. Newspapers soon picked up on the innovative gymnasium under construction. "Miss Garrett," the *Cincinnati Enquirer* noted, "of late has manifested much interest in the physical culture and developement [*sic*] of American girls." The

New York Times wrote that "[p]hysical culture is to receive as much attention as mental improvement."[59]

Not long after the school's gym construction began to garner attention, Mary was invited to attend "a conference in the interest of Physical Education" in Boston on November 29–30, 1889. Conference presenters were invited from around the world to present papers on the importance of physical exercise. One of the scholars included was "Dr. Hartwell of Johns Hopkins." Hartwell lived next door to Mary on Monument Street and served as a medical advisor during the construction of the school. Mary wrote to Carey that she was enthused about attending and bringing the latest ideas back to the Bryn Mawr School, since the conference was to discuss "what is now proposed in schools of the country."[60]

The founders hired Dr. Kate Campbell Hurd as the school's physician; it was a first in the United States for a school to have a full-time medical doctor on staff. As the new building grew, Hurd traveled throughout the country and Europe, at Mary's expense, to scout out the latest physical education movements and equipment.

The gymnasium provided the literal and physical foundation of the new building. From the basement, it rose two stories. No more would students have to exercise on a dirt floor, with a nearby noisy furnace and makeshift flying rings, as they had on Eutaw Street. At Cathedral and Preston, large windows opened up on the brightly lit, basketball court–size gymnasium. Encircling the periphery of the gymnasium, about fifteen feet off the floor, an elevated indoor track complete with a challenging incline allowed students to run and build leg muscle strength. The track space also doubled as a seating gallery when commencement ceremonies were held in the gymnasium.

Mary spared no expense in buying the latest exercise equipment. With the advice of Drs. Sargent and Hartwell, she searched near and far for rowing machines, rings, vaulting bars, dumbbells, "Indian clubs," wands, medicine balls, and ropes, since Sargent emphasized stretching and wand exercises as integral components of an exercise regimen.

Sargent also heartily endorsed swimming, and to this end, Mary approved a 50- × 20-foot tiled swimming pool to be built next to the gymnasium. She commissioned the B&O's premier architectural firm Baldwin and Pennington, who had designed the impressive Deer Park Hotel for John Work Garrett, to create the pool. She maneuvered Robert into contributing $4,268 for its construction. In the spacious new pool, advanced swimmers, as well as young tadpoles who had never dipped a toe into a pool, could enjoy its therapeutic benefits in separate areas. Locker rooms, where the students could keep their uniforms, "blue sailor blouses and dark blue bloomers," complemented the gymnasium.[61] On Sargent's advice, Mary installed modern, hygienic showers—"needle baths"—to replace the old-fashioned, unclean bathtub. After the school opened, however, parents were not enthusiastic, fearing illness brought on by daytime bathing, and the innovative needle baths went largely unused.

Mary oversaw every detail of the school's construction and, no doubt, the work-men who at first had no idea about the identity of the woman who came to "in-spect the place" soon got to know her all too well. She examined the site when-ever she was in Baltimore, making sure the correct paint and plaster were applied and the windows were positioned to allow students the most beneficial lighting. Showing up unannounced, she would climb around the muddy construction site and up the rickety scaffolding in her elegant ankle-length dresses, making sure the roof tiles she had bought in England were laid out in the exact pattern that she required. "I went to the building this morning and it is really beginning to look as if it would someday be ready for occupancy," she wrote in February 1889. "The rooms already are very attractive."[62]

Always her father's daughter, she scrutinized every bill and invoice. She drove a hard bargain with the builders, negotiating for the most cost-efficient prices and standing down any tradesman who dared to disagree with her. Her keen sense of business flourished as the building grew and took shape. In 1890, as con-struction was coming to an end, she fired off an angry letter to A. L. Bogart and Co. in New York, disputing an overcharge for the art gallery in the school. She demanded itemized accounts of their hourly wages and what she thought might be overcharges.

As the school prepared to open, Mary created a visual interior masterpiece to complement Marshall's striking architectural design. Inside, the main entrance area opened to a grand slate staircase with a wrought-iron railing, which "would have graced a palace."[63] The building eventually encompassed forty-seven rooms and fifteen fireplaces. The first floor featured Tiffany glass globes scattered gen-erously throughout the reception rooms. On the upper floors, the bright class-rooms, library, art room, science laboratories, and Mary's favorite "silent study room" allowed students to concentrate on their rigorous academic curriculum.

She filled the school's spacious rooms with countless *objets d'art*, notably the statuary that she had come to admire under her father's tutelage. Though she carefully scrutinized the costs of the bricks-and-mortar construction, no expense was spared in collecting the artwork for the interior. If a nook or cranny appeared unoccupied, Mary bought the perfect piece to fill it. Like most bric-a-brac-obsessed Victorians, who shuddered at the thought of a vacant wall, Mary found a use for every inch of space. She traveled and bought incessantly to display works of art that would fill the students' minds with an appreciation of beauty and the classics. It is likely that she also borrowed paintings and statuary from her own gallery on Monument Street to display at the school.

Carefully planning ahead, in September 1889, she asked Amzi Crane to quickly cable Carey, then vacationing in Paris, to order two Pantheon casts and any others she thought might be desirable.

Under Mary's direction, each room, many with large fireplaces, took on a distinctive character, reflecting the literary and historical figures she had read since childhood. There was the History Room, with classical paintings and bas-relief of crusaders and kings. A portrait of Galileo inspired students in the Mathematics Room. The Latin Room featured a painting of a Roman aqueduct and the Coliseum. The Study Hall boasted a shelf of busts around the periphery of the room, topped by a plaster copy of the Parthenon frieze, artistic features more than likely unique at the time.[64]

The English Room displayed portraits of Nathaniel Hawthorne, William Makepeace Thackeray, Sir Walter Scott, and Alfred Lord Tennyson. The younger students were deemed important enough to benefit from beautiful art, as well. A painting of Granada's fifteenth-century Alhambra hung near the primary classrooms. Even the school secretary's room was replete with Egyptian statuettes. "It is more than doubtful if any other preparatory school in the country has so generous a collection of Braun autotypes of the most famous paintings, to say nothing of the chromolithographs by the Arundel Society of London," an observer wrote of the school's abundance of masterpieces.[65]

Five years and two days after the Bryn Mawr School for Girls had opened in rented rooms on Eutaw Street, the splendid new building at Cathedral and Preston Streets threw open its huge front doors for the school's sixth year in business. On September 23, 1890, the *Baltimore American* announced the opening of "Miss Garrett's New School." It was a hit. "At that time," a commentator later noted, "it was probably the best school building in the United States."[66] Newspapers enumerated the impressive list of new faculty, each, as promised, with a college degree from the country's finest colleges and, most often, the Seven Sisters colleges.

The modern, groundbreaking school had the desired effect, dazzling all who walked down its brightly lit corridors and peeked into the art-enriched rooms. The *Baltimore American* reported that on opening day "[a] number of callers went through the new building on a tour of inspection. They came away delighted."[67]

Years later, a former student summed up her experience at the school. "No child could walk through that heavy iron-studded front door (which closed with a somber click—*swuush!*) without sensing the building Stood For Something. Solid and spacious, it was furnished not for comfort or charm but for serious study—and it had Status. Among the city's private schools, we knew simply and without question that Bryn Mawr was the *best*."[68]

The Friday Night had successfully turned their dream of creating a trailblazing girls preparatory school into a bricks-and-mortar reality. But by the time the school opened in Mary's innovative new building in September 1890, Mary and her compatriots already were well into a new project on a far grander scale. They were determined to break the barriers that held women back in the male-dominated profession of medicine. They set their sites on the Bryn Mawr School's former neighbor on Eutaw Street, the Johns Hopkins University, which still, more than fifteen years after its founder's death, had not opened its much-anticipated medical school.

—◆◆◆—

CHAPTER 6

THE SCHEME

COEDUCATION IN MEDICINE IS ESSENTIAL

Daniel Coit Gilman and the Hopkins trustees were not the only ones hoping to raise medical standards in the United States. Women had been working toward the same goal for more than half a century. In spite of decades of struggle, they continued to face segregation from the profession and hostility from their male counterparts. Mary Putnam Jacobi, Mary's physician and friend; Elizabeth Blackwell; and Marie Zakrzewska—the most eminent women physicians of the day—led the movement to tear down the obstacles that impeded equal medical education for women.

Women had not always been systematically excluded. In colonial times, medicine was viewed as complementary to women's traditional roles as bedside healers and nurturers. "Every woman is a born doctor," one early woman physician noted. When there was little medical training and even fewer standards, both men and women skilled in the art of healing offered a wide range of services, from surgery and dentistry and, when the need arose, veterinary treatment for the patient's livestock. Women "doctresses" were highly regarded in their communities when labor and childbirth was exclusively the domain of women attendants. Lucretia Lester, a midwife on Long Island from 1745 to 1779, was "respected as nurse and doctress to the pains and infirmities incident to her fellow mortals, especially her own sex. It is said she attended the birth of 1300 children, and of that number lost but two."[1]

Women medical practitioners began to lose ground in the late eighteenth century. The use of forceps in fetal delivery, for example, required greater skill, better education, and knowledge of anatomy. Childbirth became the purview of male physicians. Midwives soon were consigned to rural areas or the care of poor urban women. Male physicians, however poorly they may have been trained, began to dominate the profession, and women practitioners were shoved aside.

With the rise of science at the turn of the nineteenth century and a growing middle class eager to benefit from more modern treatments, medical schools sprang up around the country to keep up with increased demand. The first medical school opened at the University of Pennsylvania in 1765. By 1800, there were three more, and by 1850, forty-two medical schools conferred 11,828 degrees.[2]

But the race to open more medical schools did not mean a rise in standards; in fact, the opposite proved true. By midcentury, medical education became a free-for-all. For-profit medical schools feverishly competed with each other, opening and closing at record pace. "Any man can enter a medical college in this country without having gone through even the jest or mockery of spending a year in a private preceptor's office," an observer noted of the appalling conditions. Many students just bought their way in. The practice of medicine devolved. In the boom-and-bust industrial economy of the Gilded Age, there were far greater opportunities, status, and wealth to be made by selling stocks on Wall Street than by hanging out a medical shingle on Main Street. An eager young person with ability and potential was often viewed as "throwing his or her life away" by entering medicine. Physicians were sometimes educated (not necessarily in medicine) but not always well-respected figures in their communities. One commentator at the time wrote that being a physician was a "profession for which [he had] the utmost contempt."[3]

Medical schools were proprietary, much like modern-day vocational or trade schools, and were structured in the traditional European method of the lecture-ticket system, in which students paid by the lecture. Students were not required to have a high school or a college degree — or any formal educational background — to apply. To keep the school's bottom line profitable, the second term was often a repeat of the first. After completing a requisite number of often repetitive classes, a student might obtain a certificate deeming him or her eligible to practice medicine. But regulations were loose, and rarely was an uncertified practitioner penalized. "There are practically no legal restrictions on the practice of medicine in most States of the Union," a commentator wrote in 1876. "Rarely, if ever, are legal penalties, if they exist, enforced for practicing without a diploma or license."[4]

Even with lax academic standards, only a handful of medical schools admitted women, and then only sporadically. Coeducation *was* problematic. Victorian sensibilities about exposing women to the indelicacies of sex and bodily functions, compounded by the presumed negative effects of higher education on women, usually barred men and women from studying together. Women were considered too unstable and unpredictable: "Hysteria," one male physician commented, "was second Nature to them." And lecturing to a coeducational class might be awkward. One medical professor confessed that he would be "too embarrassed to discuss medical matters with a woman sitting in his lecture hall."[5]

Undeterred, women physicians did what women have always done—they started their own institutions. The first all-female medical school, the New England Female Medical College, opened in 1848, followed two years later by the Woman's Medical College of Pennsylvania. Over the next three decades, women organized and built numerous clinics, dispensaries, and hospitals to provide training for female physicians and care for female patients. All-female medical colleges trained not only women medical practitioners but also the faculty who provided instruction to future women physicians.

African-American women studied at black medical colleges, primarily Howard University in Washington, D.C., and Meharry Medical College in Nashville. Black colleges, often not restricted in their charters by race or gender, were open to coeducation and integration. Black—and some white—women were admitted to coeducational medical study at Howard.

The Quaker-influenced Woman's Medical College of Pennsylvania in Philadelphia, open to women of all socioeconomic and racial backgrounds, soon ranked as one of the nation's best female medical schools. It started with a faculty of six male physicians; by 1876, nine women physicians were qualified enough to join the faculty. (See appendix A, Class of 1879, the Woman's Medical College of Pennsylvania.)

Despite their preparedness for medical practice and the success of all-female medical schools, their exclusion from male medical schools still rankled many women. Male medical schools were usually better equipped and better financed, while female medical colleges were often viewed as inferior. Mary Putnam Jacobi was unambiguous in dispelling the myth of separate but equal: "There is no manner of doubt that . . . coeducation in medicine is essential to the real and permanent success of women in medicine. Isolated groups of women cannot maintain the same intellectual standards as are established and maintained by men."[6] She, Blackwell, and Zakrzewska pressed relentlessly in their campaign to integrate women into better-financed, better-equipped male medical classrooms. Jacobi started the Association for the Advancement of the Medical Education for Women, solidifying the push to coeducation and better training for women physicians. Activist Lucy Stone joined the crusade, using her fledgling *Woman's Journal*, a suffragist publication, to support the women's medical movement.

Many women physicians followed the path of Dr. Elizabeth Blackwell, who rented space in a poor area of New York City and opened the New York Infirmary for Indigent Women and Children. Early on, they recognized the value of building on special feminine, domestic attributes to assure a noncontroversial role for women in the emerging medical profession. In an era when urban poverty and disease were mounting, women physicians concentrated on family and preventive medicine and public health, areas of little interest to male physicians. They applied a brilliant strategy similar to their counterparts in women's voluntary and reform organizations, which promulgated using feminine, domestic roles to crusade for cleaner communities and healthier families, all the while inching their way forward in the public sphere. It was a safe, political compromise, one that would not encroach on male territory and stayed within the confines of expected feminine behavior.

Economics dealt another blow to women physicians. Despite their focus on family and public health, women proved to be an economic threat in the highly competitive medical job market, in which increasing numbers of physicians vied for patients. As early as 1853, the male counterattack solidified. The *Boston Medical and Surgical Journal* wrote, "It is not a matter to be laughed down as readily as was at first anticipated. The serious inroads made by female physicians in obstetrical business, one of the essential branches of income to a majority of well-established practitioners, make it natural enough to inquire what course is best to pursue."[7]

The course that "well-established practitioners" chose was to require more specialized education and more stringent legal certification for physicians, while limiting women's access to both. In a profession that seemed so compatible to women's natural roles as healers, men chose to attack female deficiencies, emphasizing, as one male physician noted in 1860, that women were unfit to practice because of "menstrual difficulties." The male offense worked. By 1890, there were 4,557 women physicians, only 4.3 percent of the nation's total.[8]

Women physicians were losing the battle for coeducational opportunities. "The habitual exclusion of women from fit opportunities," Jacobi emphasized at her commencement speech to the new graduates of the Woman's College of the New York Infirmary in 1883, "engenders a habitually low tone of confidence in their abilities, which constantly interferes to prevent any given woman from demonstrating her abilities."[9]

Women tried novel ways to break through such habitual exclusion. Starting in

1865, they began enticing male medical schools to admit women by offering scholarships. Their efforts met with little success. They targeted one of the most well-known medical schools, Harvard. The elite, all-male liberal arts college became the first battleground in the war for equal, coeducational medical training.

In 1872, the New England Female Medical College petitioned Harvard to incorporate it into the college. Harvard refused. Six years later, Marian Hovey of Massachusetts tried an innovative approach. She offered $10,000 to Harvard to admit women into its medical college "if its advantage can be offered on equal terms as men." The Harvard medical faculty actually voted eleven to seven in favor of Hovey's proposition—on the condition the amount be raised to $200,000, "a proper sum to warrant the Corporation in accepting such a proposal."[10] Hovey kept her money.

In 1880, Harvard president Charles Eliot, the same man who had advised the Hopkins trustees to forgo coeducation seven years earlier, reconsidered the benefits of commingling. Harvard desperately needed $200,000 for its new medical building. Suddenly the idea of admitting women, with the profitable tuition revenues they would generate, seemed a good one. Eliot stated that the time had arrived to raise "a round sum of money to the university in order to procure the admission of women to the medical school." The women of the New England Hospital Society, through its quick-acting network, raised $50,000 in pledges in one year. Drs. Marie Zakrzewska, Mary Putnam Jacobi, and Emily Blackwell petitioned Harvard to hold the money in trust until the full amount could be raised to expand the medical school and admit women. The board of overseers voted to accept the terms, but this time angry medical faculty threatened mass resignation if women got through the doors. Rescinding the women's offer, the overseers concluded, "It is not advisable for the University now to give any assurance, or hold out any encouragement that it would undertake the medical education of women by Harvard College at its Medical School."[11]

Getting through the front door of all-male medical schools was only the least of women's problems. Once educated, they faced even more hurdles. Jacobi noted that when universities began to dominate medical education in the early part of the century, women physicians lost the battle for equal education and equal access to hospital practice. Women physicians were often banned from advanced training and practice in large hospitals, particularly in urban areas, and were forced to take the path of Elizabeth Blackwell and practice in female clinics. Large urban hospitals were just starting to expand in the decades following the Civil War and increasingly became an essential component in medical training. The women's medical movement eagerly sought appointments for women students to study and observe with the preeminent male hospital clinicians. In one such case, a group of women students from the Woman's Medical College of Pennsylvania met with jeers and taunts—and a near riot—as they walked into their morning clinic at the nearby Blockley Hospital.[12]

Although hospitals were deemed an important step in medical training for physicians by the medical profession, the public was not yet convinced of their value. With a weak track record, hospitals often were places that accelerated death, not prolonged life. Most Americans were leery of even setting foot inside of one. One nineteenth-century commentator wrote "No gentleman of property or standing would have found himself in a hospital unless stricken with insanity or felled by epidemic or accident in a strange city."[13]

Nonetheless, the number of hospitals grew rapidly—from 178 in 1873, when the first survey of American hospitals was taken, to 700 in 1889.[14] By the 1880s, American medicine was stranded between the polarized worlds of traditional practitioners with few sure cures and the new yet untested world of science. Hospitals promised, but did not always deliver, the hope of bridging the two. The dire exigencies of the Civil War had greatly accelerated and advanced medical practice, particularly in battlefield surgery, but the medical profession still was defenseless against the killer diseases of diphtheria, yellow fever, tuberculosis, and influenza.

In the post–Civil War years, Baltimore counted sixteen hospitals and seven dispensaries. Across town from the University of Maryland's College of Medicine, through the 1880s yet another hospital was rising, this one on thirteen acres of Baltimore's abandoned insane asylum, which merchant Johns Hopkins had purchased. Despite pools of quicksand and a pesky underground stream that challenged the laying of a solid foundation, construction on the thirteen-building, $2 million complex had begun in 1877. It soon drew attention, as eager observers waited impatiently for the opening of the much-touted hospital. Baltimore's *Medical Register* announced in 1885: "This institution will, when completed, be one of the finest in the matter of appointments in the world."[15]

The Johns Hopkins Hospital was scheduled to open that year, but the day came and went with no opening. Even Baltimore's mayor implored the trustees to open the hospital, with its promising new approach to medical care. The next year, the *American Architect and Building News* made a new optimistic projection. "The Johns Hopkins Hospital has now thirteen buildings erected and finished, except the furnishing," the journal reported in February 1886. "The site is one of the most commanding possible, and the buildings, of red brick and Cheat-River bluestone, form a magnificent group, which can be seen in all directions. The Hospital will probably be ready to receive patients within the year 1886."[16]

Unfortunately, events did not go as planned. The delay was not due to quicksand or underground streams that impeded construction. Rather, the trustees faced a major challenge in laying an ideological foundation for synthesizing a new model of medical research, patient care, and training between a hospital and a university. They also had to coordinate the boards representing the two separate legal entities, the Johns Hopkins University and the Johns Hopkins Hospital. In 1883, a joint committee of three university trustees and three hospital trustees met to hammer out their differences and to discuss how the hospital and proposed medical school would jointly operate. Never before had hospital clinical care, academic instruction, and medical research been triangulated in American higher education.

The hospital trustees also faced the identical problem their counterparts at the university were grappling with: a lack of money. By 1887, after Mary's abortive plans to move the university to Clifton and Robert's futile option to buy the university's B&O stocks, the university continued its downward financial plunge. In 1888, it hit rock bottom. The decade-old university fell into a dire financial crisis, one that threatened to shut it down. The loss of stock dividend cut the university's annual income 75 percent, more than $155,000 from its operating budget of $200,000. In addition, the trustees anticipated a $98,000 deficit for the coming year. "The fiasco to the Baltimore and Ohio Railroad system threatened to paralyze the university," the *Chicago Journal* reported. The trustees briefly considered reversing the founder's directive to keep the stocks and selling the stocks for whatever price they would fetch. But they were warned that such a large sell-off might give B&O control to the rival Richmond and West Point Terminal Company and bring financial ruin to Baltimore.[17] The trustees instead scrapped plans for the new library and laboratories and raised tuition.

Although the public's perception was that of a university flush with money— its multimillion dollar endowment rivaled that of long-established universities— the reality was much different. Daniel Coit Gilman, renowned academician and celebrated university president, was forced to take on yet another role: fundraiser. He faced three seemingly impossible mandates: to keep the university open, to complete the massive and very costly hospital construction, and to establish the long-awaited medical school. All the while, he had to adhere to the founder's directive to use only the stock income—now mostly gone—and worse—hold on to the B&O stocks.

Gilman was desperate. The impending opening of the state-of-the-art hospital had generated much national attention, raising sensitive questions about the yet-unopened medical school. With most of the university's income gone and the expensive hospital construction still underway, in the fall of 1888, he sent a confidential letter to trustees George Dobbin and Charles Gwinn arguing for the need to find an outside source to fund the proposed medical school. The university had only $67,480.42 in its coffers specifically earmarked for the medical school.[18]

For a university that had been so well endowed and so associated with the founding benefactor's name, bringing in another donor was a risky step. Gilman rationalized that his plan would allow the donor to align himself with a great institution. Because of "a remarkable concurrence of events there is now an opportunity to establish in Baltimore a school of medicine, such as the world does not now possess, but it will take a considerable amount of money," he wrote on November 9, 1888.[19]

Gilman assured the trustees that the donor would be well rewarded and widely recognized for his gift. The new medical school, he suggested, could be named in the donor's honor. "This separate school should have its own name, its own funds, its own buildings, its own observations & progress—its special faculty and students." He emphasized, "There then could be established 'the _____ school of medicine' on such a basis as to benefit not one district, nor one state only, but the entire land." Reiterating his stand against coeducation, he added, "It is not too much to say that such a school ought to be of service, by its discoveries and its training of superior men, to all the world." Gilman concluded in his letter to the trustees: "Only a man of large means and large views will be very likely to appreciate the situation; but if such a man can be found willing to consider a plan in detail it will be easy to show him that a like opportunity to be of service to mankind has never been presented."[20]

Gilman had faith that one donor would contribute the entire amount for the medical school—originally estimated to be $100,000—an asking price that would increase fivefold over the coming years. Perhaps he had in mind two recent major contributions to medical schools. In 1884, industrialist Andrew Carnegie donated funding for a laboratory in his name for research and teaching in pathology and bacteriology at Bellevue Hospital Medical College in New York. In the same year, New York Central Railroad president William H. Vanderbilt—the same man who would die during the meeting with Robert in 1885—contributed $500,000 to expand the College of Physicians and Surgeons in New York.[21]

As Gilman would soon discover, aside from gifts such as Vanderbilt's and Carnegie's, medical education was not a major philanthropic priority for most wealthy Americans who could afford to give $100,000 or more. Philanthropists then, as now, invested in causes that had a good chance of transforming society for the better. There was little reason to think that medicine in the 1880s would offer such change. Its future seemed uncertain. Medical education, still unproven, was not of much interest to major philanthropists. Few were willing to gamble on its future.

As Gilman frantically searched for a major donor to fund the medical school, the university concurrently embarked on its first major fundraising campaign, the Emergency Fund of 1889, to replenish the coffers left near empty after the B&O debacle. Baltimore businessman William Wallace Spence stepped up to direct the appeal. The campaign quickly raised $108,700 from thirty-two donors, mostly Baltimore businessmen who were targeted for the appeal.[22] Mary enthusiastically supported the urgent fundraising appeal with a $5,000 contribution, although only two years earlier, Gilman and the trustees had rejected her offer to move the university to Clifton and had voted down Robert's bid to buy the university's stocks. Her continued interest in the university in light of her many rejections from it ironically was an encouraging sign to the trustees that Mary's largess might be increased to an even greater amount to alleviate the financial crisis.

There were other encouraging signs as well. On May 7, 1889, a beautiful, balmy spring day, the long-awaited Johns Hopkins Hospital in East Baltimore finally debuted—sixteen years after its benefactor's death and twelve years of construction. "The Great Hospital—Ready for Its Mission," the *Baltimore Sun* exclaimed in a front-page banner headline. Many agreed that it was well worth the wait. A new age of hospital care in the United States began on that spring day. Huge crowds gathered early on the streets, eagerly waiting for the festivities to begin. "Lines of private carriages, doctors' buggies and other conveyances stood on both sides of Broadway for several squares," the *Baltimore Sun* reported. Visitors were issued tickets: yellow for VIPs, white for out-of-town guests, green for medical professionals, and pink for ladies, who were allowed "to enter through the central door." More than eight hundred guests "poured into the main gateway on Broadway," and were heartily greeted by the trustees waiting inside. The president of the board, Francis T. King, Bessie's father, presided over the ceremonies, which frequently invoked the good name of the hospital's benefactor. "The example of Johns Hopkins will not be lost upon this country," King emphasized in his welcoming speech.[23]

After sitting through the requisite inaugural speeches—women were relegated to watch from the gallery—the guests toured the grand pavilion of the hospital with its splendid rotunda and the brightly lit wards with a total of 220 beds. The buildings were arranged at a distance from each other to prevent the spread of disease. The corridors were sunny, bright, clean, and open. Modern incandescent electric lamps lit the rooms. There were telephones and, for the winter months ahead, there would be central heating—a first for an American hospital. "All possible improvements in ventilation, heating, isolation, all that modern medical science can suggest for the study and relief of disease, were included in the plan," the *St. Louis Republic* pronounced. "For example," the article continued, "the temperature of a single bed can be made to differ nine or ten degrees from the surrounding beds in the same ward."[24]

Guests marveled at the other buildings as well—the bathhouses, the apothecary, the pathology building, the 280-seat surgical amphitheater, all surrounded by spacious manicured lawns. The large outpatient ward provided ample waiting room for as many as four hundred patients, since benefactor Johns Hopkins had stipulated in his final instructions that the hospital should open its doors to "the indigent sick of this city and its environs, without regard to sex, age or color, who may require surgical or medical treatment." The *New York Times* pronounced the Johns Hopkins Hospital "the best institution of its kind in the world."[25]

On the day the hospital opened, a much-relieved Gilman concluded the gala by announcing the success of the Emergency Fund's campaign: "The university will now be enabled to continue its work without contraction."[26] That year, 1889, marked a watershed moment in the university's history. Gilman and the trustees had averted a financial catastrophe and opened the most advanced hospital in the nation. And the university had remained open, in spite of all its difficulties.

In the midst of the celebration—the open house for public viewing lasted a week before the hospital admitted its first patients—Gilman lamented that an integral component of the founder's vision was still missing to tie the great hospital to the academic university. "Is there anything wanting?" Gilman asked rhetorically. "Yes, there is still a great want to be supplied, an arch to rest upon these pillars: an institute of medicine and surgery, a college of physicians and surgeons, a medical school."[27] The medical school was proposed, planned, and somewhat underway, but far from becoming a reality.

With Johns Hopkins University still in financial straits in 1888, as Harvard medical college had been a few years earlier, and sensing a weak chink in the trustees' armor, Mary and the Friday Night began plotting their move to have women admitted. After nearly a decade of being rebuffed and rejected, of trying to break through the impenetrable wall of the trustees' reluctance to make the university coeducational, the emboldened young women saw a vulnerability: the medical school. It was a financial weakness—and an opportunity—that Mary understood all too well.

The five women, who had first organized themselves as the Friday Night in the mid-1870s and evolved a decade later into the founders of the pioneering Bryn Mawr School, were now prepared to take on a much larger challenge. They had pushed for separate but equal education for girls at Bryn Mawr School. Now, they hoped to dismantle the centuries-old tradition of separate medical training for men and women and to break down one more societal barrier that stood in the way of women's advancement and, as Mary Putnam Jacobi had stressed, "women's real and permanent success in medicine." They would force Gilman and the trustees' opposition against coeducation out into the open. They would attempt to take the women's medical movement to its logical and successful conclusion. Their new campaign would prove a far more formidable ambition than they had imagined and would produce very unexpected results.

EVERY DAY COUNTS

It did not take long for the Friday Night to make their move. Within days of Daniel Coit Gilman's November 9, 1888, letter to trustees Charles Gwinn and George Dobbin explaining the urgent need to find " a man of large means" to endow the medical school, the five friends began plotting. They dreamed a daring dream—to organize a national network of women to raise $100,000 to open the medical school. But they would insist on one very specific condition: that women students be admitted to the new school on the same terms as men. They knew they faced enormous odds in raising the exorbitant amount, but mostly they feared Gilman would find the money first. "I am nervous about waiting because I am so afraid [of] the med. school getting money before their promise has been given," Carey wrote hurriedly to Mary after learning of Gilman's letter.[28]

There were other formidable obstacles, as well, namely Gilman and the majority of trustees who remained firmly opposed to coeducation. Worse, they knew other women had tried and failed such a tactic, notably Marian Hovey's $10,000 bid in 1878 and the New England Hospital Society's $50,000 offer two years later to make Harvard Medical College coeducational.

This was not an ideal time for Mary to take on yet another major volunteer effort, especially one with such potential magnitude. She was still reeling from Harry's death and Robert's breakdown earlier that summer. She was now the primary executor of her father's estate and already dealing with the opposing interests of the other Garrett heirs. She usually spent about half of each day poring over her father's accounts and was actively agitating to gain access to his estate records at Robert Garrett and Sons. The extensive renovations of 101 West Monument, started after her father's death four years earlier, were ongoing. And, she had just purchased the lot for the new Bryn Mawr School and was making preparations for the building's construction.

Mary hardly had a successful track record of persuading the university trustees to see matters her way. In 1876, Gilman had rejected her request to attend the university and, in 1887, the board had roundly rebuffed the financially enticing proposal to move the university to Clifton. She knew the trustees would not easily acquiesce on the controversial issue of medical coeducation. But this was a once-in-a-lifetime moment she could not resist. She had very personal reasons for wanting the medical school to open. Women physicians, particularly Dr. Mary Putnam Jacobi and others who treated her, and their crusade for coeducational medical training had long been of personal interest to Mary. It represented yet another opportunity in her self-proclaimed goal to "help women."

Perhaps as important to Mary was her family's long association with university founder Johns Hopkins and the memory of her father's displeasure with the trustees' inability to establish the medical school. He had resigned in anger from the board and later publicly condemned the trustees' failure to open the medical school in a timely manner. Five years had passed since her father's outburst at the YMCA anniversary event in January 1883 and fifteen years since Hopkins's death. Still, the medical school, as the benefactor had envisioned it, was nowhere in sight. And she was not the least bit cowed by Gilman or the trustees.

Although already proven as astute organizers and promoters with their Bryn Mawr School success, the women needed to test their newest idea—their "scheme" as they soon began to call it. Carey found sympathetic counsel next door to her at Bryn Mawr College. She met with George Childs, a Bryn Mawr College neighbor, who often helped the struggling college out of fiscal emergencies and happened to be one of Philadelphia's wealthiest publishers. She told him of Hopkins' financial predicament and the pressure to open the medical school. She explained the Friday Night's scheme to raise the endowment. Childs was skeptical. "To me personally he was charming but [toward] the plan he is not very well disposed," Carey reported to Mary. Childs warned her that "the people who wd [would] be most interested wd not have money and 100,000 (or 150,000 as I told him) was a very large sum." He suggested that they talk with Anna Hallowell, a pivotal activist in Philadelphia. Carey did, and Hallowell, too, urged caution, adding that it was important "to get a promise [from the trustees] before any general attempt is made."[29]

These were the first, but not the last, times the Friday Night's idea would be discouraged and dismissed. Undaunted, they forged ahead. Mary, always the grounding counteraction to Carey's impulsiveness, also was cautious. "Just as soon as I have made up my mind about the Johns Hopkins plan of action, I will write to you," Mary wrote back immediately to Carey's report about Childs. Although Mary wanted to keep the plan clandestine until it was more fully developed, Carey soon let the idea slip during a meeting with Gilman. Mary was mortified, perhaps thinking the trustees would be suspicious of yet another Garrett proposal so quickly on the heels of the last one just a year earlier. "I *did* say in so many words," Carey confessed repentantly to Mary, "that a certain number of us would 'undertake to raise the $100,000 if the Trustees would vote to accept such a gift subject to the condition that women be admitted to the medical school on the same terms as men.'" Carey tried to ease Mary's fears. "I can't tell you *how genuinely* nice Mr. Gilman was. I have never really liked him before and I fear I reported him very badly."[30] Carey's glowing affection for Gilman would be short-lived.

By New Year's Day, 1889, the news was out and the embryonic scheme was launched. It soon accelerated into a four-year, often acrimonious, race to the finish line between two oppositional forces. As Daniel Coit Gilman searched for his single donor, a Carnegie or a Vanderbilt, the five women searched for the pot of gold that would endow the medical school on *their* terms. Fortunately for the ambitious and eager women, as they moved ahead in their planning and organizing, they had a direct pipeline to the internal machinations of the university and the trustees' activities. Carey's, Mamie's, and Bessie's fathers—James Thomas, Charles Gwinn, and Francis King—were on the university board, and King also served as president of the hospital. Charles Gwinn, an executor of the Hopkins estate, had helped to draft the articles of incorporation for the university and the hospital. Although outnumbered by other trustees, Thomas and Gwinn, in particular, favored making the proposed medical school coeducational. They often telegraphed their daughters, then living at Bryn Mawr College, about an impending move on the part of the trustees, allowing the women to preempt the trustees' decisions. The fathers became trusted advocates of their daughters' scheme to push for coeducation.

The women established their scheme on a fundraising and public-relations model that most modern-day fundraisers would easily recognize. They first conducted the "quiet phase," in which they lined up powerful allies across the country who could promote their cause. Then they went public, aggressively pushing to reach their monetary goal.

The first job at hand was to rally the most prominent women in the country, "names of influence" as Mary wrote, who could muster their social standing and connections to raise public awareness about coeducational medical training—

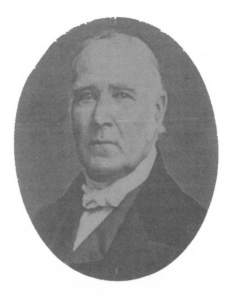

Family patriarch and Irish immigrant Robert Garrett arrived in Baltimore in the early nineteenth century around the same time as did Johns Hopkins, George Peabody, Enoch Pratt, and other merchants who would shape Baltimore's commercial and cultural future. Courtesy of the Evergreen House Foundation at Evergreen Museum and Library, The Johns Hopkins University.

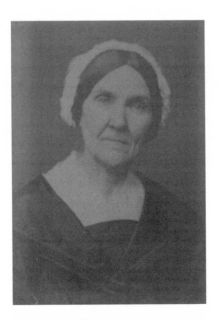

Mary's grandmother Elizabeth Stouffer Garrett set an example of antebellum women's voluntarism through her work with many Baltimore charities. Courtesy of the Evergreen House Foundation at Evergreen Museum and Library, The Johns Hopkins University.

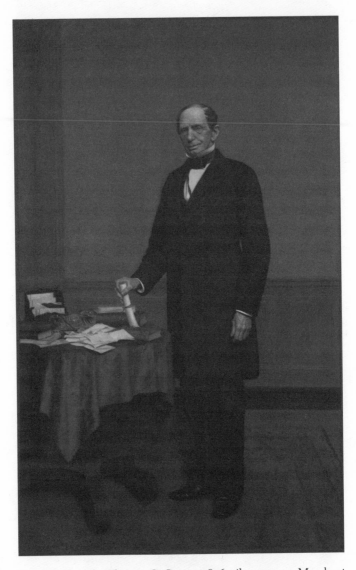

Johns Hopkins, by Thomas C. Corner, 1896, oil on canvas. Merchant and banker Johns Hopkins became the majority stockholder of the B&O Railroad and successfully lobbied for John Work Garrett's election as its president in 1858. Courtesy of the Alan Mason Chesney Medical Archives of The Johns Hopkins Medical Institutions. Photo by Aaron Levin.

As president of the B&O Railroad, John Work Garrett became the most powerful man in Maryland and a dominant influence on his daughter. Courtesy of the Evergreen House Foundation at Evergreen Museum and Library, The Johns Hopkins University.

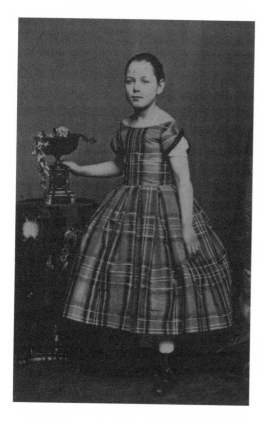

Mary's fashionable hoop skirts and high-top shoes hid her leg braces and the ankle injury she had suffered as an infant. Courtesy of the Evergreen House Foundation at Evergreen Museum and Library, The Johns Hopkins University.

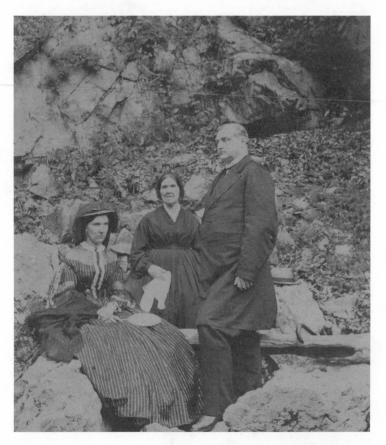

Mary's uncle Henry Garrett, pictured here with his sister Elizabeth
Barbara (left) and mother Elizabeth, exemplified the meaning of the
"Brothers' War" as he worked against John Work Garrett's efforts to
preserve the Union. Courtesy of the Evergreen House Foundation at Evergreen Museum
and Library, The Johns Hopkins University.

(*Opposite*) In 1872, twenty-five-year-old Robert married twenty-
one-year-old Mary Sloan Frick in the social event of the season.
John Work Garrett gave the couple an elegant townhouse on Mount
Vernon Place, now known as the Garrett-Jacobs Mansion. Courtesy of
the Evergreen House Foundation at Evergreen Museum and Library, The Johns Hopkins
University.

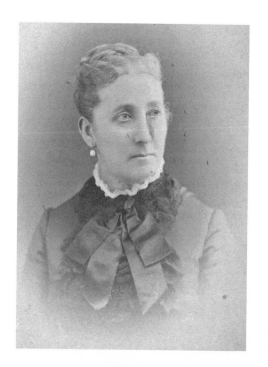

Mary's mother, Rachel, "a lady of most amiable disposition," helped the Garretts to weather the tumultuous years of the Civil War and guided the family's subsequent rise to social prominence. Courtesy of the Evergreen House Foundation at Evergreen Museum and Library, The Johns Hopkins University.

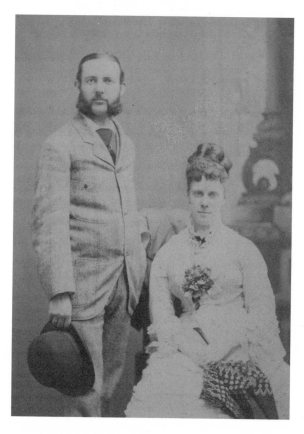

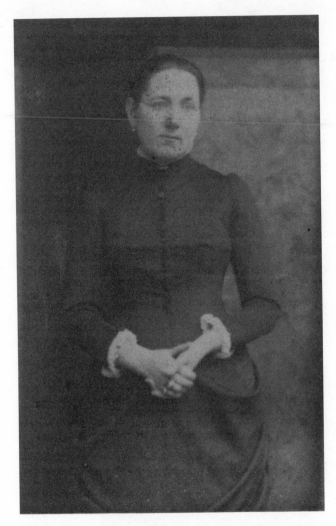

By early adulthood, Mary had become a slender, attractive young woman and an excellent equestrian who loved the out-doors. Despite her shyness, she became a competent business-woman as "Papa's secretary." Photograph by G. C. Cox, courtesy of Bryn Mawr College Library.

(*Opposite*) In 1878, Harry, Alice, and their three sons moved into Evergreen House on North Charles Street. Harry soon added a modern gymnasium and a bowling alley. The mansion gained fame for its "Gold Bathroom," a symbol of Gilded Age extravagance. Courtesy of the Evergreen House Foundation at Evergreen Museum and Library, The Johns Hopkins University.

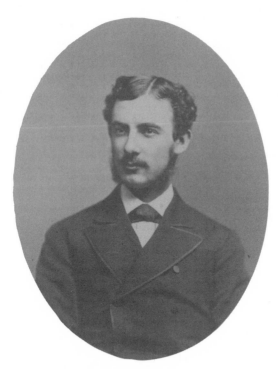

T. Harrison Garrett became head of the family business, Robert Garrett and Sons, and a collector of rare books and coins. Courtesy of the Evergreen House Foundation at Evergreen Museum and Library, The Johns Hopkins University.

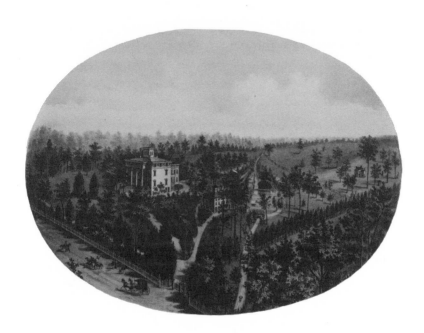

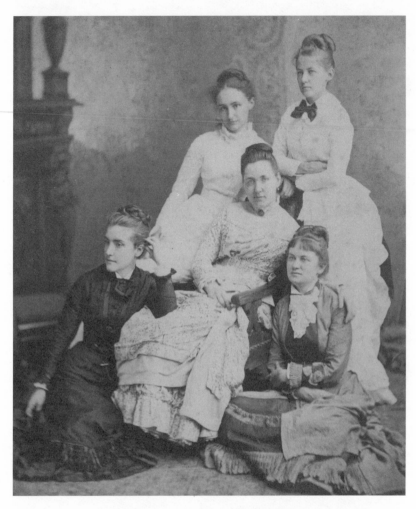

In her early twenties, Mary's circle of friends included the lively Friday Night, which incited her rebellious side. Pictured here, Mary is at the center, and clockwise from upper left are Mamie Gwinn, Bessie King, Julia Rogers, and Carey Thomas. Courtesy of Bryn Mawr College Library.

(*Opposite*) Widowed in 1888, Alice Whitridge Garrett and her sons, Horatio, Robert III, and John Work Garrett II (left to right), moved to Princeton, New Jersey, while the boys completed college. Courtesy of the Evergreen House Foundation at Evergreen Museum and Library, The Johns Hopkins University.

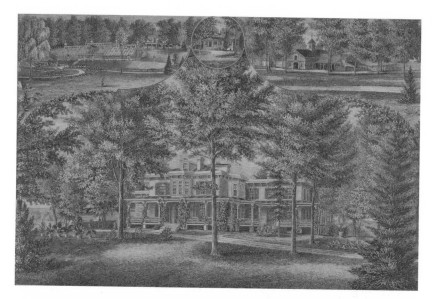

John Work Garrett lived the "life of a nobleman" at his fourteen-hundred-acre Montebello estate, with its Arabian stables, racetrack, lake, and two mansions. He converted the old Stirling mansion, pictured here, into a rustic retreat where he entertained lavishly. Courtesy of the Evergreen House Foundation at Evergreen Museum and Library, The Johns Hopkins University.

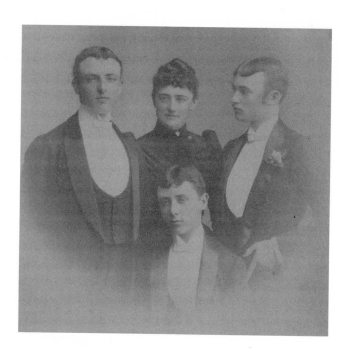

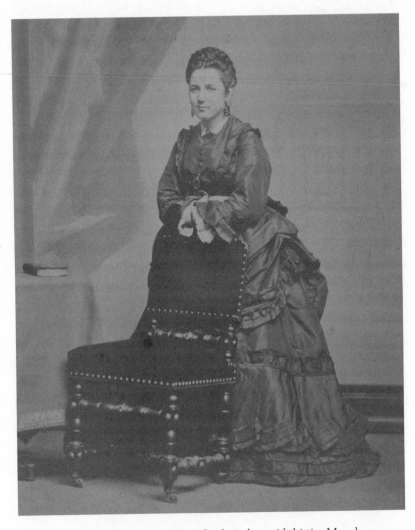

After Robert's breakdown and Harry's death, in her mid-thirties Mary became the primary family executor of her father's estate and began wielding behind-the-scenes influence at the B&O. Courtesy of the Evergreen House Foundation at Evergreen Museum and Library, The Johns Hopkins University.

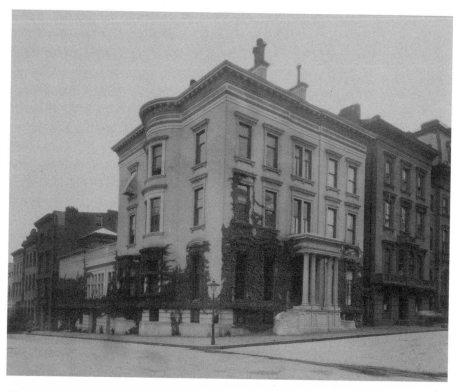

The Garrett mansion on Mount Vernon Place. Mary completed her late father's domed art gallery, which was at the back of the house. The thirty-room mansion also featured the extraordinary "East Indian Room" designed by Lockwood de Forest.

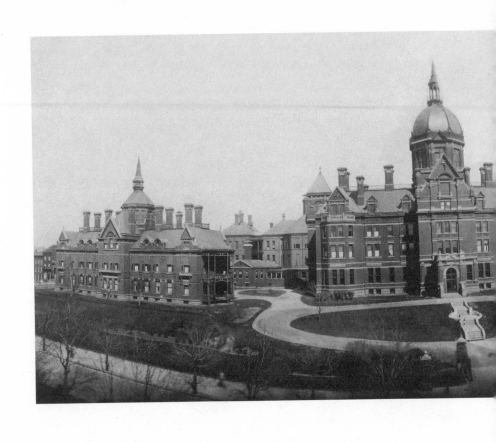

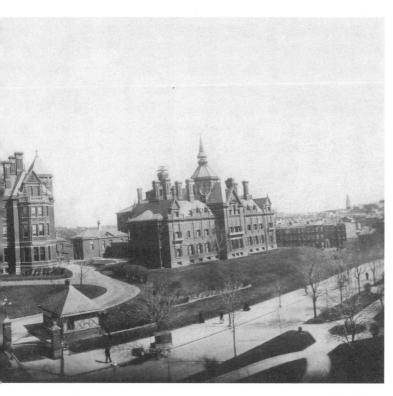

After twelve years of construction—battling underground streams, quick-sand, and unsettled finances—the Johns Hopkins Hospital opened in May 1889. "It is the best institution of its kind in the world," the *New York Times* announced. Courtesy of the Alan Mason Chesney Medical Archives of The Johns Hopkins Medical Institutions.

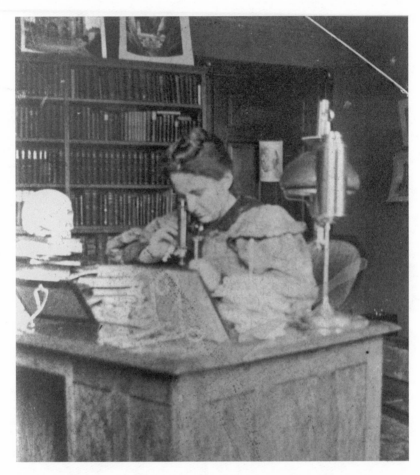

While a medical student at Hopkins, Gertrude Stein conducted impressive scientific research, but she dropped out of school months short of graduating. She went on to achieve great fame as a writer, penning a fictionalized version of the titillating *ménage à trois* among Carey Thomas, Mamie Gwinn, and Alfred Hodder. Courtesy of the Yale Collection of American Literature, Beinecke Rare Book and Manuscript Library.

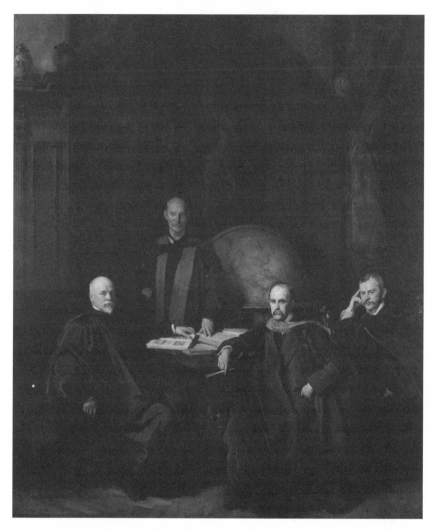

The Four Doctors, by John Singer Sargent, 1906, oil on canvas. "We have got our picture!" John Singer Sargent exclaimed after months of working on the difficult composition of *The Four Doctors,* which Mary commissioned in 1905 to commemorate the founding physicians of the Hopkins medical school. Courtesy of the Alan Mason Chesney Medical Archives of The Johns Hopkins Medical Institutions. Photo by Aaron Levin.

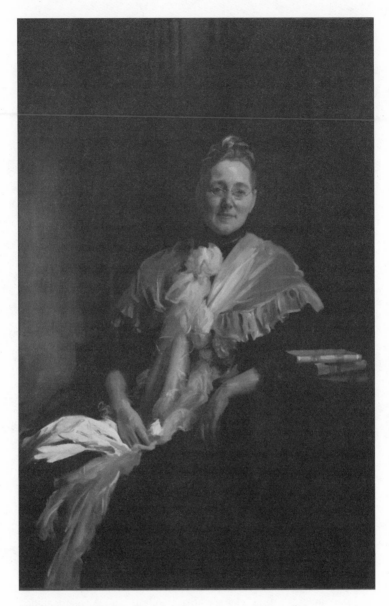

Mary Elizabeth Garrett, by John Singer Sargent, 1904, oil on canvas.
John Singer Sargent's portrait captured Mary's serenity and "the
peace which comes with the years" after a lifetime of highs and lows,
accomplishments and disappointments. Courtesy of the Alan Mason Chesney
Medical Archives of The Johns Hopkins Medical Institutions. Photo by Aaron Levin.

and give lots of money.[31] Carey and Mary regularly conferred about potential candidates and strategized about how to build the regional committees. They tapped
into the strong national network of women's organizations and interconnectedness
built over many decades of community activism. Mary took charge of writing
dozens upon dozens of recruitment letters. Through most of 1889 and early 1890,
as she was overseeing the construction of the Bryn Mawr School, she wrote many
letters each day to friends far and near who, in turn, asked their friends far and near
to join the committees. By mid-1889, the first regional committees were organized
in Baltimore, New York, Boston, and Philadelphia, with 123 members in all. Additional committees were planned for Chicago, San Francisco, and other areas with
high concentrations of wealth. With Mary's vast family connections and Carey's
national academic network, the organizers identified potential members.

To recruit members to the committees, the organizers developed a "General
Circular" and printed five hundred copies. It appears from an early draft of the circular that the organizers expected to raise the $100,000 within a year, by spring
1890. Having written similar publicity for the Bryn Mawr School, Mary and Carey
had honed the fine art of persuasion. Appealing to the special concerns of
women, the circular assured that "the object thus proposed will seem of the greatest importance to the friends of the medical education of women in all parts of
the country." However, the organizers were careful not to offend those who favored single-sex medical schools, diplomatically explaining that the proposed coeducational medical school would not "take the place of the medical schools for
women now in existence." If the fundraising campaign failed, "and the medical
school open[ed] without women among its students, it would be difficult to secure their admission later," the organizers stressed.[32]

Aside from targeting wealthy women and well-known suffrage activists, the organizers also identified leading women physicians who had long been involved in
the women's medical movement for coeducation. Mary felt women physicians
would lend credibility to the campaign. "Please ask about graduates of the Philadelphia Medical School," she wrote in December 1888 to Carey. Prominent
among such physicians was her own, Dr. Mary Putnam Jacobi. Mary visited Jacobi in New York early on to solicit her help and that of the vast network of women
physicians of the Association for the Advancement of the Medical Education of
Women, which Jacobi had established in 1872. Drs. Elizabeth and Emily Blackwell joined the effort as well. Carey, too, felt it important for women physicians
to give "their names to a larger committee . . . to show their approval."[33]

From the start, the campaign organizers recognized, as did Gilman, the need
to find donors who could contribute substantial amounts—thousands of dollars,

not nickels and dimes—to meet the required endowment. Mary immediately began to think of wealthy women, particularly unmarried or widowed women unencumbered by marital restrictions or family obligations, who could give large contributions. This would have been an important consideration for the campaign and one of which Mary, as a wealthy, unmarried woman, was well aware. In many states, laws prevented married women from controlling or disbursing large sums of money, an obvious impediment when trying to find a female major donor to underwrite the medical fund endowment. Although women generally contributed annual subscriptions of five or twenty-five dollars with much enthusiasm to their favorite causes, married women often did not control the family's finances to the extent that they could make more substantial gifts.

Mary recommended women who could make large contributions, such as a woman she knew in Boston from a wealthy publishing family, "a widow of considerable means, very philanthropic and very liberal in her ways." Carey also thought she had hit the jackpot. "I have secured $10,000 toward our plan," she excitedly wrote to Mary. Carey had made inquiries about donors in Boston and had found intriguing rumors about "$10,000 left by Mr. Huvey for the Med. ed. of women."[34] More than likely, "Mr. Huvey" was Marian Hovey, whose 1878 offer of $10,000 to make Harvard's medical school coeducation was rejected.

Mary and the other organizers left few records about their early fundraising efforts in 1889, but, apparently, their initial attempts to find substantial funding were unsuccessful. They had gathered enthusiastic, influential women to lend their names to the regional committees, but major funding proved to be elusive. In a meeting during the summer of 1889, Gilman pressed Mary about the progress of "the campaign." She wrote to Carey "I argued [with Gilman] that money was difficult to raise."[35] Gilman faced the same problem in his hunt for "a man of large means."

By mid-1889, the campaign moved into high gear. Spurred on by the initial success in recruiting members to the first four committees, the organizers expanded the campaign nationwide. Through the end of 1889 and into 1890, their activities—letter writing, hastily convened meetings, more anxious letter writing—revealed the sense of urgency and desperation they must have felt to outpace Gilman and the trustees. In September, Carey saw Gilman and could no longer describe him as "genuinely nice," as she had done just a few months earlier. "Mr. Gilman is now totally opposed to the scheme much more opposed than I realised [sp]," Carey reported to Mary. The good news was that two key faculty, "Dr. Hurd and Dr. Osler [are] vehemently in favour of it."[36]

By early 1890, the national press picked up on the campaign. Since the Fri-

day Night already had contracted with several clipping services to gather national news about the Bryn Mawr School, they similarly started collecting news
snippets of their fledgling effort to raise funds for a coeducational medical school
at Hopkins. They wanted to make certain that each stage of their struggle was
well documented.

On March 30, the *Nation* published an article favorable to women's equal
medical education and the efforts of the fundraising campaign. It was no accident
that Mrs. Edwin L. Godkin, wife of the *Nation's* editor, was an enthusiastic member of the New York committee. The article noted that the Johns Hopkins University was still lacking the endowment to open its medical school. But, "women
need not despair," the article's writer encouraged. "The trend of university movement and development is on their side. It is in the interest of the public to hasten
this development by such additional endowment as will secure for its medical
servants, irrespective of sex, the best training."[37] The organizers already were
learning to astutely use the press to their advantage.

Despite the favorable publicity, the organizers worried. Publicly, they continued to expand their national coalition of prominent women in regional committees and to seek major funding. They put a positive face on their progress. Behind the scenes, however, like the organizers of most fundraising campaigns then
and now, they desperately worried. The committees were shaping up nicely
around the country, but the wealthy "names of influence" were not contributing
the necessary amounts. The hope of finding major contributors began to fade.

In the midst of all of her other obligations, in spring 1890, as she busily prepared
to open the new Bryn Mawr School, Mary made an important trip. She traveled
to New York to hunt for donors. Mary was not shy about approaching men, many
of them her father's former business associates, for major contributions. In New
York, she met with Peter Cooper Hewitt, of the Cooper-Hewitt Union, which his
grandfather Peter Cooper had founded in 1859 to provide free industrial-arts training. Sixty years earlier, Cooper had opened the Canton Iron Works on three thousand acres on the Baltimore waterfront and in 1830 had revolutionized American
railroading by building the first steam locomotive, the *Tom Thumb*, for the B&O.
The New York Coopers and Hewitts ranked among the country's greatest philanthropists; Peter Cooper, in fact, served as the philanthropic model for Andrew
Carnegie. "No one could be possibly any kinder or nicer," Mary wrote of her visit
with Hewitt, "but he said that in view of the Cooper Institute and what they [the
family] had done, it would be impossible for them to do anything towards the
endowment of another institution." Hewitt said he thought the "chances for success in New York were especially small unless we could get some of the people who

are interested in medical study." Hewitt suggested "old Mrs. Vanderbilt." Mary wrote, "He is going to write to her to tell her about the scheme."[38]

During the meeting, Mrs. Hewitt came into the room. Mary later noted that after Peter Hewitt had declined Mary's request for funding, she did not ask Mrs. Hewitt to join the New York committee, stating, "I don't think the names of wealthy people, if they don't give, will do much."[39] It was a highly accurate prediction.

The next day, Mary met with her father's old friend Andrew Carnegie to ask for his support. She knew him from his trips to Montebello. Carnegie, who six years earlier had funded a research laboratory at Bellevue Hospital Medical College in New York, seemed a likely candidate to contribute to the women's fund. "Yesterday Mr. Carnegie came to see me and he does not think he could say no to me about anything in the world," Mary recalled in a light-hearted note to Carey, "but his care is libraries & he has pledged all he has for two years to come and a good deal more." Their meeting, Mary added whimsically, "was interesting and entertaining." Mary noted that Carnegie "thinks women should do it themselves" — an idea already underway.[40]

She also approached George Childs, who had offered his advice to Carey early in the campaign, for a major contribution. Writing to the Dear Girls, Mary described her visit with Childs and her "gentle" solicitation for $10,000. "He exclaimed that he was interested & that he told us he would be very happy to contribute $1,000 toward. As nice as I could, I told him that we should very much like him to help it very early . . . of how much good it would do if he wd start the Phila Fund with a very early subs. I indicated that the $10,000 basis w'd be a very delightful one that it w'd influence not only in Philadelphia but all over the country . . . He w'd of course have preferred not to be asked for . . . the ten thousand, but he was really as nice as possible . . . I am inclined to think he will increase his subscription."[41]

Mary visited James Cardinal Gibbons, the revered and influential Catholic spiritual leader in Baltimore, not to ask for money but for support. He assured Mary that she "was entirely at liberty to say that he was fully in sympathy & would throw all the weight of his influence on our side." Cardinal Gibbons addressed the subject often whispered in hushed, polite Victorian parlor conversations, that of "the possible desirability of separate dissecting rooms for men and women and the desirability of treating a few classes of disease separately," Mary reported. "He felt equally as strongly that some classes of disease should not be treated by men as he did that some of the classes of disease should not be treated by women, but all these things he thinks are questions of detail and can be arranged when the time comes for actions."[42]

During her fundraising trip to New York, Mary realized the difficulty she and the campaign faced in raising the large endowment through both small contributions and large gifts, which had yet to materialize. Despite her many family connections, Mary wrote, "I am now more than ever convinced that I am not the right person to beg."[43] But beg she did, for many months to come, to try to raise the money. Mary's friend Julia de Forest wondered if "they should let men do the asking"—a technique that many women's groups at the time employed to reach wealthy businessmen. They did not pursue that option. The women directly solicited male friends and colleagues themselves as the campaign progressed.

After returning from the New York trip, and perhaps feeling the first pangs of desperation that the major funding might not materialize, Mary's letter writing intensified. Within two days of being rebuffed by Carnegie and Hewitt, she accelerated her efforts to recruit new members to the committees.

One by one, the regional committees shaped up. The wide-ranging appeal reached prominent women from coast to coast, grande dames and longtime activists alike. Mary was pleased with the news that the San Francisco committee was coming together. "Mrs. George Hearst was most cordial & sensible in her suggestions for the San Francisco committee," Mary wrote on April 18.[44]

Mary especially wanted to include Marian Hovey, whom Carey had misidentified as "Mr. Huvey." Hovey, still holding on to the ten thousand dollars rejected by Harvard, eagerly contributed the full amount to the Hopkins fund. Katherine Loring, chair of the Boston committee, was often away, but Mary enticed thirty other prominent women from the area, including her friends writers Sarah Orne Jewett and Annie Fields and reformer Julia Ward Howe, writer of "The Battle Hymn of the Republic," to join, along with women from the Quincy, Cabot, and Lowell families. Despite the stellar lineup of names, Carey was "inclined to think the Boston scheme will fall through," since the wealthy members had yet to contribute a significant amount.[45]

Julia de Forest and Dr. Mary Putnam Jacobi helped to organize the New York committee. While in New York to visit with Carnegie and Hewitt, Mary talked with Dr. Emily Blackwell to ask for "names [of women physicians] . . . to show their approval" for the fundraising effort.[46] Jacobi also was instrumental in lining up fellow physicians in other cities, including Dr. Marie Zakrzewska. Mrs. John Wanamaker of department-store fame joined the New York committee, as did "Frankie" Cleveland, who had spent her honeymoon at Deer Park four years earlier. Her husband was between his two inconsecutive terms as president of the United States.

The Washington, D.C., committee was of special concern, given its national clout. Mary was careful to list the names on the roster according to what she thought was the proper political pecking order. First Lady Caroline Harrison headed the Washington committee. Mary knew her from when the Harrisons vacationed at Deer Park. The first lady's endorsement was important, lending the campaign credibility and national visibility. "Mrs. Harrison Accepts," the *Washington Post* proclaimed. "She is interested in creating a fund for a medical school [and] a chance for women doctors." Others from Washington included the wives of cabinet members and Mrs. Alexander Graham Bell. "Mrs. Harrison and Other Washington Ladies Use Their Influence," the *Chicago Daily Tribune* announced. Mary carefully reviewed each Washington name, striking out one she felt might bring a hint of scandal to the campaign. "The woman is hard working and capable," Mary wrote to the Dear Girls of one such possibility, "but her husband is a defaulter."[47] The unfortunate candidate did not make the cut.

The grandest of the country's grande dames, Mrs. Potter (Bertha) Palmer, *the* absolutely essential member of any late-century women's effort, reigned as treasurer of the Chicago committee. She was an important ally to have on board, lending cachet and giving the campaign the ultimate seal of approval. Mary formed committees in Annapolis and Port Deposit in Maryland; Madison, Wisconsin; Springfield, Massachusetts; Milwaukee; St. Louis; Buffalo; Philadelphia; Essex County, Massachusetts; and The Kennebec, a wealthy resort area in Maine.

Baltimore counted the largest committee with 106 members. Visibly absent from the committee were Mary's sisters-in-law—and not surprisingly. Mary already was embroiled in heated family squabbles over her father's estate. After Harry's death, Alice and her three sons moved to Europe and lived abroad for most of the fundraising campaign. Mary Frick did not approve of the effort to force coeducation and did not give her support, moral or monetary. She let her displeasure be known to all, trying to dissuade her wealthy friends around the country from joining as well. Her influence was widely felt. Mamie Gwinn later recalled, "The New York chairwoman Mrs. Richard Irving was intimate with Mrs. Robert Garrett and correspondingly slack in her New York work when she found Mrs. Robert Garrett disapproved of the campaign."[48] Mary did not write of her sister-in-law's counteraction to the campaign, although it more than likely contributed to the ongoing estrangement between the two women.

Many women sided with Mary Frick's perspective. Not everyone jumped at the chance to support the campaign for medical coeducation. Much as Mary had noted the "prejudice of the community" when starting the controversial Bryn Mawr School in 1885, she also encountered resistance with the medical school campaign. Mary recalled visiting one potential committee member, "[but] she refuses to serve on a committee, saying simply she is not in sympathy with women studying medicine . . . Prejudice is certainly the most difficult thing to meet," Mary noted.[49]

Another challenge was time commitment. Prominent women, often over-committed and over-worked in voluntary activities, were inundated with requests to support worthy causes. They often did not have the time or energy needed take on yet one more fundraising obligation. "The difficulty is they are all busy," Mary lamented.[50]

In the midst of her hurried recruitment letters to expand the committees, Mary dashed off an intriguing letter to Carey in April 1890. The letter reveals that she and the other organizers already knew the trustees had upped the ante consider-ably beyond the original $100,000. Gilman had suggested the revised amount at a trustees meeting a few months earlier, on October 7, 1889. "They [the trustees] say they now need $500,000 to $600,000 in order to make the medical school what it should be," she wrote. "Mr. Gilman is unwilling to open it without that amount. I want you to tell me in as much detail as you can just how they would propose to use that money—how much for buildings, how many and what build-ings are needed, etc., etc." Mary continued, "I have a reason for asking you and you need not be afraid to give me every item of information that you can. Although it may lead to nothing, it will do no harm."[51]

We are left to speculate about Mary's reason for asking for "every item of in-formation" at this moment, for she did not again elaborate on her query. Was she unsure of the campaign's success and outcome? Was she thinking of following Carnegie and Vanderbilt's philanthropic examples in giving the full amount her-self to start the medical school? Did she see a safety net in her own inheritance?

Carey, who had direct access through her father to information concerning the trustees and their discussions about the medical school, responded immediately to Mary's request for details. Carey agreed that $500,000 would allow the uni-versity to open not simply a good medical school, but a "great one." In a detailed letter, Carey reiterated the university's loss of income from the failure of the B&O stocks, which would force the trustees to "either close the univ. or . . . raise enough money to go on." This had spurred the first fundraising campaign, the Emergency Fund of 1889. There were salaries to be paid and laboratories to be fi-nanced, particularly those related to Welsh, Osler, Kelly, and Halsted, since the university already had committed to an embryonic medical faculty. "At present," Carey continued, "the univ's hands are tied tight—they have no money. To erect buildings, the Hosp pays all salaries and stands like a dog in the manger prevent-ing all action. The strain of affairs is so great that I think our $100,000 wd. prob.

enable the Univ. to begin in some small way; but of course it will not enable it to begin right. It needs $500,000 sep. endowment." Carey enumerated the salary commitments: Welsh, $5,000; Osler, $2,500; Kelly, $2,500; Halsted, $2,500; and listed the costs of assistant lecturers in the various disciplines: eye, $1,000; ear, 1,000; skin, $1,000; and nerves, $1,000.[52]

Carey expressed the organizers' desperation should they fail. "I should feel unable to hold up my head again if after we have aroused everyone, the trustees refuse it," she wrote to Mary. "It would do harm to women's medical education. We simply must carry it through, no matter what happens. They must *not* refuse it."[53]

The $500,000 endowment—five times the campaign's original target— seemed unreachable, insurmountable. The women were struggling mightily to meet the $100,000 goal. Writing daily to committee chairwomen, Mary prodded and pushed to keep the fundraising going. Fearing that Gilman might be closing in on his own donor, Mary urgently wrote, "Every day counts."[54]

Emboldened by the article in the *Nation* yet concerned about the lackluster level of contributions, members of the Baltimore committee gathered in Bessie's parlor on May 2, 1890, for a show of force. They officially kicked off the "public" phase of their campaign. The "scheme" adopted an official, more sophisticated, name: the Women's Fund for the Medical School, or the Women's Medical School Fund (WMSF), as it has been called since.[55] After working for more than a year and a half behind the scenes, the fund organizers reaffirmed that the campaign would continue until it reached its goal. With the $100,000 not yet raised, Mary discreetly revised the first version of the "General Circular." "I have omitted 'an attempt will be made to raise the money before June 1890,'" she wrote on May 22, a week from the original, failed target date.

After the May 2 meeting at Bessie's house, contributions stepped up. The organizers felt a surge of hope. Mary carefully tracked the responses: "Notes are pouring in about the parlor meeting," Mary wrote. "Even those who are not prepared to give time to the matter give warm sympathy & even money. Subscriptions amount at the moment to $21,950."[56]

Working at odds with the goals of the women's committee, Gilman continued in earnest with his own search. In August 1890, he sent a confidential memo to the trustees. He reiterated his hope that "some individual will give the entire amount required for an endowment, or thus associate his name permanently with the institution as its founder." Trustee George W. Brown concurred. "I believe, as you suggest, that some of the trustees are not without hope that some individual will give the entire endowment and thus associate his name with the institution and I can only pray that the hope is well found," Brown wrote. He added that the "plan of the Ladies in their General Circular 'to raise the sum of $100,000 and as much more as possible' was I think unfortunate and the result has been that the sum mentioned has not yet been raised."[57]

Always looking over their shoulders, the WMSF organizers stepped up their campaign. With the regional committees solidified, they moved into the active fundraising phase of the campaign. They cast a larger net, expanding their fundraising to a general audience. Committee members were expected to solicit donations in their communities. (See appendix B, Analysis of the Women's Medical School Fund Campaign.)

By fall, contributions once again dropped off. The scheme was not materializing as expected. While the fund's efforts had opened the floodgate of public debate and enthusiasm, it hardly opened the pocketbooks of the four-hundred-member committee or other willing contributors enough to raise the required $100,000, much less the new target of $500,000. The enormous family wealth and prestige represented on the roster provided the "names of influence" the organizers had wanted but not the needed cash. "I fear we cannot hope that there are very many large amounts of which I have not heard," Mary lamented in August.[58]

With little more than half the amount raised from the committees and the campaign already a subject of national publicity, there was but one way out to save face. Mary stepped up to the plate. She had already contributed $10,000, but increased her gift to $47,787.50, the balance needed for the $100,000 target. Finally, with Mary's major infusion of cash, the fund reached its goal.

A NOTABLE GATHERING OF WOMEN

The women were at last in a position to ask for the trustees' "promise," as Anna Hallowell had encouraged at the start, to admit women students when—or if—the medical school ever opened. Trustee Charles Gwinn, Mamie's father, assisted the fund with the precise legal wording he felt would be amenable to his fellow trustees. On October 28, 1890, Nancy Morris Davis, chairwoman of the Baltimore committee, presented the fund's offer, not yet the money, with a letter reiterating the caveat that women "shall be admitted to the school, when it shall open, upon the same terms which may be prescribed for men." The trustees accepted the offer, resolving "to the terms upon which the money was contributed by its donors."[59] The trustees' resolution to accept women on the same terms as men was a giant leap for womanhood.

Gilman, who had been traveling in Europe when the women presented their offer in October, later stated it was a "noble act" and one "that will result in great good." Unfortunately, as the fund organizers had feared, and as Mary had expressed in her letter a year and a half earlier, the trustees had increased the amount required for the endowment to $500,000. The trustees stated the gift from the fund would be accepted as the "foundation" for the required $500,000. "Then, and not until then, will a Medical School be opened by this University," the trustees emphasized.[60] It was a "promise"—of sorts.

Their acceptance of the Fund's offer put the trustees in a delicate situation. They had to defuse public reaction to the perception that a possible coeducational medical school at the Johns Hopkins University meant women's full-court press into the male-dominated medical profession, an issue of grave economic threat to male physicians. The trustees emphasized that Hopkins women medical students would focus on traditional female medical fields, such as "in penal institutions, in which women are prisoners, in charitable institutions in which women are cared for, and in private life, when women are to be attended." The new medical school "would make provision for the training and full qualification of such women for the abundant work which awaits them in these wide areas of usefulness."[61] The trustees' statement came as no surprise to the women. Even advocates such as James Cardinal Gibbons had expressed the need for such limitations of female study during Mary's visit with him.

Controversy aside, the fund organizers had firmly planted a collective foot through the door of the male-dominated medical profession. It was time to celebrate their victory. It was also time for the fund to once again grab headlines.

On November 14, 1890, a date selected by First Lady Caroline Harrison, members of the regional committees convened in Baltimore to celebrate their milestone and to take a firsthand look at the object of their hard work over the past two years: the new Johns Hopkins Hospital, which had opened a year and a half earlier. As hoped, newspapers scrambled to top each other in reporting on the glamorous guests—and the occasion's significance.

Baltimore had never seen such a parade of feminine glitz and glamour. "One of the most notable gatherings ever occurring in Baltimore of women nationally prominent in philanthropic work took place yesterday at the Johns Hopkins Hospital," the *Baltimore American* raved. The *Baltimore Sun* bested its rival. "Through the lofty doors of the Johns Hopkins Hospital crowded such a notable gathering of women yesterday as has seldom been seen in the country before. No movement started for years has so generally enlisted the sympathy of women throughout the nation as this plan for the medical education of their sex."[62]

Caroline Harrison presided over the event. Smiling trustees greeted the committee members as they filed through "the lofty doors." The women toured the hospital for an "inspection and luncheon." They met the famed doctors and the scientists. They peered into labs to look at intriguing medical research in progress. Dr. Mary Putnam Jacobi, "a pleasant-faced lady in middle life, with thoughtful dark eyes," pronounced the day "a great occasion."[63]

But the best was yet to come. At nine that evening, Mary threw open the doors of her spectacularly refurbished thirty-room mansion on West Monument Street for a grand celebration for fifteen hundred guests. "Nearly every citizen of Baltimore known to society responded to the invitation," the *Baltimore Sun* reported. Carriages lined Mount Vernon Place, waiting to discharge their fashionable occupants. A footman escorted the guests up the double marble staircase inside to the grand foyer with its magnificent carved staircase and Tiffany windows. Mary, with the first lady, Bessie, Carey, and Mamie at her side, cheerfully received her guests. Not as accustomed to welcoming hundreds of guests, Mary "laughingly reminded her [Mrs. Harrison] that she had more experience in receiving so many people."[64]

The newspapers jumped at the chance to describe Mary, the shy, elusive philanthropist and millionaire. She wore "a magnificent crepe costume of a delicate shade of blue, cut V-neck back and front and filled in with point lace and pearls. Around her neck she wore a superb Oriental necklace of inlaid gold, from which hung a magnificent gold ornament, from which sparkled numerous diamonds. Her dress was cut short sleeves, en train. She also wore long white gloves, which came to her elbow."[65]

With bountiful candles sparkling in the background, the first lady, too, looked resplendent. She wore "a handsome dress of seal-brown velvet, with a front of point lace and trimmed with pearls."[66] Cardinal Gibbons, whose support had been integral to the campaign, was dazzling in his scarlet robes. Vicar-General McColgan accompanied him.

The orchestra, discreetly hidden from view behind a row of palms, played while guests dined "in the second parlor on the left." The enormous buffet table was decorated with "glass, silver and a display of roses four-feet in diameter. It was one of the most brilliant events of the season," the *Washington Post* concluded the next morning.[67]

The event had been a spectacular success and a public relations coup for the languishing fund. But, Mary did not comment on the irony of the evening. The well-heeled women—the fifteen hundred guests who drove up to her home in their liveried broughams and poured into her house bedecked in their jewel-encrusted gowns—had contributed just slightly more than half of the $100,000 goal.

The glorious moment of the November festivities soon faded. Within weeks, the campaign again faded and vanished from the front pages. Mary continued to host "at homes," small fundraising parties at her mansion, to keep the dream alive.

As contributions slowed to a trickle by the fall and winter, the organizers once again stepped up their public-relations campaign. Again, as with the *Nation's* endorsement the year before, it helped to have a well-placed editor's wife on board. In this case, it was Mrs. Richard Watson Gilder, member of the New York committee and wife of the editor of the *Century Illustrated Magazine*, one of the most widely read publications at the time. In February 1891, *Century* published a series of "open letters" entitled "The Opening of the Johns Hopkins Medical School to Women." Respected writers, including Josephine Shaw Lowell, Carey Thomas, Cardinal James Gibbons, and Dr. Mary Putnam Jacobi contributed to the forum. Hopkins' physician-in-chief Dr. William Osler, an essential advocate for the fund, gave a strong endorsement, stating, "if any woman feels the medical profession is her vocation, no obstacles should be placed in the way of her obtaining the best possible education; every facility should be offered, so that, as a practitioner, she should have a fair start in the race."[68]

The constant anxiety of the roller-coaster campaign took its toll on the Friday Night. The cracks in the relationships that had started to appear in disagreements over the management of the Bryn Mawr School grew irrevocably wider. Old relationships faded as new ones blossomed. The group that had sustained the young women in their formative years began to disintegrate. Julia Rogers and Mary, whose intimate friendship dated back to Miss Kummer's School in the years following the Civil War, grew apart as Mary and Carey began to dominate the Bryn Mawr School and Women's Medical School Fund activities. Julia eventually resigned from the Bryn Mawr School Board, a result of her anger over Mary and Carey's intensifying relationship and being shut out of important school decisions. Julia was noticeably absent from the receiving line during the WMSF November 14 gala at Mary's house. Before going their separate ways, Mary and Julia mutually agreed to expunge many of the letters that had passed between them for more than twenty years.

Why did they do this? We are left to wonder why Mary, who had saved boxes and boxes of letters, receipts, official documents, and random memorabilia since childhood would choose in her mid-thirties to destroy the record of her most valued female friendship. Were there aspects of their relationship Mary felt were better left untold? Did the letters hint at a physical relationship beyond an intimate friendship? After this, Mary did not mention Julia in her letters, nor is there any indication the two women saw each other again. The destruction of their letters remains as mysterious as the true nature of their friendship.

With Julia finally removed from Mary's life, Carey's long-simmering interest in Mary—and as important, in Mary's money—heated up. Mary, always circumspect and mindful of social propriety, did not openly reciprocate the feelings. She wrote a reproachful letter to Carey, chastising her for outward displays of affection. At a Garrett family gathering, Carey had unexpectedly kissed Mary in front of the family. Mary admonished her: "I was surprised by your offering to kiss me goodnight before all the family. I showed a little embarrassment and hesitation," Mary wrote. "[It was] destructive to our friendship so I think we must be on guard."[69]

Mary also grew impatient with Mamie and often criticized her judgments about the Bryn Mawr School and medical school fund campaign. Bessie was often ill and removed from the day-to-day anxiety of the campaign. She was slowly being expelled, or extricating herself, from the group. When her father died in 1891, in the midst of the campaign, Bessie withdrew her support, feeling the goals of a coeducation medical school at Hopkins ran counter to the wishes of her father, who had been president of the hospital board.

By early 1891, the pressures of managing the Bryn Mawr School, the sadness of the disintegration of her family, the rancor over her father's estate, keeping the floundering Women's Medical School Fund afloat, and sorting out the intrigues of the Friday Night, overwhelmed Mary. Carey, who immersed herself in her work at Bryn Mawr College, wrote to her, warning that if Mary didn't "break through this ever contracting net of personal differences and friction and nervous strains your health will certainly break down and you will lose all possibility of real goodness."[70]

Mary's health did break down. She began to display the familiar symptoms of sleeplessness and anxiety prevalent in her previous breakdown fifteen years earlier during her twenties. She lapsed into what would become a two-year period of depression, personal reflection, and self-imposed solitude and exile.

As she had learned from her father, during difficult times the best remedy for illness and despair was to put many miles between herself and her troubles. In February 1891, she traveled to Mountain Park Hotel in Hot Springs, a curative spa in the mountains of North Carolina. She could not sleep. She felt anxious. The least activity exhausted her. "I was so tired after walking about 200 yards that I came back and subsided into a chair in the sun," she wrote to Carey. The damp, dreary mountains of North Carolina in the midst of winter seemed an unlikely spot to raise the spirits. "It has rained two-thirds of the time," Mary complained. There were "only five days in the last three weeks in which it has not rained."[71]

Her days took on familiar, mundane routine and tragic loneliness. Breakfast at nine; mail at noon; a short walk, a curative bath, massage, nap, dinner at quarter of three; another walk, another nap, one more walk ("unless it's raining & there is nowhere for me to go"); five o'clock, "a solitary cup of tea"; letter writing, "but it's tiring"; supper at 7:45; mail, again; "back to sitting room at 10:15 or 10:50"; hair washed and "a treatment before going to bed."[72]

As with her failure to pass the Harvard entrance exam, she felt despondent. As the prime fundraiser and organizer of the fund's regional committees, she held herself responsible for the medical campaign's failure to reach the new $500,000 goal.

She felt especially desperate about the university's possible, and perhaps imminent, counteraction to open the medical school without admitting women if Gilman found his donor. "Daniel [Gilman] has concluded that we now have had enough time & he will move forward," she wrote fearfully that winter. She still questioned why the trustees had raised the amount so significantly, from $100,000 to $500,000. Carey agreed, writing, "Gilman would rather not open the medical school than open one with women."[73]

Hope was fading for any additional help from the regional committees. "The New York Committee [says] its work is over . . . and has done nothing since it sent its [letter] in October]."[74] March 15, the date for the formal conclusion of the Women's Medical School Fund campaign, was drawing near.

In a last-ditch effort to jumpstart the moribund campaign, a Washington, D.C., newspaper columnist lent her support in March. "That no reader of this review may be ignorant of the chairwomen of these committees," famed journalist and rabble-rouser Kate Field published names and addresses in the *National Independent Review* where contributions could be sent. And, lest her women readers fail to understand where the blame should be assigned for the inferior training of women physicians, Field admonished women to look only at themselves: "Their worst enemies have been among the very women whose support would have given them the schools necessary for thorough education." But, "times have changed. Thanks to Miss Mary Garrett, Mrs. Henry Winter Davis, and leading women of Baltimore, the blot upon our intelligence will soon be removed, and at Johns Hopkins University it will be possible for women to procure the most advanced medical education."[75]

Field added that on March 15, the national campaign would be concluded and the regional chairwomen were due to submit the final tallies of their fundraising. "It is hoped that the distance between one hundred thousand and five hundred thousand will be much less than it was last October." Carey, too, hoped the committees would save the day with last-minute contributions, writing the women "had already secured one-fifth the sum requisite for opening the medical school.

The proportion should be . . . largely increased by March 15 [with] the fullest measure of financial support."[76]

But, unfortunately, the figures at the campaign's conclusion fell well below the "fullest measure of financial support." When the chairwomen submitted their final tallies, the news was bittersweet. The fund had met its original goal of $100,000, but fell far short of the trustees' revised goal of $500,000. The fund's final amount totaled $111,300. Of that amount, Mary had contributed nearly half, $47,787.50. The "scheme," while a public-relations success in stirring controversy about prevailing low standards of medicine and women's educational inequality, had failed to raise the needed endowment. Counting its own holdings of $81,723 and the fund's gift of $111,300, the university now had $193,023 earmarked for the medical school, less than half of the required amount.[77] The trustees still needed more than $300,000 to meet their self-imposed endowment goal.

By the spring of 1891, the echo of John Work Garrett's long-past rhetorical question, "Where are the medical classes?" could still be heard. The two-and-a-half-year race between the Women's Medical School Fund and the Johns Hopkins University had yet to produce a winner—and it was far from over.

—◦∿◦—

CHAPTER 7

A PLEASURE TO BE BOUGHT

MISS GARRETT'S PRINCELY GIFT

"The ladies' work is finished," the *Baltimore American* announced in spring 1891.[1] After more than two years of countless moments of anxiety and elation, the Women's Medical School Fund had reached its original $100,000 goal, far short of the trustees' revised $500,000 endowment requirement. But Mary was not quite ready to admit defeat in the battle to open a coeducational medical school at Hopkins.

As Baltimore chairwoman Nancy Morris Davis prepared to present the Fund's $111,300 gift to the university, Mary made yet another jolting proposal to the trustees. By this time, the trustees should have been accustomed to her surprise financial enticements. In a letter dated April 27, 1891, to "Hon. George Dobbin, President of the Board of Trustees of the Johns Hopkins University," Mary offered an additional $100,000 to sweeten the deal. But as was becoming her trademark, she attached a few strings. In order to receive her money, she required that the trustees themselves raise the balance to meet the $500,000 endowment by the following February. Should the balance be raised, she also insisted, the medical school must open in October 1892.[2]

Mary's proposal put the trustees in an awkward situation. With no other offers of their own on the table, they officially but reluctantly accepted the WMSF gift and Mary's stringent conditions for her own offer. They responded by stating "members of the board would endeavor individually to obtain, before February 1, 1892, from persons interested in higher medical education additional contributions to the amount of $221,219.58." Bessie's father, Francis King, president of the hospital board, stated in regard to Mary's offer, "the amount is not exceedingly large, but it is a very neat sum."[3]

Once again, the trustees, who were unable to raise the money themselves, downplayed the women's roles. The press, however, found the gift much more than a "very neat sum" and was far more impressed with Mary's offer than the trustees had been. It did not take the papers long to enthusiastically report the news. Not only was the fund's contribution an enormous amount in itself from a women's group, but Mary's $100,000 added incentive was an unprecedented philanthropic offer to a university from one of the country's wealthiest women. To most Americans at the time, the amount would have been incomprehensible. It was more than quadruple what the average male wage earner in the United States could expect to earn in a lifetime.

Just as two years earlier, when she financed the modern Bryn Mawr School and supervised the construction of its $500,000 building, Mary's name made headlines across the country. With her additional $100,000 offer to Hopkins, her reputation as one of the country's preeminent philanthropists was solidified.

"Miss Garrett's Gift to Science," the New York Telegraph proclaimed of the gift. The Sunday Herald announced that "Her Royal Gift" signified that "Johns Hopkins University will get a school of medicine for men and women." In Cincinnati, where the Garrett name was well known from the B&O lines that had run through the city for half a century, the Cincinnati Enquirer lauded "Miss Garrett's Munificent Gift," noting the successful opening of the medical school depended "upon the Trustees having in hand by February 1892, the remainder of the sum necessary to complete the endowment." The Baltimore American commented, "No estimate can be too high for the permanent and far-reaching value of such a school. It will be national in its scope, universal in its benefits to medicine and to humanity."[4]

The St. Louis Republic, noting that city's paltry contribution of only $550, felt compelled to chastise St. Louisans for their lackadaisical response to the fund's campaign. "St. Louis has yet contributed very meagerly."[5] The article provided the names and addresses where contributions from St. Louisans could be sent to add to the endowment.

Within days of making her enticing $100,000 offer, the always-mysterious millionaire immediately left town, leaving the trustees to ponder how to meet her terms of raising more than $220,000 within ten months. Still despondent over the WMSF's failure to raise the needed endowment, Mary set sail on the SS Servia for brighter weather, far away from the struggles of the campaign and the seemingly endless impediments of the trustees. She traveled to Europe, where she spent eighteen months. Always a prolific letter writer, she wrote often of the places she visited and the friends she saw. She continued to manage the Bryn Mawr School from across the Atlantic and to buy her beloved statuary and paintings to fill her art gallery. But she seldom mentioned "the scheme" that had occupied much of her time for the past three years. Late in the summer, she met with her family in Oxford, England. The rendezvous did little to lift her spirits. "I have been far down in the depths in spite of the pleasure of seeing Alice and the boys . . . I had gone back to my old way of not sleeping." She felt "tired and restless."[6] She moved on to Rome, always one of her favorite cities, where she lived for several months.

The latest impasse with the university, the second since her 1887 proposal to Gilman to relocate the university, hung heavily over her head. It made her physically sick and emotionally distraught, particularly given the national publicity the campaign—and she—had received. In January 1892, as her imposed February deadline for the trustees to raise the additional money approached, Mary wrote to trustee Charles Morton Stewart to bring up the issue. She reminded him of the fund's gift and her own still outstanding, unresolved offer. Much to her credit, she did not withdraw her offer; in fact, she gave the university an indefinite amount of time to come up with the additional funds. She stipulated only that she would give the trustees a year's notice if she decided to withdraw the offer. The *Baltimore Sun* explained, "The action of Miss Garrett, one of the trustees says, will give the university 'full time to consider in all its bearings the questions of the opening of the medical school.'"[7]

Stewart's response was chilly and unpromising. Yes, he wrote simply, the trustees would give her notice if they decided not to make good on her $100,000 offer, affirming her "instructions in case any future withdrawal will elicit the appreciation of all the trustees." It was hardly an enthusiastic reply. Still no decision. The campaign had died and the negotiations were hopelessly stalled. Most frustrating for Mary, the trustees could not raise the balance. Mary wrote that she was "filled with despair." Aside from Carey and Mamie, other fund organizers were not pulling their weight to keep hope alive. "We cannot expect Bessie to do anything, although she certainly has the power," Mary wrote.[8]

Although she had requested that the trustees raise the additional money, Mary continued to search for a donor to meet the $500,000 goal. Finding a philanthropist interested in contributing a major gift to medical education continued to prove elusive. "I'm afraid this imaginary person does not exist." She had heard a rumor that an elderly relative of Bessie's had died and left money for the medical school, but realized "it was just another house of cards."[9]

She was angry with the trustees for not holding up their end of the bargain. "So much emphasis was put on my share in the matter and, in fact, the university did not pledge itself to raise any of the money and has not done so," she wrote to Carey in February 1892.[10] That month marked the deadline by which the trustees were to have raised the balance of the funds. The campaign, once so promising, had become an embarrassment to Mary, her family name, the Women's Medical School Fund, and the university the fund had unwittingly dragged into the national spotlight.

By late fall 1892, Mary returned to Baltimore. After spending most of the past year and a half in the sunny climes of southern Europe, she returned to face a brutally cold winter on the East Coast. For the first time in over a century, Niagara Falls froze. But events were beginning to heat up in East Baltimore.

In November, Carey sent a distressed dispatch to Mary. The "outlook is infinitely worse than I had thought," Carey warned in a detailed memorandum entitled "Hospital Notes." More than likely, this was a verbatim account of the trustees' latest meeting, clandestinely conveyed by James Thomas to his daughter. Carey related that the university and the hospital, two separate legal entities, were engaged in a power struggle over which one would open, and thereby control, the proposed medical school. "If the university got the big money then it—not the hospital—would have to appoint the faculty." Carey warned "Mr. King's old plan has been revived by him [Stewart] in order to give the hospital control of the medical school." The women must act immediately, Carey urged, before the trustees' next meeting in mid-December, when the decision was to be made. "No words can say what I should think of such a medical school," Carey added, "Mamie will write to her father to tell him to postpone the meeting."[11] Carey encouraged Mary to write yet another letter to Stewart, reminding him of the outstanding offers.

Although reporting erroneous information or misinterpreting it—Johns Hopkins had stated unambiguously in his will that the medical school should be part of the university and not the hospital—Carey's frantic letter spurred Mary into instant action. Mary's fortitude was once again restored and her anger piqued. She desperately wanted the long, bitter race between the WMSF and the university to end. She took matters into her own hands. She had been so much identified with the campaign that the failure of the fund and the university to raise the endowment required that she step in to save face for all involved.

She decided to contribute the balance—more than $300,000—herself.

With her inheritance inextricably tied to the precarious B&O, the same company that had caused the university's fortunes to fall, she did not make the decision lightly. She met with Charles Mayer, a co-executor of her father's estate, and told him of her plan. "I am representing all with whom I had acted in the Women's Fund," she explained of the meeting in a letter to Carey. Mayer made arrangements with Charles Gwinn to present Mary's offer to the trustees. Consulting with Carey, Mary outlined a draft of the letter Gwinn would present to the trustees: "I am so much interested in the establishment of the medical school on the right basis that I am prepared to make a proposition to complete the endowment." Mary explained to Carey the strategy for presenting the offer to the university: "Mr. Gwinn is willing to present this proposition with the trustees."[12] On December 22, 1892, Gwinn presented her offer to the board.

Mary offered to give the university $306,977. Her annoyance and impatience with the trustees showed. She offered not one penny more than the precise amount needed to complete the endowment level, the astronomical $500,000 that had been so far out of the reach of the WMSF campaign to raise. She stipulated she would pay annual installments of $50,000 each, beginning in January 1894, the year after the school opened, and continue through the final payment of $6,977, to be paid on January 1, 1899.[13] Since the university would not receive the full endowment until the final year, she offered to pay 5 percent interest each year.

When the trustees looked at Mary's final terms on that cold December day, they might have wished they had opened the medical school with her $100,000 offer—and less stringent terms—a year and a half earlier. Mary, too, had upped the ante. Just as she had done in April 1891, before leaving for Europe, Mary set forth unprecedented terms, this time six rigorous conditions for acceptance of her gift. She had expanded considerably upon the fund's original caveat to simply admit women medical students "on the same terms as men." She had more far-reaching goals in mind for the new medical school.

First and foremost, the woman who had completed the construction of the innovative Bryn Mawr School building just two years earlier designated that a building be erected at the new medical school to honor the vital role women had played in calling attention to the sorry state of American medicine and in revolutionizing medical education and training. She knew the importance of a bricks-and-mortar monument to the women's accomplishments. She did not seek the spotlight for herself. Rather, she instructed that the building be named the "Women's Fund Memorial Building." Although the fund, with its roster of some of the nation's wealthiest women, was rescued from embarrassment when Mary contributed the lion's share of the endowment, she nonetheless insisted that the women's efforts be recognized. She stipulated that $50,000 of the $500,000 endowment should be "expended on a building or buildings . . . in memory of the contributions of the Committees of the Women's Medical School Fund . . . [and it] shall be known as the Women's Fund Memorial Building."[14]

Reacting to the trustees' October 28, 1890, public assurance that women medical students would limit their studies to female-oriented medical fields — "in penal institutions, in which women are prisoners, in charitable institutions in which women are cared for, and in private life, when women are to be attended" — Mary made a subtle, but significant stipulation. Rather than limiting women medical students' scope of study, she instead insisted that women "enjoy all the advantages on the same terms as men" as well as "all prizes, dignities, or honors" that were afforded male students.[15]

To make certain future generations would not forget the Women's Medical School Fund, Mary instructed that the Resolution of October 28th, 1890, in which the trustees agreed to the terms of the Women's Medical School Fund to accept women students on the same terms as men, "shall be printed each year in whatever annual or semi-annual calendars may be issued announcing the courses of the Medical School." She handpicked the first members of the oversight committee: "Mrs. Henry M. Hurd and Mrs. Ira Remsen, both of whom were active members of the Baltimore Committee of the Women's Medical School Fund; Mrs. William Osler; Miss M. Carey Thomas and Miss Mamie M. Gwinn, the two friends who have been most closely associated with me in promoting the opening of the Medical School, both of whom are daughters of Trustees of the University; and myself."[16]

Of most significance to the future of medicine, Mary stipulated unprecedented academic terms that would equal those of the great, centuries-old European universities. She insisted that the "Medical School of the University shall be exclusively a Graduate School . . . [and] shall form an integral part of the Johns Hopkins University . . . [and] shall provide a four years' course, leading to the Doctor of Medicine." She required that students have knowledge "imparted in the preliminary Medical Course," which meant that they would have a background in the sciences as well as be fluent in French and German. She also required that students successfully pass examinations based on the preliminary medical course as well as their studies in the medical school before receiving their degrees.

Gilman had first recommended such standards in 1876, when he proposed a specific curriculum, as he noted, "for one who looks toward a course in medicine," by including courses in chemistry, physics, modern languages, and philosophy. Dr. William Welch had similarly enumerated many of the academic requirements years earlier, never imagining that such lofty standards could actually be implemented. "She naturally thought this is what we wanted," Welch later commented on Mary's gift. "It is one thing to build an educational castle in the air at your library table, and another to face its actual appearance under the existing circumstances."[17]

Perhaps of greatest surprise was Mary's deadline for the opening of the medical school that had taken so long to establish. She insisted that it open in less than a year—by "autumn of 1893 and notice of such intended opening shall be given on February 22, 1893." That date would commemorate the seventeenth anniversary of the inauguration of the Johns Hopkins University in 1876. Carey was thrilled with Mary's firm decision and the trustees' sudden flurry of activity. "Dixon [a trustee] was simply charmed to see father & now he is talking to Gilman," Carey wrote. "Good night, my dear," she added, sending "kisses of congratulations."[18]

Two days later, on Christmas Eve 1892, nineteen years to the day after Johns Hopkins had died, the trustees met at a hastily convened meeting at the home of Charles Gwinn to officially accept Mary's "munificent gift." Their resolution provided "a memorial of her liberality to this University and . . . its obligations to her." Johns Hopkins's dream for a medical school came one step closer to reality—thanks to Mary's "holiday gift," as her contribution has since been called. Charles Gwinn telegrammed Gilman, then staying in New York at the Fifth Avenue Hotel, informing him of the board's decision.[19]

Gilman was mortified. He rushed back to Baltimore, shocked at the trustees' acceptance of the terms of the gift. He feared the wording on Mary's admissions stipulations restricted academic freedom, was too binding, and might one day cause embarrassment if the 1892 standards were applied in perpetuity. He also worried about the language requirements of fluency in French and German. Carey felt that was a weak excuse. Bryn Mawr College, she coyly pointed out, had 170 students at that time, "everyone of whom has passed our examination for reading French and German. It is folly to suppose that men cannot do the same at a much more mature age."[20]

Gilman had good reason to be apprehensive. Years earlier, when the University of Pennsylvania and Harvard had tried to raise their academic standards, admissions and much-needed revenue dropped off. With the Johns Hopkins University still in fragile financial health, he could not afford a similar dilemma. And then there was the issue of coeducation. How would the faculty respond? He could not risk a repeat of Harvard's experience when, in 1878, Marian Hovey's $10,000 offer to make the medical school coeducational stirred great controversy among Harvard's faculty.

Gilman and Welch tried to convince Mary to lower, or at least compromise, her terms for admission. Every day, a university trustee, a faculty member, or Gilman trekked to Mary's Mount Vernon Place mansion to plead for a concession. On January 26, a month after Mary had made her offer, Welch reported that he could find "no indication that she was willing to modify those terms." The medical faculty voiced their own concerns about academic control. On February 9, they submitted a document stating, among other concerns, that the university should have the right to determine under what conditions students could be admitted and have the right to change the conditions when mandatory.[21]

But they greatly underestimated Mary's resolve. Her years of sitting in on railroad meetings, listening to her unbending father strike deals, and, not least, having her previous proposals rejected, finally paid off. She refused to budge. Carey described the ongoing negotiations with her usual dramatic flair: "The trustees get so angry they [fling] brickbats at each other's heads."[22]

The debates dragged on through February. Finally, when all parties appeared to reach consensus, Mary raised minor objections, among them finding fault with an aspect of the entrance examination and one of the course offerings, "a chemical-biological course that required too little skill knowledge for the medical students."[23] The entire arrangement, so near to closure, was suddenly thrown into jeopardy.

It was touch and go, with neither side quite sure of the outcome. Mary fretted fitfully. "Heaven only knows what new difficulties will have been hatched and have attained their full growth by that time," she wrote as she waited for Gilman's and the trustees' final decision. She put her faith in Charles Gwinn to argue for her conditions. "Mr. Gwinn has been our counselor as well as our advocate," she reminded Carey, who also worried about the down-to-the-wire negotiations. To calm her nerves, Mary often rode out to Montebello in the afternoons. "The ride made me feel a little better . . . my heart has been beating in quite such a suffocating fashion." In the final weeks, when Mary's nerves frayed almost to the breaking point, Carey dashed down to Baltimore from Bryn Mawr as often as twice a week to keep the negotiations on track. "I sat up all night preparing campaign broadsides," Carey later recalled.[24]

At long last, on the day before Mary's February 22 deadline and after nearly two months of nonstop discussions and debates, all sides—the trustees, the faculty, Gilman, and Mary—reached an agreement. To satisfy the faculty's concerns over academic freedom, Mary modified two paragraphs of her original letter to allow for special circumstances, to "bring the terms of her gift into entire accordance with the statement of the requirements for admission to the Medical School which had been formulated by the Medical Faculty and approved by the Board of Directors."[25] Finally, she agreed to sign the documents.

With a stroke of her pen, Mary made the long-awaited Johns Hopkins University School of Medicine a reality. It had taken four years, but finally Daniel Coit Gilman had found a donor willing to invest in medical education. But it was not the "man of large means" he had hoped for. Instead, it was a Baltimore heiress, whose father had helped the university benefactor develop his philanthropic plan a quarter of a century earlier in the family's home on Mount Vernon Place. Although Gilman's 1888 letter to trustees George Dobbin and Charles Gwinn had suggested that the school would be named for the donor, only the endowment, not the medical school, was named the "Mary Elizabeth Garrett Fund."

Mary was thirty-eight years old when she joined the ranks of the country's most renowned philanthropists, the same age her father had been when he made his first major step in the world as president of the B&O.

The day after the agreement was signed, the university joyfully commemorated its seventeenth anniversary with a convocation and celebration at the Peabody Institute, where two years earlier famed Russian composer Pyotr Ilich Tchaikovsky had performed. At the convocation, the Peabody Student Orchestra played and the chorus sang. President Angell of the University of Michigan, who had helped to advise the trustees in the formation of the university twenty years earlier, delivered the address.[26] There was much to celebrate. At last, all the parts of the benefactor's great dream—the university, the hospital, and the medical school—were complete.

The trustees held a luncheon in honor of the Women's Medical School Fund members and Gilman wrote a warm and complimentary acknowledgment letter to Mary. "Medical education for women and for men will at once receive an impulse as a consequence of your generosity, which will be felt throughout the land for years and years to come." He added that "you have won the acknowledgements not only of all the friends of the University and Hospital, but of a much wider circle of persons who desire to see improved methods of study introduced into medical colleges of the country. I beg you to accept this personal expression of most hearty gratitude." Commenting on the unparalleled academic standards, Osler joked to Welch, "It is lucky we got in as professors. We could never enter as students."[27]

Mary had required that a "Preliminary Announcement" be distributed by the required date of February 22, giving public notice of the new medical school. The announcement stated the new medical school "will be opened for the instruction of properly qualified students, October 2, 1893. Men and women will be admitted on the same terms."[28] The announcement reiterated Mary's terms, that candidates for the medical school be "Graduates of approved colleges or scientific schools" and have "a knowledge of French, German, Physics, Chemistry and Biology."

The simple, four-page announcement, with its unprecedented terms and standards, revolutionized medical education in the United States. It provided a final vindication of the often-agonized and polarized race between the university and the Women's Medical School Fund. Unfortunately, the announcement failed to mention one important point: the name of the benefactor who worked tirelessly for four years to make it all possible.

But the press did not overlook this important part of the story. Once again, Mary's name was splashed across the headlines. Unlike the earlier publicity in the spring of 1891, announcing her $100,000 offer, when the status of the medical school remained unresolved, she might have felt easier with the new wave of public accolades. "Enlarges Woman's Sphere," the *Chicago Herald* pronounced. "Miss Garrett's Princely Gift," the *San Francisco Examiner* weighed in. Rev. C. T. Weede, pastor of Baltimore's Exeter Methodist Episcopal Church, in a Sunday sermon in early 1893 felt compelled to thank a higher authority that the protracted impasse was finally solved. "And who in our fair city has not felt during the past week a thrill of pardonable pride that Baltimore has one woman like the noble Miss Garrett who lays almost $400,000 at the altar of science in connection with our beloved Johns Hopkins?" The *Baltimore American* succinctly summed up the twenty-year effort to open the medical school: "Miss Garrett's Gift Solved the Problem."[29]

Much of the publicity focused on the unprecedented, rigorous academic terms that accompanied the gift. The *Baltimore Sun* wrote "Miss Garrett, in her letter, sets forth the conditions of her gift clearly and explicitly, not only that women shall be admitted, but that their rights and privileges in the school shall be for all time the same as those enjoyed by men, and further, that the school shall be exclusively a graduate school. She is [unwilling] to contribute at any time to the maintenance of an undergraduate or partly undergraduate school."[30]

Mary suddenly found that publicity placed her in the company of the great male philanthropists of the day. "Never in the history of the world were there such general and grand donations to charitable, benevolent and educational purposes," the *Philadelphia Call* wrote. "The example set by Mr. Childs and Mr. Drexel has been followed by P. D. Armour and John D. Rockefeller. Now it is announced that Miss Mary E. Garrett of Baltimore has contributed over $300,000 to the endowment fund of the Johns Hopkins University. The world at large is made better by the existence of such donors."[31]

The *New York Review of Reviews* wrote an article entitled "What Baltimore's

Rich Men Have Done." In Baltimore, the article noted, "we find about fifty-five large Baltimore fortunes listed as equal to one million or more . . . and their wealth has been accumulated slowly and by old fashioned business care and sagacity. Just one-half of the names [belong] to men of a recognized disposition to be generous. . . The most noteworthy of recent benefactions in Baltimore is Miss Mary E. Garrett's check for $350,000 to the trustees of the Johns Hopkins University." The *Philadelphia Ledger* found that "for a long time it seemed left to men alone, like Matthew Vassar and Henry M. Sage, to remember that women also had wants of knowledge."[32]

Not everyone was impressed. Delaware's *Wilmington Journal* found little would change in medical education. "Women will now have the opportunity to learn how to give breast pills or listen sympathetically to a dear patient's enumeration of all the diseases the human flesh is heir to."[33]

Within six months of striking the deal, the university appointed additional faculty—in pharmacology, anatomy, physiology, obstetrics and gynecology, and surgery—to round out the medical faculty in preparation for the school's imminent opening. Years later, physician-in-chief William Osler jadedly commented to then–university president Ira Remsen on Mary's blatant bribery of the trustees: "We are all for sale, dear Remsen," Osler quipped. "You and I have been in the market for years, and have loved to buy and sell our wares in brains and books— it has been our life. So with institutions. It is always a pleasure to be bought, when the purchase price does not involve the sacrifice of an essential—as was the case in that happy purchase of us by the Women's Medical Association."[34]

It had taken three tries, but Mary finally had "bought" coeducation at the Johns Hopkins University.

A NEW MODEL OF MEDICINE

But what did Mary's "princely gift" mean to medical education and medical science? How would the gift affect women medical students and women physicians? Would the extraordinary efforts of Mary and the Women's Medical School Fund vastly improve American medicine, as they had hoped?

Although many feared Mary's rigid academic standards would limit applicants to Hopkins' class of 1897, the opposite proved true. Word quickly spread of the innovative medical school with its demanding curriculum, modern laboratories, and renowned faculty. The quality of the first applicants exceeded all expectations. Only one-third of the first class of eighteen students had graduated from Johns Hopkins; the others represented colleges from across the country.

There were other, more profound differences that would influence the future of medicine. For the first time, students were not seen simply as revenue-generators, as had been the case with the traditional proprietary, for-profit system of medical education. Instead, the abundant annual income generated from the $500,000 endowment provided much-needed budget relief from day-to-day money woes, as well as funding for the "extras"—purchasing modern equipment for laboratories and expanding the faculty. Students could learn the best science and faculty could teach the best practices without worrying about the bottom line of profit making. The first class, in fact, filled every seat and provided an added bonus for the university: $27,000 in income, $2,400 more than expenditures.[35]

Perhaps most important, the Hopkins medical school offered an entirely new prototype for higher-education relationships. Over the coming decades, it provided a model to bridge not only hospital clinical care with academic coursework of the university but also science and research with patient care. Scientific discoveries would no longer be confined to the laboratory but would be put to practical bedside use in treating patients and educating students in the latest scientific breakthroughs. The medical school–hospital relationship had a ripple effect, as early graduates of the school eventually spread across the country, instilling the Hopkins model of "clinician-scientists" and transforming American medical study and practice along the way.

Mary Putnam Jacobi thought the greatest benefit of the Hopkins coeducational medical school would be that it would "open the doors of various hospitals to ladies pursuing the field of medicine and admit them on their respective staffs." Jacobi, along with the Blackwell sisters and other early women physicians, had for the most part been banned from practicing in the larger, better-equipped urban hospitals. The greatest impediment for women physicians, Jacobi noted, was that "no lady physician is admitted to the staff of any of the New York hospitals, although probably half the patients are women and from the nature of their diseases require the aid of a member of their own sex."[36] Hopefully, the day would come when women physicians, such as those at the Woman's Medical College of Pennsylvania, would not have to endure the shouts, jeers, and near-riot of their male counterparts when making clinical rounds at a hospital.

As Jacobi had predicted, the higher academic standards lent credibility to women physicians and eventually helped to open the doors for them to practice in the larger hospitals. After the turn of the century, hospital clerkships increasingly opened in New York, Philadelphia, and Chicago and several states began appointing women as clinicians or superintendents at female state asylums for the insane. Women physicians initiated their own publications, notably the *Woman's*

Medical Journal, which published scientific articles and material focused specifically for women physicians.[37] Women physicians also began to expand their professional networks and to establish their own medical societies.

In the midst of the seemingly endless public debate over the impact of her gift, Mary turned to a more practical matter, the construction of the Women's Fund Memorial Building. Dr. Kelly met with her to discuss it. "Beginning at once in the most cheery and enthusiastic way to discuss [the] medical school and how busy they all have been in [making] plans," Mary wrote of Kelly's visits. "He was delighted to hear that I had spoken to Mr. Dixon [the new president of the board] about the necessity for the building."[38]

There already was one academic building, the Pathological Building, next to the thirteen-building hospital complex. Mary insisted that construction start immediately on the Women's Fund Memorial Building. Dr. Franklin P. Mall, the university's first professor of anatomy, was selected to design it. He hoped to create an environment where students could learn by actually performing dissections, not just by watching them. The building also provided laboratories for histology and embryology. The building's ample space for dissection led to a change in medical pedagogy, as anatomy assumed a prominent place in the overall curriculum, rather than just being relegated as "the handmaiden of surgery."[39]

As Mary had stipulated in the terms of her gift, classes began on schedule on October 3. The country once again was mired in a devastating economic depression, the Panic of 1893. In a historical moment, three women took their places beside fifteen male students in the nation's first coeducational, graduate-level medical school.

Although the first women students might have been admitted "on the same terms as men," once in the door, they hardly were treated equally. Many suffered from the "rougher influences" of the male population, as expressed by Gilman at the founding of the university. The first three women—Cornelia O. Church, Mabel Glover, and Mary S. Packard—endured relentless taunts and teasing. The women's dorm was dubbed the "Hen House." Male students chided, "Are you a lady or a doctor?" Even the eminent William Osler, proponent of the WMSF, remarked that humanity is divided into three categories: "men, women and women physicians."[40]

The women also faced enormous expectations for their success. They had graduated from Wellesley, Smith, and Vassar, but despite their stellar academic credentials, they did not all succeed. Church dropped out in her third year to become a Christian Scientist, Glover married her anatomy professor, and Packard was the only one of the three to graduate with her male classmates in 1897. Osler quipped, "As to the women students, 33⅓ percent of them were engaged to their professors by the end of the first year."[41]

Nor did life improve for women interns. They continued to face exclusion and hostility from many of the male students and faculty. Dorothy Reed, class of 1900, chronicled her years as a Hopkins medical student and intern in a series of journals. On her first day of class in 1896, Reed recalled, a "distinguished middle-aged man" approached her and asked her if she was on her way to a medical class. "Are you entering here?" the man asked. "Yes," she answered. "Don't," was the reply from none other than the eminent Osler.[42]

His advice was ominous. Florence Sabin was in the same class as Reed, and the women's experiences at Hopkins reveal the unending hurdles women interns encountered. The best research projects, laboratories, and hospital internships were usually awarded to men. At the completion of their medical degrees, the two women vied with their male classmates for coveted internships in the Department of Medicine. Both were accepted; Sabin was assigned to the white women's ward and Reed to the wards for black men, women, and children. Reed accepted the assignment with grace but was soon ridiculed by the hospital superintendent, the omnipotent Dr. Henry Mills Hurd, for being a "sexual pervert"—rejecting acceptable female behavior—to accept such a position. Reed was infuriated. "He thought—and all of my classmates and the medical staff would think—that only my desire to satisfy sexual curiosity would allow me or any woman to take charge of a male ward."[43]

Revenge and anger kept Reed working at Herculean pace through the grueling year. She and Sabin finished successfully, eventually banishing criticism of their work. "Something Dr. Hurd had said of a woman's being irresponsible and not to be trusted to see things through, kept me at my post," Reed later wrote.[44]

Their hard work paid off—for a while. Both women went on to become two of the great scientists of the twentieth century, but only after their departures from Hopkins. After her internship, Reed accepted a fellowship in the laboratory of Dr. William Welch and, with a colleague, discovered the lymph cells that characterize Hodgkin's disease. After doing trailblazing research, she was passed over for a teaching position in favor of a male colleague who had done no research. When asked for an explanation, Welch simply explained that no woman had ever held a teaching position and, no doubt, there would be great opposition to it. Reed soon left Hopkins. She continued epidemiological studies on infant mortality and during World War I became a medical officer in the U.S. Children's Bureau, working on behalf of war orphans in Europe.[45]

Sabin met a similar ignoble ending at Hopkins. Dr. Franklin Mall guided Sabin in her early career, and her research in histology led to the discovery of the lymphatic channels. In 1917, she was the first woman awarded a full professorship in the School of Medicine. When Mall died a few months later, Sabin was passed over for a promotion to the head of the Department of Anatomy in favor of one of her male students. In 1925 she defected from Hopkins to the Rockefeller Institute and later became the first woman member of the National Academy of Sciences.

It did not help that Mary and other members of the Women's Medical School Fund scrutinized the women students' every move. Mary often hosted the women medical students and interns in her home. But her hospitality and endless prying about the students' progress was not always welcomed. Dorothy Reed noted that she and others came to "dread the invitations of Miss Garrett to her huge home on Mount Vernon Place."[46]

On a more positive note, interested Baltimore women aided and supported the women students, particularly in their research efforts, by offering fellowships. One such source of funding was the prestigious Naples Table Association for Promoting Laboratory Research by Women. Carey had first lobbied to obtain a research position—a "table"—for women scientists at the zoological station in Naples, Italy, in 1896. She became president and continued on as a board member and Mary contributed generous financial support to the organization.

One of the medical school's first women students went on to achieve great fame—but not in medicine. Gertrude Stein entered with the class of 1903. Stein proved to be an inquisitive medical student, enjoying scientific discovery and conducting research on the development of the human embryo's brain. By her third year, however, her interest in medicine faded. She was riding out a stormy love affair with a fellow student, May Brookstaver. Worse, wanderlust stirred. She found clinical rotations—particularly, as she noted, "the delivering of babies"—to be especially unpleasant. Stein dropped out of medical school in the middle of her fourth year. Her brother, Leo, lamented that "the first person in the family to have gone so far should fall back on it." Her feminist friends thought "she had done harm to her sex."[47] Stein soon sailed off to Europe and on to an iconoclastic, legendary literary career, coming to epitomize the "Lost Generation" between the world wars.

Not everyone sailed off to such bright futures. The opening of a coeducational medical school at Hopkins proved to be both a blessing and a curse to the future of women's medical education. By 1900, the number of women medical students at Hopkins increased to fourteen out of forty-three students. Although the Women's Medical School Fund "General Circular" had assured that coeducational medical schools "would not take the place of medical schools for women now in existence," just such a scenario played out. While the Hopkins model had elevated academic standards, it also sounded the death knell for female medical colleges. Within a decade of Hopkins' opening, fourteen of seventeen female medical colleges closed in favor of the coeducational model.

Within a decade, a backlash struck. The number of women medical students nationally began a precipitous reversal, from 1,280 in 1902 to 992 out of a total of 18,840 in 1926, a trend that continued for the next seventy years.[48] Several factors contributed to the decline. Once-stringent Victorian sexual taboos were disappearing, and women patients, the guaranteed market niche for women physicians, were no longer reluctant to be examined by male physicians. Also, by the 1920s, after the passage of the Nineteenth Amendment giving women the right to vote, women's push into the public sphere declined as many women felt their political enfranchisement was the ultimate victory necessary for their full inclusion in mainstream society.

But, more profoundly, women physicians were left behind at a time when the field of medicine virtually exploded into its modern form. Women continued to be confined to their traditional nineteenth-century specializations at a critical time when medicine rapidly changed into a more scientific and specialized profession. Once again, male physicians dominated the more profitable fields, while women physicians were excluded. "My experience . . . has taught me that the day has not yet come for men to yield to us equal ground with them," a woman physician lamented in 1918.[49]

Aside from keeping an eye on the women medical students, Mary, the woman who had climbed over the construction site to inspect every detail of the new Bryn Mawr School in the 1880s, similarly kept close watch over the progress of the Women's Fund Memorial Building a decade later. When the building was completed in the fall of 1894, Gilman, still uneasy with the idea of a commingling at his university, insisted that the Women's Fund Memorial Building sign be discreetly placed inside away from public view. Welch advised him to temper his views, suggesting that Mary might someday give more money or worse, withdraw the money she already had given. The sign was soon placed outside for all to see.

Gilman soon misstepped again. The university's 1894 catalogue listed the new Women's Fund Memorial Building as the Anatomy Building. Angered, Mary wrote a terse note to him expressing indignation that the building was not appropriately named in the catalogue. Gilman insisted it was an oversight. Mary demanded the university "have a new issue of the Directory published and sent out and destroy what remains undistributed of the present one."[50] Gilman complied.

A year after the medical school negotiations were settled, Carey looked back to the controversial "scheme" the Friday Night had launched in 1888 and how the medical school might not have materialized at all, given its volatile political nature. Carey wrote that Mary had offered her final gift "to *force* the trustees to open. Many of them, and President Gilman, above all, preferred never to have the medical school at all rather than to have one to which women were admitted." Carey divulged that the trustees did not fight publicly, but "in the dark with treachery and false reasons. Trustees, doctors, professors (Mr. Gwinn and Father leading our forces) became involved in a tangle of hatred, malice, detraction that beggars description."[51]

But for the future of medical education and research, Mary's victory at Hopkins was worth the tangle of hatred. Her gift not only revolutionized medical education but also medical philanthropy, which had been sorely missing in the nineteenth century. In the years ahead, her gift greatly influenced other notable philanthropists. In 1901, John D. Rockefeller Jr. established medicine as a major philanthropic priority with the establishment of the Rockefeller Institute for Medical Research in New York. Frederick T. Gates, head of the Rockefeller family philanthropies, was much impressed by the Hopkins "bench-to-bedside model," citing William Osler's textbook on medicine as the prime inspiration for the creation of "the Rockefeller," as it has since been called. After the 1904 Great Fire of Baltimore destroyed many of the income-producing real estate buildings in the Hopkins bequest, Rockefeller contributed $500,000 to assist the university, a move that fostered a close affiliation that continues to this day. William Welch, considered to be the world's most preeminent pathologist, became the first president of the Rockefeller's Board of Scientific Advisors, and Hopkins-trained physician Simon Flexner its first director, a position he held for thirty-two years.

In 1910, seventeen years after the Hopkins medical school opened, the Carnegie Foundation issued a report, *Medical Education in the United States and Canada*, by Simon Flexner, that would soon become the barometer of medical education. Flexner analyzed the state of modern medicine in 174 medical schools in 98 cities. Although the Hopkins model was slowly replicating throughout the country, Flexner found most medical schools still dirty and backward, with only five worthy of any commendation; of those, Hopkins ranked at the top. Medical education was still in a state of transition; by 1900 only 15 to 20 percent of medical schools required a high school diploma. Flexner noted of Hopkins that "this institution, fortunate in its freedom from all entanglements, in its possession of an excellent endowed hospital, and above all, in its wise and devoted leadership, set a new and stimulating example precisely when a demonstration of the right type was most urgently needed."[52]

Flexner's report of 1910 soon attracted the attention of major philanthropists such as Paul Mellon, Julius Rosenwald, and George Eastman. The success of the Hopkins medical school model, bolstered by the revelations of the Flexner report concerning the abysmal conditions of medical care in the United States, established medical education and research as major funding priorities. From that point forward, university presidents would no longer be forced to desperately search for years to find a "man of large means"—or a woman—to fund important medical initiatives.

For Mary, the prolonged and often painful scheme to start the medical school proved bittersweet. She had at last broken through one more barrier in the path of women's advancement. She had made good on her father's concern for the university. She had fulfilled the wish of her family's longtime friend Johns Hopkins to establish his medical school. But, the protracted ordeal had taken a toll on her health and her longtime, cherished relationships with her family and the Friday Night. By the time the medical school opened, the group that had been together for two decades had splintered, with Julia and Bessie angrily severing ties with their old friends.

Mary and Carey had weathered the storm together—two storms, in fact: the launchings of the Bryn Mawr School and the Hopkins medical school. Their shared sense of accomplishment and commitment to their feminist goals and to each other strengthened their emotional bonds. Mary, who had once scoffed at Carey's overtures, now began to embrace Carey as an intimate friend, cherished companion, and powerful ally in her mission to "help women." Carey wrote to Mary of the final challenges of the medical school campaign and the disintegration of the Friday Night. The situation is "hopeless, hopeless . . . & so let us leave behind this heartbreaking chapter & close it past."[53] It was advice that Mary sadly accepted as the high price she had to pay for her success.

THE HELPING HAND

As Mary drafted her letter offering to complete the medical school endowment in December 1892, Carey received startling news that would soon steer their lives in an unanticipated direction. Dr. James Rhoads, founding president of Bryn Mawr College and supportive mentor to Carey's deanship since the mid-1880s, announced his retirement after seven years of presiding over the Quaker women's college.

Rhoads had been instrumental in shaping the new college with founder Joseph Wright Taylor, a physician. The fifth of the eventual famed Seven Sisters women's colleges in the Northeast, Bryn Mawr was chartered in 1877 to educate Quaker women of "the higher and more refined classes of Society." The college's founders and advisors, who included Bessie's and Carey's fathers as well as Daniel Coit Gilman, spent several years gathering ideas on academic standards and architectural concepts. They visited Mount Holyoke, Vassar, and Smith colleges. With its "cottage plan," Smith proved to be their favored ideology, emphasizing a central academic building surrounded by smaller cottage-style dormitories for students. As Smith's president L. Clark Seelye explained to Taylor, the college in Northampton, Massachusetts, hoped to create an environment that would replicate a "refined home" promoting "desirable moral and social influences." The small, homey cottages would give women students "greater comfort and less nervous excitement," Seelye added.[54]

While many of Bryn Mawr's trustees argued to locate the college adjacent to its male counterpart, Haverford College, Rhoads encouraged a physical and ideological separation between the two, allowing "more untrammeled and vigorous growth of both institutions."[55] The women's college eventually was located on a thirty-two-acre site five miles away from Haverford. Quaker architect Addison Hutton, who had created Haverford's austere Barclay Hall, designed the first buildings. Taylor Hall, not quite finished on opening day in 1885, housed the academic classrooms and administrative offices. The nearby dormitory, Merion Hall, provided seventy-five spacious rooms and suites for students. Both sat on a high hill, a *bryn mawr*. The college adopted the Welsh name of the nearby station of the Pennsylvania Railroad and the surrounding town.

Rhoads had nurtured the brilliant young Carey Thomas in the first steps of her career, always encouraging her while trying, often unsuccessfully, to temper her demonstrative and dramatic impulses. He had fought for Carey's appointment as Bryn Mawr's first dean in the year before the college opened. Though her impetuousness and strong will often clashed with the conservative male trustees, Rhoads's endorsement proved to be a solid decision. Notwithstanding the trustees' and the president's own vision for the new college, Carey, with her impressive new PhD, saw the yet-unopened college as a blank slate on which to imprint her grand, groundbreaking ideas about women's higher education. Concurrent with planning Bryn Mawr College, Carey, Mary, and the Friday Night were busy organizing the Bryn Mawr School in Baltimore, which opened just days before the college in 1885. The two plans, for female preparatory education at Bryn Mawr School and female higher education at Bryn Mawr College, held identical, complementary goals: to break with past restrictions on women's education and debunk notions of women's intellectual and physical inferiority.

Despite her youth and relative inexperience as dean at the age of twenty-seven, Carey was a driving force in shaping Bryn Mawr College. She was determined to make Bryn Mawr, in her own words, "the very best woman's college there is."[56] She wanted to give Bryn Mawr students free reign of serious scholarship and freedom from overprotectiveness, as she had enjoyed while pursuing her doctorate in Europe.

Carey, too, made the rounds of women's colleges in the Northeast. Unlike President Taylor and his advisors, Carey was disillusioned by Smith, where she disliked the notion of cottage-style family living that she felt counterproductive to nurturing young women's sense of independence. She concluded that at Smith the students' "education is in the hands of men who *do not care*." She was enthralled by Vassar, but loathed the "Lady Principal's" blind obedience to rules and regulations. Wellesley most impressed her, with its five hundred students and "not a man's influence to be seen or felt."[57]

She found fault that none of the women's colleges emphasized original scholarship or research, elements that Carey, who had studied in the European system, found essential to higher education. By the end of her tour of the Northeast, she had perfected a visual image of the model women's college, drawing from examples of all she had seen. But, Carey added an unexpected influence to her ideal: the Johns Hopkins University. While the Bryn Mawr trustees imagined a "female Haverford," a liberal arts college, Carey had other ideas. She envisioned a female Johns Hopkins, insisting that Bryn Mawr offer a graduate school emphasizing original, scholarly research, a requirement then limited to elite male colleges. Not only would this expand students' education, she reasoned, but it would keep faculty current in their own fields of scholarship. Perhaps another, more personal motivation fueled her insistence. Graduate education had been denied to her several years before, forcing her to study in Europe to complete her doctorate. She held her ground against the trustees' opposition. Bryn Mawr opened as the only women's college to offer graduate education. Its high scholastic standards soon earned it the monikers "Jane Hopkins" and the "men's college for women."[58]

Carey thrived in her new role as dean. She tended to her administrative duties, always improving the curriculum and hiring bright young faculty when the college's modest budget allowed. She played both taskmaster and den mother, hovering over the students—thirty-six in the first year—all the while keeping a close eye on their personal and academic growth.

As dean, Carey was assigned to live in the Deanery, one of three small Victorian houses—the others dubbed the Betweenery and the Greenery—provided for faculty housing. She shared the five-room residence with Mamie and often invited students, faculty, and college visitors to dinner and tea. In 1885, Carey began to expand and renovate her unpretentious quarters, adding a fireplace on the first floor and a sitting room on the second. She soon could write to Mary, "I already like my little cottage, and I think I can care for it when it has been filled with a few year's memories."[59]

Mary expressed great pride in her friend's meteoric academic ascent and envy in Carey's absorption in academic activities. While traveling in Europe during her self-exile in 1891, Mary wrote in response to Carey's usual litany of complaints about the trustees, that "even with such possibilities before me, how I envy you the doing of the work!"[60]

With her strong personality and unflappable determination, Carey more often than not stood down the trustees over her grand plans for the college. She hoped to convert what she thought were the trustees' stodgy, old-fashioned conventions of a "Quaker Lady" college into a more sophisticated, secular, urbane institution, with no hint, in either curriculum or architecture, of feminine vulnerability.

But the battles often left Carey wondering if she should simply give up all she had worked for and walk away. Mary would have none of it. Carey's unique academic potential was not to be thrown away at any cost. Mary always offered an encouraging word to remain resolute. During one of Carey's particularly difficult disagreements with the trustees, Mary, recognizing the great good Carey could do for women's advancement, wrote "I am not unsympathetic about yr. [your] college reluctances, and I recognize how much you are giving up, but that chained woman does so strongly need the helping hand—the very strongest—& needs it now at once." The plight of that "chained woman" was one that Mary knew all too well. "You can do so much where you are, that I can not help feeling as if you ought to stay there a few years longer."[61]

Mary had every intention of helping Carey to stay there at least a few years—and longer, if she had her way. Carey began to take on particular importance for Mary. Carey's work in shaping a model of women's higher education, of pushing women one step further to rise "above the dull commonplace of their lives," proved of ultimate importance, and these were goals very compatible to Mary's. By this point, Mary and Carey had proven to be a forceful, effective team, essentially a no-nonsense business partnership in forging women's advancement. Carey, too, understood the soundness of their mutually beneficial relationship—her own academic credentials paired with Mary's wealth and social status. Carey found the combination unbeatable, "the very rarest thing in the world for anyone with your and my views."[62]

Carey also began to fill a void in Mary's life left hollow from the absence of her once-close family and breakup of the Friday Night. Although Carey wrote to her frequently, sometimes three letters a day, Mary increasingly craved to be around Carey's magnetism, excitement, and emotional assurance. When Mary's energy flagged and her demons consumed her, Carey put her on a strict regimen: helping her to find household staff, prodding her to keep up with business affairs, and weaning Mary from her overdoses of medical advice. Still, Mamie always remained at Carey's side, with a geographical proximity and emotional intimacy that Mary did not have.

Now, the vacancy of the Bryn Mawr presidency and Carey's possible candidacy provided another philanthropic challenge for Mary and the chance to create a unique status in Carey's life. She wanted the presidency for Carey as much as Carey did. Mary needed to be part of Carey's academic success. Association with her longtime friend gave Mary the intellectual and academic legitimacy she craved and could not achieve on her own.

Carey felt uncertain about her chances to succeed Rhoads as president. She faced many hurdles. She was young, thirty-five when Rhoads announced his retirement, and she was a woman, although Quakers espoused equality of the sexes. More detrimental to the traditional-minded trustees, she had long since abandoned the fundamental Quaker beliefs that the trustees greatly valued as the philosophical foundation of the college. She was always at odds with the thirteen male trustees who collectively held her future in their hands. Each month at their meetings, the trustees, disbelieving of Rhoads's resignation and with no likely successor in sight, implored him to stay on "for the sake of harmony" but a while longer.[63] Each month, the elderly and ailing Rhoads reluctantly agreed.

By the early spring of 1893, Mary had much to occupy her time. She had two boards to worry about, the Hopkins trustees, who were preparing to open the medical school, and now the Bryn Mawr trustees, whose path in selecting a new president for the college seemed uncertain. She kept careful watch over the construction of the Women's Fund Memorial Building, making sure that Gilman and the trustees followed the exact terms spelled out in her December 22, 1892, letter. She also kept a tight reign on Bryn Mawr School, attending the teachers' meetings, consulting with Amzi Crane about financial matters, and screening student and teacher applicants.

At the same time, she prodded Carey to reach for the brass ring, the Bryn Mawr presidency, a coveted position they both wanted for Carey. Mary sympathized that Carey's fate was in the hands of the changing temperament of "the trustees [who] all belong to the older generation."[64] Mary had no intention of allowing the "older generation" to derail her friend's exceptional academic trajectory. In March, just two months after standing firm with the Hopkins trustees to accept the full terms of her gift to the medical school, Mary again put her persuasive philanthropy to work. Once again, she saw a financial vulnerability in a male-run institution and took advantage of it.

Mary moved into her well-tested proactive mode. She carefully and secretively formulated a philanthropic plan for the college. The nation was reeling from one of its worst financial depressions in history, and Mary's personal finances proved no different. Her financial battles with her family over her father's estate were intensifying, with no resolution in sight. Her income, now depleted from the lack of the annual $200,000 B&O cash dividend, was always tenuous. Over the next months, she sold her inheritance of Chesapeake and Ohio Canal stocks, netting her $510,000, a much-needed infusion of income into her coffers.

She had much to consider, given her many major financial obligations and the tottering B&O stocks. She was committed to paying Hopkins $50,000 a year through 1899 to complete the medical school endowment, money that dearly mattered to the school's survival in its embryonic years. The Bryn Mawr School building, although finished in 1890, still required constant maintenance and new equipment, which Mary financed at approximately $10,000 annually. She already had given several $1,000–$2,000 contributions to Bryn Mawr College's English Department, where Carey, in addition to her duties as dean, held the rank of professor. She also generously augmented Carey's $5,000 annual dean's salary with frequent infusions of spending and entertainment money.

Not least, and at enormous expense, Mary maintained three expansive estates, Mount Vernon Place, Montebello, and Deer Park, with a full contingent of servants at each. She traveled extensively and entertained lavishly. She was living on the economic edge, with annual financial and philanthropic commitments nearly equaling her annual $86,000 from rental properties and income from other investments.

Yet she desperately wanted the Bryn Mawr presidency for Carey, who was ready to resign the deanship and sideline her promising career if the decision did not go her way. If all else failed, Carey was ready to throw in the towel, to spend her life traveling in the lap of luxury with Mary—on Mary's money. But Carey did not understand that such a plan would not have appealed to Mary. Mary was not interested in Carey as a traveling companion. She had other friends who served that role. Instead, she coveted, as Mamie later described, Carey's "careerist, active side."[65] The Bryn Mawr presidency represented a visible and critical position for women's advancement, and Mary was willing to risk making yet another long-term financial commitment to assure the prestigious position for Carey.

Mary thought about it for several weeks, "going over my accounts carefully," as she wrote to Carey before making her decision public.[66] She finally decided that she would offer the college $10,000 annually, for her lifetime, if the trustees would not only *appoint* Carey to the presidency, but also *retain* her in the position.

In March, Mary discreetly presented her idea by letter to Carey, not knowing how Carey would react. Mary argued that Carey's appointment as president was the only logical choice, given Carey's contributions to the college's success. "It would be perfectly clear to everyone who was interested in educational matters that your not being elected as Dr. Rhoads' successor meant a change of policy and c'd [could] mean nothing else, as the success under his and your policy had been so brilliant and solid." She explained her terms. She would give the college "$5,000 next year and each succeeding year that you remain president in the same way, $10,000." To Mary, this caveat assured that Carey would be appointed—and would be given time to prove herself over an extended period. She added, "You know how happy it would make me." It also made Carey happy. She was delighted, praising Mary's offer to use her family's wealth for such a cause, to, as she wrote, "use Mammon for righteousness."[67] They planned the best, most diplomatic way to present the offer to the trustees.

Once again, the timing was right for Mary's particular brand of bribery. In March, Rhoads became so ill that Carey took over most of his duties. Carey was now center stage, proving her value to the college in full view of the trustees. Mary made the most of it.

There was an even more critical factor in Mary's favor: the college desperately needed income. Even before Bryn Mawr opened in fall 1885, the trustees realized the college faced an uncertain financial future. Like the Johns Hopkins University one hundred miles to the south, Bryn Mawr was restricted from spending the principal of the founder's endowment. Like Hopkins, the new college would have to subsist on tuition revenues and endowment income. And, like Hopkins, it soon faced financial difficulties. It was struggling to get by on its limited revenues. The college counted approximately $98,000 in resources from tuition and endowment income and each year quickly spent every penny of it.[68] The college had a small income from a few private donors, most of whom gave from $35 to $100. Mary's offer would add a significant, much-needed 10 percent increase to the college's coffers.

At the trustees' April 14, 1893, meeting, "a communication from Mary E. Garrett was read offering a certain contingency connected with the Presidency of the College to pay the trustees the sum of $5,000 for the next academic year and $10,000 thereafter during her lifetime permanently for the benefit of the English department and then for other departments, but not to be used for building purposes." Mary's letter stated her intentions "whenever Miss M. Carey Thomas should become President of your College, to pay into her hands the sum of ten thousand dollars yearly so long as I live and she remains President, to be used at her discretion." Mary added that were Carey not to be appointed president, "the greatest misfortune that could befall the education of women in this country" would occur.[69]

The trustees gave an anemic answer, a response that after years of quibbling with the Hopkins board must have seemed all too familiar to Mary. They unenthusiastically noted in the minutes that "the Secretary was directed to acknowledge to Mary E. Garrett the high appreciation of the Trustees of her liberal offer and for her added evidence of her interest in the higher education of women."[70]

Aside from their probable surprise at such a significant and financially enticing offer, the trustees were unsure of its political implications. They feared the imbalance of power it would give to the president. The gift would, as Rhoads explained, put "great power in the hands of an officer, which would be wholly beyond the guidance of the board."[71]

Nonetheless, Mary began in earnest to work behind the scenes to bolster her credibility and to prove her philanthropic value to the college. She bailed the college out of minor financial jams, often contributing $3,000–$4,000 to bring the college's account books back into the black. Between 1893 and 1897, she gave $79,300.[72] She donated twenty-six marble busts of classical figures to the college's library. She and Bryn Mawr neighbor George Childs, the same Philadelphia publisher who had contributed $1,000 to the Women's Medical School Fund campaign two years earlier, helped the college out of an anxious situation when each paid $950 to purchase a much-needed parcel of land adjacent to the expanding college.

Mary's "Mammon," her great family wealth, was proving valuable to the young college. But once again, she found herself in the middle of a stalemate with a board of trustees. The Bryn Mawr board tabled her offer while they turned their attention to the matter of the role of Quakerism in the college's curriculum. As with her $100,000 offer to Hopkins in the spring of 1891, her proposal to Bryn Mawr languished, unresolved.

To distract themselves that agonizing summer, Mary, Carey, and Mamie traveled to the World's Columbian Exposition in Chicago. They had eagerly planned the trip for months. The grand World's Fair, the first American fair since the Philadelphia Centennial of 1876, marked the 400th anniversary, albeit a year late, of Columbus's "discovery" of the New World.

On May 1, opening day, 350,000 visitors rushed through the gates to see the dazzling displays at the famed "White City." More than 21 million visitors followed throughout the summer. The fairgrounds, sprawled out across 633 acres in Jackson Park, a former swamp on Chicago's south side near the Lake Michigan shore, promised visitors a fantastic voyage to another world, with spectacular, futuristic sights. For the first time, Americans saw moving pictures, a dishwasher, a zipper, and an all-electric kitchen. A full orchestra, playing live in New York five hundred miles away, transmitted a symphony by long-distance telephone. Henry Adams wrote of the fair, "The first astonishment became greater every day."[73]

Much of the fair's astonishment was a result of the efforts of Bertha Honore Palmer, "Mrs. Astor of the Middle West," famed hostess, socialite, arts patron, and, not least, feminist activist. She served as president of the Board of Lady Managers of the fair's Woman's Building and was a driving force behind the fair's success. Mary knew Palmer from the earliest days of the Hopkins Women's Medical School Fund campaign, when Palmer eagerly signed on as treasurer of the Chicago committee. Palmer contributed $250 to the medical school endowment, nearly a quarter of the $1,140 raised from Chicago donors.

Mary, Carey, and Mamie made the rounds of many of the fair's twenty-eight buildings. Maryland was well represented with the state's and the Johns Hopkins University's exhibits. There was another Maryland exhibit of special interest to the three women. Always anxious to showcase the Bryn Mawr School's innovative curriculum and the modern building that she had financed, Mary had arranged an exhibit for the school in the Liberal Arts Building.

At the entrance to the exhibit, a picture and a large sign boldly announced "The Bryn Mawr School, Preparatory School for Girls, Opened 1885, Baltimore, Maryland." The exhibit featured architectural blueprints and photographs of the school's design and amenities. Visitors could sit in a simulated modern Bryn Mawr School classroom, complete with chairs and desks. The exhibit walls were covered with photographs of Dr. Sargent's up-to-the-minute gymnasium, the art-infused classrooms, a sampling of some of the science and physical education equipment, and the statuary that Mary had purchased for the school over the years.

The exhibit was a hit, winning a blue ribbon in the education section. The certificate commended the school as "a comprehensive system [with] good results."[74]

Mary made a point to visit the B&O's "World's Railway" exhibit, the most expansive and impressive of the fair's transportation displays. Occupying an enormous area, nearly an acre in the center of the fair's "Department of Transportation," it won several awards. Mary most particularly wanted to see if a statue of her father was on display. In February, she had received an artist's rendering of the statue. It distressed her. She found it unacceptable. "It is atrocious," she wrote to Carey.[75] "It has no possible resemblance to my father." She wrote to the exhibit coordinators demanding that they not show it. It is unknown if they complied.

With the excitement of their trip to the World's Fair over, by fall, Carey and Mamie settled back at Bryn Mawr, and Mary returned to Baltimore. The question of the presidency dragged on, with Mary's financial offer still unresolved. By November, with no viable alternatives in sight, the trustees had no choice but to consider Carey's candidacy. A familiar pattern was emerging. As with the Hopkins trustees, who had no other choice but to accept Mary's offer when no male donors stepped forward, so, too, did the Bryn Mawr trustees accept her offer when no other candidate met the required presidential standards. On November 17, by a vote of seven to five, the board elected her to the presidency.[76] As Carey anticipated, two trustees resigned in protest. The long wait was finally over. "P.T.," as the students soon called President Thomas, was on her way.

Within days of the announcement, Carey and the trustees put Mary's guaranteed annual contribution, named the "Mary E. Garrett Fund," to good use. Thus began a twenty-year pattern of major gifts from Mary that kept the young college a step ahead of its less endowed sister colleges. Within days of her election, Carey learned that one of the finest private library collections in Europe, belonging to Professor Sauppe of the University of Göttingen, was up for sale. Carey desperately wanted it, as did several other colleges, including Yale. Mary advanced $5,000 immediately. The collection, sixteen thousand books, "probably *the* finest in America," Carey boasted, soon found its way to Bryn Mawr. By December, the trustees also voted to use $1,500 of Mary's gift "toward the cost of a swimming pool in the basement of the gymnasium."[77]

In the years ahead, Mary's gifts, which far exceeded her promised annual $10,000, supported an impressive range of programs: graduate scholarships, fellowships, modern science equipment, even an investigation room at the Woods Hole Marine Laboratory in Massachusetts. Each year, the college's annual reports dutifully reported how Mary's gifts were put to use: books—Greek, Latin, math, and science; magazine subscriptions; updated architectural plans; caps and gowns for faculty; archaeology digs in exotic locales; support for distinguished visiting lecturers; encyclopedias; original research support in chemistry and physics.[78] Mary's funding provided the extra financial edge during the college's critical formative years, helping to bring to life Carey's dream of creating "the very best woman's college there is."

As president, Carey could finally unleash her grand, secular architectural plans for the college. Within two years of her election, the college commissioned Central Park designer Frederick Law Olmsted to review the earlier plans of architects Cope and Stewardson. The famed landscape architect, with his stepson John C. Olmsted, created a visual, graceful masterpiece that did far more than beautify and expand the small campus. The new campus plan, with its unyielding granite academic buildings and spacious dormitories, reflected Carey's ideals of fostering independence and self-determination in young women and were reminiscent of the stately buildings in which she had studied in Europe. The dormitories, with their luxurious single rooms and suites, soon attracted wealthy, non-Quaker students—just what Carey had wanted. Carey also secularized the curriculum of the once "Quaker Lady" college. Within four years of Carey's election as president, only two students were Quaker.

As if her finances had not been stretched enough, to reflect her friend's great accomplishment, in Carey's inaugural year, Mary redecorated the president and secretary's offices in Taylor Hall for $7,000. She carefully transported some of the most treasured pieces of art from her gallery at 101 West Monument to Carey's office. "I cannot tell you how different these long days have been spent in the office because of its beauty," Carey wrote to Mary in gratitude.[79] Mary made sure that Carey had ample funds to entertain in a style befitting her new position. She then turned to redecorating the sitting rooms of Pembroke Hall, the long, fortress-like granite dorm that represented one of Carey's earliest visions for the campus plan.

Carey's move up from dean to president also meant a requisite step up in living arrangements. The new architectural plan situated the Deanery, once relegated to the edge of the embryonic campus, to a central location, where it, and its charismatic young president, would become the locus of campus life. In 1894, Walter Cope oversaw the second expansion of the Deanery after Carey's earlier more modest expansion in 1885. The original living room was converted to Carey's study. What once had been the dining room became Mamie's study. Another dining room was added, with a pantry and kitchen, and the second and third floors were expanded to include guest and servant quarters. To help the college, and Carey, elevate the modest Deanery to presidential stature, Mary augmented Carey's salary by as much as $5,000 a year.

Not surprisingly, Mary's abundant gifts to the college were dangerously straining her already shaky financial resources. The great weight of her benevolence, particularly her new and ongoing gifts to Bryn Mawr, hung heavily over her. Many of her assets were still tied up in the fallout of the B&O and generated no income, only stock dividends. "The B&O dividend is passed," she wrote in early 1895. "I really must seriously review the situation and decide from an economic standpoint as well as for other reasons what is best to do in regard for the next years."[80]

Desperate to fulfill her philanthropic pledges and always suspicious that her father's estate had not been managed prudently and profitably, Mary found "what is best to do" was to finally force a full accounting of her father's estate. She soon began a course of action that would forever sever ties with her once-beloved family.

CHAPTER 8

THE HAPPINESS OF GETTING
OUR WORK DONE

GARRETT *V.* GARRETT

"The attitude of those men (J.G. and R.G.) (how I hate to have them bear my name) simply makes my blood boil—How much more has to be done before women's position is what it should be!"[1] Mary wrote the stinging attack in March 1893, just two months after her gift to Hopkins had been finalized and she was scraping together her finances to present her offer to Bryn Mawr College to assure Carey's presidency. Her latest grievance was not against her brothers; Harry was gone and Robert debilitated, nor her sisters-in-law, with whom she had been battling in one form or another for years. Rather, her new anger turned toward her nephews, Harry's sons, John Work II, twenty-one, Horatio, twenty, and Robert III, eighteen.

As her philanthropic commitments mounted and she became more desperate to increase the cash flow from her inheritance, Mary's suspicions about her family became an all-consuming and destructive obsession. She had been agitating since her father's death in 1884 to review the accounting books of Robert Garrett and Sons, which controlled the purse strings of the Garrett estate. For twenty years, she had seethed over the opportunities that had been freely handed to her brothers when they were younger, as Robert easily followed in the footsteps of their father in the B&O and Harry glided into the leadership of Robert Garrett and Sons. She, on the other hand, was forbidden to marry, attend college, or pursue her independence during their father's lifetime. She was left to tend to her father during his repeated illnesses and to care for her handicapped brother.

Yet, she had proven to be a valuable business assistant for her father and he had recognized her abilities by naming her an executor of his estate and depending on her business judgment. In turn, she had become a vigilant watchdog of his name and legacy. She had become in the eyes of many people an astute businesswoman and behind-the-scenes influence at the B&O. And, against all odds, she was making her mark as a respected and nationally recognized philanthropist and activist. And now, in Mary's mind, a new generation of Garrett men was coming along to undermine all she had worked for.

Despite her status as the remaining family executor, she feared her young nephews would collectively usurp her position and influence. She feared that if her nephews entered Robert Garrett and Sons, they would surreptitiously conspire to drain what was left of her accounts. She wondered if they would assume that because she was a woman without a formal education, she was unable to execute the estate. Could she hold her own against her three Princeton-educated nephews?

Mary held little hope for sustaining a strong bond with her nephews who, as children, she had adored. They had spent happy holidays at Evergreen and Montebello and traveled abroad together. The young boys had often scribbled little notes and drawings to her, which Mary kept among her lifelong treasured possessions. But those relationships, too, had frayed over time. "The chances for my nephews are not very great," she concluded.[2]

The three boys' feelings toward their aunt appeared to be mutually pessimistic. They increasingly pulled away from her. The oldest, John Work II, tried to distance himself from the escalating family money squabbles, writing in his diary, "I do not represent the Garrett interests or even a large part of them . . . If I knew whom to believe I would be bubbling over with suppressed merriment and could I but find out whom to trust, then laughter and roundelay would hold sway." He found both his aunts—Mary and Mary Frick—to be "troublesome."[3]

Carey added fuel to the fire. Directly and indirectly, she encouraged Mary's estrangement from her family. Always enthralled with and increasingly dependent upon Mary's wealth, Carey learned early how valuable Mary's money could be in financing their mutual ambitions. Years earlier, Carey had been seduced by the glamorous world that Mary inhabited, a world of luxury, extravagance, and material possessions well beyond the reach of her modest Quaker upbringing. Mary's $10,000 annual gifts to Bryn Mawr College had guaranteed Carey's presidency and Mary's ongoing largess to Carey's personal coffers provided an irresistible lifestyle. Carey felt protective, perhaps covetous, of Mary's money. At Mary's most vulnerable moments, the domineering Carey kept Mary's paranoia and suspicions about her family alive.

By 1895, with little settled to her satisfaction, Mary stepped up her efforts. She officially hired another attorney to her lineup, her longtime friend and advisor Robert de Forest, the seasoned, hard-hitting New York railroad attorney, to secure "a final settlement and division of estate." "I am in a very great perplexity & trouble about the affairs of my father's estate and my own financial affairs," she confided to de Forest in September 1895, "and I have come to the conclusion that the only hope of settling things satisfactorily lies in your being able to act for me." De Forest made one last-ditch attempt before starting legal action to get at the books, asking William Frick that a third-party accountant be able "to see these accounts of the late Mr. John Work Garrett in the firm books and to make sure whatever examination of these books is necessary to inform himself respecting them."[4]

To add to Mary's "perplexity & trouble," in 1896 the B&O entered receivership, joining a host of other railroads in the same predicament. Seven other major companies, representing forty thousand miles of track, faced similar circumstances.[5] Several factors contributed to the B&O's latest insolvency, not least the lingering disastrous financial crisis of 1893, exacerbated by the company's skyrocketing debt and high interest rates. To compound its problems, the company had not fully implemented the short-lived President Spencer's much-needed reforms. In 1887, the federal government had established the Interstate Commerce Commission to attempt to bring some regulation to the free-for-all railroading business. It proved to be ineffective against powerful railroading interests.

Of more concern to Mary was that more than a decade after John Work Garrett's death, his management, deal making, and public accounting of the B&O's true financial state were still under intense investigation. Despite her behind-the-scenes machinations at the B&O to purge Garrett adversaries from the ranks, the controversy surrounding her father's tenure did not fade with time. In fact, investigations into Garrett's "tricks of book-keeping," as the B&O report had stated the year after his death, increased as the company veered toward another insolvency. For years, taxpayers had cried foul, demanding an accounting of how Garrett, on an annual president's salary of $4,000 to $6,000, could amass a $17 million fortune, mostly from company stocks, and how a handful of major stockholders could similarly grow rich.

But by the closing decade of the nineteenth century, Gilded Age cronyism and corruption came face to face with formidable forces—reform, public outrage, and federal investigations—that would soon demand accountability and answers to a quarter century of fortune-grabbing in many national corporations at taxpayer expense.

The United States Circuit Court in Baltimore took over the management of the B&O. Shareholders stood by helplessly as the value of their stock plummeted to $13 per share, a far cry from the near $200 at the time of John Work Garrett's death a decade before. Charles Mayer, who had been supported in his B&O presidency by Mary and the Garrett factions in 1888, was soon shown the door. Although Mary had agreed to appoint Mayer as an executor of her father's estate after Harry's drowning in 1888, supported the early years of his B&O presidency, and depended on his legal advice in settling her father's estate, she and other Garrett interests came to distrust his management of the railroad. John K. Cowen, a member of the U.S. House of Representatives, the B&O's general counsel since 1876, and a Princeton classmate of Robert's, was elected the B&O's eleventh president. Cowen, along with Oscar Murray, a vice president of the B&O, would guide the B&O through receivership.

The court also appointed the Baltimore Reorganizing Committee to help restructure the company. Mary was named to the committee, but resigned within a month when the committee was faced with the inevitable: continuing to probe her father's presidency. "Miss Garrett Drops Out, Displeased with Inquiry into B&O Financial Deals," the *Chicago Daily Tribune* explained.[6]

She was probably even more displeased when in December 1896, Stephen Little, a no-nonsense railroad accountant, issued what would become the infamous "Little Report." The report stated that over a period of years, B&O leadership had been guilty of a host of misdeeds and deceptions, including overstating net income, paying unearned dividends, and understating liabilities.[7] Although some in the railroading business dismissed the report, it gained credibility and vindicated the efforts of earlier reformers and critics, such as Robert's successor Samuel Spencer.

As the B&O wound its way through the federal courts to regain solvency, there was still plenty left in John Work Garrett's vast estate for the family to fight over, notably the huge tracts of undeveloped and profitable land that he had owned throughout Maryland. As the B&O drama unfolded and the company the Garretts had identified with for half a century was slipping away, Mary tried to clarify the escalating family financial battles to her nephew John Work II. She wrote to him, reassuring that, "if at all possible, all public appearances of differences of opinion be avoided," wishful thinking for a tantalizing family feud that increasingly grabbed headlines. She reiterated the futility of her father's will, which, written in 1884 with such optimism, now seemed hopeless to execute. "The affairs of the railroad became involved in very great confusions and the business transactions of the firm of Robert Garrett and Sons were so closely bound up with the railway that it proved impossible to disentangle them at once . . . Uncle Robert took the presidency of the railroad and his health rapidly gave way under the strain."[8]

Mary continued, explaining that she had persistently asked for an accounting of the estate in the years between her father's death in 1884 and Robert's breakdown three years later. It was only in 1892, she stated, while in Rome awaiting the final word from the Hopkins trustees, that she received the first statement from Robert Garrett and Sons. That was when she discovered $30,000 charged against her portion of the estate. This greatly increased her concern about the accuracy of the accounting. Her brother Harry, Mary explained, "did not watch for details" and "Mr. Mayer has not attempted to follow them in detail." To placate her nephew, Mary concluded that the "examination of accounts in winding up so large an estate is a simple business transaction and does not imply distrust of anyone," although she blamed Charles Nitze, president of Robert Garrett and Sons, for the ongoing and irresolvable crisis.[9]

There were other, long-festering, far more menacing problems among the Garretts, specifically Mary and her sisters-in-law, that could not be explained away in a pacifying letter. The three women—Mary, Mary Frick, and Alice—were the ones left to untangle the family's money matters and the decision could not have been left to three more discordant, incompatible women. The intensifying hostility over the estate settlement gave the three women ample opportunity to air their grievances with each other. The money battles that began after John Work Garrett died in 1884 and would continue through the early years of the twentieth century only served to underscore the ferocity of Alice's and Mary Frick's dislike of Mary. Over the years, the three women were publicly cordial and companionable, for appearances greatly mattered among the Gilded Age elite. But the women had different tastes, different activities, different social circles—and very clashing personalities. Each was strong-willed, determined, and opinionated. "The attitude taken by Miss Garrett's sisters-in-law at this time is shown by a voluminous correspondence (all the letters being in their hand-writing) between them and Miss Garrett," Charles Mayer wrote to William Frick, adding, as any good attorney would, that "Miss Garrett's letters were the only calm and good tempered ones."[10]

Mary Frick had burdens to bear beyond settling her father-in-law's estate. Despite the allure of her ever-expanding mansion on Mount Vernon Place, her husband, Robert, suffered debilitating mental and physical frailties. Within a year of Robert's breakdown in 1887, Mary Frick hired Dr. Henry Barton Jacobs, a recent Harvard Medical School graduate, to care for her husband. Robert's health became increasingly fragile. He often fell seriously ill. The family tried in vain to protect his privacy, but each new lapse of health made headlines. "Mr. Garrett Takes Ill at Club," the *Baltimore American* reported after Robert suffered a brief fainting spell at the Maryland Club in 1890.[11] The progress of his recovery from such a relatively minor incident stayed in the papers for days. While visiting the World's Fair in 1893, he became too ill to return to Baltimore. Traveling with Carey and Mamie to the fair, Mary stayed on with her brother to be by his side, helping to nurse him back to health.

But she felt little affection for Mary Frick. Perhaps it was their proximity on Mount Vernon Place, just a few doors away from each other, that most exacerbated their pronounced personality differences and competition as Baltimore's grande dames. "Robert's house is dark," Mary noted in 1895 after Robert and Mary Frick had decamped from Mount Vernon Place for the spring social season at Uplands. "What a relief!" Robert was the common denominator between Mary and her sister-in-law. With his gradual decline, that tie became more tenuous. "Mary [Frick] and I are bound together in our love for Robert and even my little share of that she has always been jealous," Mary wrote. With Robert's death, which seemed all too imminent, "our community of interest will also die," Mary speculated of the almost-certain disintegration of her family.[12]

Mary's nephews appeared to have had little interest in sabotaging their aunt's inheritance. While affiliated with the family business of Robert Garrett and Sons, their interests extended well beyond commerce. They centered their lives at Evergreen, which vied with Mary Frick's mansion as a Baltimore showcase. One by one, over the next years, they graduated from Princeton, their father's and Uncle Robert's alma mater.

John Work II proved to be the family's entrepreneur and future diplomat. Although a childhood injury after a fall from a pony cart had left his leg deformed, he dedicated his life to adventure. After graduating from Princeton in 1895, he traveled with the Princeton Geological Expedition to Yellowstone. En route, Indians captured his group. Mary read the news in the morning paper. Panicked for her nephew's safety, she wanted to ascertain the validity of the article. "I telegraphed the Secretary of War and the Commissioner of Indian Affairs asking if there was any truth to the story," she wrote Carey in July. "They had no news except what they had read in the paper."[13]

Despite his harrowing adventure, or perhaps because of it, John stayed out West for a while to try his hand at the insurance business. Unlike his father and uncle, who had little choice but to follow in the family business, John, as a young man, knew other adventures awaited him. "How can I ever settle down to be a business man, a banker or a railroader? There is a splendid business [Robert Gar-

rett and Sons] waiting for us and we 3 are none too many, for it's hard work to enter without a father to show us what to do." Within a few years, his wanderlust
lured him into a life of diplomatic service. "Banking, railroading, even birds do
not interest me as much as politics now," he wrote in 1893.[14]

The middle son, Horatio, nicknamed "Ray" or "Ratio," married Charlotte Dore-
mus Pierson in October 1895, the year he, too, graduated from Princeton. Horatio immediately entered the family firm. Alice commissioned architect Lawrence
Aspinwall to build a splendid Tudor house for the newlyweds, at the cost of
$85,000, on the southeast edge of the Evergreen estate. The stylish mansion soon
acquired the name Evergreen Jr.

For the youngest, Robert III, or "Rob," years of activity in Dr. Sargent's modern
gymnasium at Evergreen paid off. He became the star of Princeton's track team,
qualifying for the U.S. Olympic Team in 1896. He won gold medals in the discus
throw and the shot put at the Olympic Games. Robert's outstanding showing at
the games and his membership on Princeton's Olympic Committee eventually
led to the establishment of the university's Department of Physical Education. He
also was elected president of his class at Princeton.

Rob graduated from Princeton the year after the Olympics and, like his oldest
brother, soon headed off for adventure. He traveled to Syria with the American
Archeological Expedition to excavate in the ancient country. From his travels, he
penned a scholarly book, *Topography and Itinerary*. Unlike John, however, Robert
returned to build his career in Baltimore. He revitalized Robert Garrett and Sons,
reorganizing it to admit non–family members as partners and expanding it to its
former international scope.[15]

With the B&O in receivership and the estate's finances hopelessly logjammed,
Mary began to think where she could cut down on expenses. Her philanthropies
remained her priority. "I want to do all, of course, that I have agreed to do," she
wrote.[16] Her solvency was important not just to maintain her standard of living.
The new institutions she started or helped to finance depended on her financial
support.

Cutting back on entertaining seemed a logical first step toward economizing.
"I have been going over last year's account today to see where retrenchments c'd
[could] be made," she explained to Carey. "Even if I lived in this house [101 West
Monument] next year without entertaining, except the Bryn Mawr School Christmas party, I c'd spend $30,000 less." But there was still 1,400-acre Montebello and
the stables. She also was concerned about the servants at Deer Park, who remained on the payroll despite her infrequent visits there. "The servants at Deer
Park want to know whether they are to be kept for the summer." She advised the

servants at 101 West Monument to cut corners wherever they could. "All the household expenses must be watched as carefully as possible," she wrote.[17] Presents, in particular, presented a problem for economizing. She frequently showered gifts on friends, family, and beloved servants, selecting shawls, jewelry, or a small piece of statuary for special occasions.

Economizing was difficult for a generous and hospitable woman who eagerly welcomed guests to her beautiful homes. Her "at homes," held during the Women's Medical School Fund campaign, had fine-tuned her entertaining skills. She hosted lavish dinners for friends or visiting dignitaries to Baltimore. She often invited the Hopkins faculty to her social events, and the Rowlands were great favorites. "Would you and Mr. Rowland come next Sunday . . . to have a cup of tea," she wrote to Mrs. Rowland in January 1895, from 101 West Monument. "I am asking only a few small number of friends and a few strangers who are either living in Baltimore or are spending the winter here."[18] Constantly entertaining longtime friends and "a few strangers" did not help Mary's attempts for economic retrenchment.

Nor did her national visibility as a philanthropist. Amzi Crane kept careful watch over Mary's impulse to send off gifts, large or small, to charities. As her major financial commitments increased in the 1890s, he worried. He often admonished her to restrain herself. "My understanding is that you agree that it is not desirable to add *any* new institutions than we already have on the list," he wrote sternly to Mary in March 1893. Little did he suspect that at that very moment, she was secretly devising yet another major gift, this time her lifetime commitment—$10,000 a year at the minimum—for Bryn Mawr College. By the next month, after Mary's plan for Bryn Mawr became public, Crane, probably throwing up his hands in exasperation, suggested that she at least cut back on her annual $500 contribution to another favorite, the Baltimore Charitable Organization Society, making only a $300 gift that year.[19]

Not surprisingly, given her endless charitable contributions and seemingly deep pockets, the press continued its fascination with Mary's money, however inaccurate its appraisals. "Old Maids of Wealth," the *Washington Post* headlined an article in 1896, which erroneously estimated Mary's estate at $13 million. "Miss Garrett is not the only millionaire spinster that the country can boast of, although she is the richest by several millions. The number of unmarried women beyond the allotted age of girlhood who have a fortune of at least $1,000,000 is not small." The four women—the others included "Miss Gwendoline Caldwell of Kentucky, Miss Anna Leary of New York, and Miss Grace Dodge of New York"—each managed her own money and "have done more good in the world by far than the four

richest married or unmarried men in the country," the paper pronounced, adding
that "they have charming personalities, have wide circles of friends and probably
would not exchange places with any married woman the world over."[20]

Despite her good deeds, there were few pleasures for Mary during this time.
Her philanthropic commitments, the B&O debacle, and, particularly, the increasing estrangement from her family troubled her. "I find that the worry of having my affairs in this condition is affecting my health very seriously," she wrote to
de Forest in 1895. Her health had been slowly improving over the years, "uphill
work," she noted, but the "miserable fuss with my sisters-in-law" had once again
made her sick. She suffered from bronchitis and was hospitalized. Her familiar
pattern of despair and despondency once again set in. She could not sleep and felt
chronically tired. Her symptoms became more noticeable—and noticed. Judge
William Fisher, another of Mary's many attorneys, advised Carey that Mary's behavior appeared odd and was causing public comment. Many people feared her
an eccentric. Her nephew John worried about her state of mind and the "gossip
that Aunt Mary is crazy."[21]

Mary's confrontations with her family escalated. In an angry but articulate
fifteen-page letter to Mayer, she tallied her grievances, real or perceived. The document reveals a complete breakdown in communications and eruption of Mary's
long-suppressed anger. First, she demanded, if her nephews were to enter Robert
Garrett and Sons when they came of age, "that an immediate change be made in
the management [of the estate]." Her list continued, citing a range of problems,
from disappointments with Robert Garrett and Sons' management of the estate to
failed investments. Most pointedly, she faulted Alice and Mary Frick "in regard
to the H.S.G. matter." H.S.G. was Mary's invalid brother, Henry, who lived with
her at Montebello and 101 West Monument. Her father's will set aside $3,000 per
year for Henry's care. Mary insisted that it was her accounts, not her nephews' or
brothers' estates, that were being charged for Henry's upkeep, a point which, however petty, represented to Mary how she was being cheated out of her fair share of
her inheritance. "The whole matter is so complicated," she concluded. To prepare for the worst, Mary inventoried all of her homes and possessions. She listed
furniture, artwork, jewelry, china—anything that could eventually come under
legal dispute. She already had distributed much of the family jewelry in her possession to her nephews.[22]

Mary's timing to threaten legal action against her family could not have been
worse. In 1896, family tragedy struck not once but twice. Mary was vacationing on
Montauk, Long Island, in July 1896, when she received word that Robert had died
in the early morning hours of July 29 at Deer Park in the cottage next to where

their father had died twelve years earlier. He was forty-nine. Robert died as the company he and his father had presided over for three decades entered receivership and faced the worst financial crisis of its sixty-eight years.

The papers reported that Robert's death came as a "profound surprise." But the family knew that he had been in desperately poor mental and physical health since well before his complete breakdown in 1887. Since that time, he seldom had been seen in public. "He sought no society and saw only members of his family or very intimate friends." Except for two trips to Europe and stays in Newport or Uplands, Robert had been confined to his Mount Vernon Place mansion. "He was frequently morose and melancholy, but could be induced to converse upon social topics," the *Baltimore Sun* reported.[23] In the month before his death, Robert and Mary Frick had been at Uplands for the spring social season; they removed to Alice's cottage in Deer Park in late June. Alice was spending the summer in England. Robert's personal, full-time physician, Dr. Jacobs, recommended the move, thinking the change of scenery and cool mountain air would improve his patient's deteriorating health. But the familiar setting of Deer Park did not provide the needed rejuvenation. Robert's condition slowly declined.

By early July, his mental health worsened. He "suffered from much mental depression and melancholia," the papers reported. He had gone riding three days before his death, and his appetite was good. But suddenly, he was "seized with alarming symptoms of heart failure and began to sink rapidly." Dr. Jacobs reported Robert's sudden "high fever and weak pulse."[24]

He died at three in the morning. His funeral was held in Baltimore on August 1 at Grace Protestant Episcopal Church at the corner of Monument Street and Park Avenue. The church was filled to capacity, with crowds spilling over outside. As the funeral cortège wound its way north to Green Mount Cemetery, "the streets were blocked in all directions and hushed crowds lined the path." He was buried in the Garrett family plot.

Later, when Dr. Jacobs reported the details of the death to Mary, "the dr. broke down and cried. He said it was hopeless," Mary recalled. The cause of death was listed as "chronic nephritis"—kidney failure—the same affliction that had been reported as John Work Garrett's cause of death.[25]

The papers again dredged up all the old stories about Robert's failed career with the B&O and his subsequent resignation and breakdown. "A Millionaire's Sad Career," the *Louisville Courier Journal* reported. Some were kind enough to recognize the B&O's untenable financial condition when Robert succeeded his father in 1884. "The condition of the company's finances and the disastrous rate war then prevailing made his task an extremely difficult one," the *Chicago Trib-*

une acknowledged. The *Baltimore American* similarly concluded, "Contrary to the belief in some quarters, he accomplished much during his short career." The papers sensationalized the Garretts' wealth. The *Chicago Tribune* reported, "Mr. Garrett's wealth is estimated at between $12,000,000 and $15,000,000."[26]

Once again, Mary felt that her family, however estranged she was becoming from them, was under attack. The articles outraged and upset her and dragged up what she thought were the same biased, cruel remarks about her family that were written after Harry's and her father's deaths. "The newspaper articles are most unkind & also full of falsehoods like when my father died," she wrote to Carey the day after Robert died. "They said he had been in an asylum for years," Mary wrote despairingly.[27]

As the family grappled with Robert's death, yet another heartbreak slowly unfolded. Horatio, just twenty-three and newly married, was diagnosed with bone cancer early in 1896. He and his wife and Alice traveled to England to a clinic known for its specialized treatment of the disease. Young Ray suffered in excruciating pain for ten months, while his family at his side could do little to help. He died in November. In her son's memory, Alice commissioned a stained glass window at the magnificent Princeton University Chapel.

Alice had lost a husband and son within a few years; Mary Frick, her husband of twenty-four years. Mary Frick carried on, focusing many of her charitable activities on children's causes. Always philanthropic, she had begun to memorialize her husband the decade before, soon after his retirement from the B&O. In 1888, she had founded the thirty-bed Garrett Sanitarium for Children in Mt. Airy, Maryland, and in 1889 had established the Robert Garrett Fund for the Surgical Treatment of Children, which laid the groundwork for the juvenile cardiac research center and the Children's Medical and Surgical Center at the Johns Hopkins Hospital.

After Robert's death, Mary was left with her two sisters-in-law to bring resolution to her father's complicated estate. Given the three women's inability to even attempt an amicable peace, Mary felt there was only one course: legal warfare. Despite her years of agitating to see the accounts of Robert Garrett and Sons, she had been hesitant to bring formal legal action against the company for fear it would suggest malfeasance and bring public ridicule to a company founded by her grandfather, continued by her father, uncle, and brother, and in which her nephews were now associated.

But now, her brothers were dead, her nephews estranged, and worse, Mary Frick was exerting greater control over the estate through her powerful father, William Frick, co-trustee of the estate. All combined to dash any hope of civility.

Mary's lingering suspicion of being shortchanged by her family's business of Robert Garrett and Sons, the company's continuing refusal to allow her to personally examine the books, and her rancor with her sisters-in-law finally exploded. In December 1896, one month after Horatio's death, she filed suit. She asked that the money that had been taken from her accounts to support her invalid brother be restored and that John Work Garrett's $150,000 bequest to "the betterment of the condition of the poor" be reinvested and the income given specifically to his favorite charity, the Baltimore Association for the Improvement of the Poor. "Heirs of John W. Garrett in Court," the *Chicago Tribune* announced of the eruption of the family feud.[28] Mary's hope "to keep up public appearances and avoid differences of opinion" proved to be sheer folly.

Nor was there any hope of keeping up optimistic public appearances about the B&O. After fifteen years of tenuous solvency followed by calamitous insolvency, all hopes of controlling "Garrett's Road" within the Garrett family were lost. This time, the Garretts would not come out on top. Six years before John Work Garrett's twenty-year plan to retain thirty thousand shares of stock to stabilize the company and keep it in Garrett hands would have expired in 1904, his heirs sold off their controlling shares at tremendous loss to all. In 1898, Mary began to sell off blocks of her greatly devalued B&O shares, worth not much more than Civil War–era Confederate bonds. She sold twenty thousand shares at ten dollars per share, according to the *New York Times*. She also sold five thousand shares of Consolidated Coal at thirty-five dollars a share. "All sorts of rumors were in circulation as to the cause of the sale," the *Times* reported, "but it is understood that Miss Garrett unloaded her stock because she was unwilling to hold assets that paid so poorly."[29]

But why would Mary and the other Garrett factions have abdicated their three-generation stronghold on the company at such an unpropitious, unprofitable moment? The illogical move has long baffled railroad historians. Traditionally, receivership offers a prime buying opportunity for a devalued stock, as a company is carefully restructured and brought back to profitability. Indeed, over the years that followed, the B&O re-emerged from receivership stronger than ever.

But in 1898, there were factors well beyond Mary's or any Garrett's control. Mary's reasons for cutting the emotional and financial strings from the B&O in the late-1890s more than likely superseded economic considerations. Railroading was entering a new phase, one much different from John Work Garrett's midcentury autocratic rule of the company. The Garretts could not compete with the big syndicates dominating turn-of-the-century railroading. Mary also had fought to keep her father's name and legacy sanitized in the eyes of the public. Now her efforts were failing, as the B&O receivership and the Little Report unearthed possible improprieties. She could no longer protect her father or defend his presidency. And who in the family would have run the company? Mary, who might have taken over and certainly done less harm than Robert, was forbidden by social restrictions to enter the bastion of male-dominated railroading. Her nephews had no interest in continuing the family's leadership. There no longer was a Garrett able to "inherit" the mantle of Railroad King—or queen. As important, by 1898, Mary was probably worn down by fifteen years of fighting a futile battle. It was time to bow out of the B&O, as gracefully and discreetly as possible.

John Work Garrett's unswerving belief, like that of Johns Hopkins's, in the infallibility of the B&O, had been shortsighted and disastrous. Had Mary and her brothers been able to sell the thirty thousand shares of stocks held in trust at two hundred dollars a share in 1884, had they been able to emotionally divest themselves from controlling the company, had Johns Hopkins also not directed his trustees to hold onto declining stocks, had the company been able to implement much-needed reforms, the fates of the B&O, the Johns Hopkins University, and the Garretts might have evolved much differently.

The B&O, the little railroad started in 1828 with big dreams to put Baltimore on the map and assure its future prosperity, the line that had helped President Lincoln claim victory over the Confederacy, the company that had enabled John Work Garrett "to live the life of a nobleman," finally passed out of Garrett and Baltimore hands. After its 1896 receivership and subsequent reorganization three years later, a new generation of tycoons, Marshall Field, Philip D. Armour, and James J. Hill, among others, purchased the majority stock. In 1886–87, the board of directors had all been Baltimoreans. By 1901–2, only one Baltimorean served on the board; the others represented interests in New York, Philadelphia, Chicago, and Pittsburgh.[30] The Baltimore and Ohio no longer "belonged" to Baltimore—or to the Garretts.

Divested from the B&O, Mary still needed to resolve one sizable chunk of John Work Garrett's estate: her father's land holdings. In 1899, "without previous notice," according to her nephew Robert, Mary took the final, irrevocable step to bring an end to her father's estate and to divvy up the contested land.[31] After years of getting nowhere in her attempts to arrive at a consensus among her co-executors to discreetly and privately divide the tracts of land among the heirs, she went public. She filed a "bill of complaint," against her sisters-in-law for adjudicial partition of her father's estate, asking for the court to divide the remaining assets and land.

Her nephews were angered and astonished that their aunt's actions again had escalated so publicly. Robert thought they had all agreed on a course of action. "This was wholly unnecessary," he fired back, pointing out that the suit "brought yet more expenses on the estate." Robert wondered why she hadn't talked with him and his brother first, "to make some effort to agree with us before proceeding against us." He felt her actions would cause the valuable Garrett properties "to be sold at public auction."[32]

But her final action could not have been too much of a surprise, not after her suit three years earlier, her decade-old attempt to audit the books of Robert Garrett and Sons, and the hateful words that had volleyed back and forth within the family for years. All outward signs of propriety were vanquished. The scintillating feud over the family's millions was just the kind of copy that appealed to gossip-hungry Gilded Age newspapers. "Fight Over Garrett Estate," the *Washington Post* broadcast. "Garrett Estate in Court," the *Syracuse Standard* echoed. The defendants, Mary Frick and Alice, held their ground, rebutting that the best way to proceed would be through "private sale and partition" of assets.[33]

Mary had publicly forced the issue to bring a resolution among the three executors to resolve the long ordeal of dividing the estate and letting the heirs go their separate ways. John Work Garrett's twenty-year plan had unalterably torn his family apart, never to be put back together again. Mary's breach with the Garretts was complete. She would seldom again personally communicate or socialize with her sisters-in-law or nephews, except for resolving lingering legal issues. The ill will generated by her legal proceedings against her family, the animosity of her sisters-in-law toward her, and her unshakable conviction that she had been cheated out of her fair share of her inheritance, irrevocably slammed the door on her family ties.

As her family relationships soured, Mary turned to the ever-present Carey, who never failed to offer advice on medical treatments, daily health regimens, and fiscal administration, despite her inability to manage her own accounts. By 1896, Mary was spending long weekends at the Deanery, often tending to Carey's business matters. She would try to make sense of Carey's haphazard accounting, often making corrective notations in the margins of Carey's "untidy jottings" in the account books.[34]

With Julia Rogers out of the picture, Carey thrived on the intrigue of the developing *ménage à trois*, as Mary and Mamie vied for her attention. All were hopelessly dependent on each other. Mamie needed Carey to assure her position on the Bryn Mawr faculty. For Mary, Carey was the conduit to achieve her own feminist goals. And Carey needed Mary's abundant gifts and generosity. Mary agonized over the conflicted relationships, which only exacerbated her despondency over her family.

In the late 1890s, Mary rented another apartment in New York, this time at "The Ava" at 9 East Tenth Street near Lockwood de Forest. Carey often escaped for extended stays away from the college. Forgetting her self-pledge for economic retrenchment made years earlier, Mary again decorated and bought with abandon so that she and Carey could live luxuriously in the New York getaway that Cary referred to as "our flat."[35]

Mary was lost between two worlds. When not in New York or abroad with friends, she rattled around in Baltimore, now vacant of longtime friends. Her ancestral roots and once-cherished relationships in Baltimore held only painful memories. In the wake of her 1899 lawsuit, she began a slow geographical and emotional detachment from her family home. She wanted to stay far away from Baltimore during the final, painful settlement and distribution of her father's estate. Broken-hearted but resilient, Mary would find new opportunities and solidify relationships with her wide circle of friends. They were her family now.

THE LOVES OF WOMEN

In late spring 1899, as she awaited the final distribution of what was left of her father's estate, Mary followed her usual routine, as she had for most of the previous twenty-five years. She went to Europe to spend the summer traveling and taking her annual cure at her favorite hotels and spas. But she was not so much sailing away from her difficulties, as she had so often done in the past. Rather, this time her course was clear. She was moving forward, toward a fresh life and a future that increasingly would include Carey, Bryn Mawr College, and a new living arrangement.

Following the spring semester at Bryn Mawr, Mary and Carey set sail on the SS *Elektra*. The two women had an important mission. The year before, Bryn Mawr alumnae had undertaken a fundraising drive to commission a portrait of Carey. Mary had at first suggested Cecelia Beaux, a Philadelphia-born, European-trained portraitist favored among the East Coast elite. Mary also thought James McNeill Whistler, the Massachusetts-born expatriate artist living in London, would be a good choice, with his beautiful paintings inspired by the seventeenth-century Dutch Great Masters. But the hands-down favorite, approved by the alumnae and applauded by Mary and Carey, was John Singer Sargent, the most renowned portraitist of his day.

Born in 1856 to American parents living in Florence, Italy, Sargent had trained in the French school of Impressionism. He had grown up among the ancient wonders of Europe, where his mother had regularly taken him to all of the great museums. He painted everything he saw—landscapes, cityscapes, scruffy street urchins, gypsies, and vagabonds. But his greatest fame came as the portraitist to the rich and famous from both sides of the Atlantic. He had reigned at the top of Paris society until the 1884 outrage over what would become his most famous painting, a highly sensual, sexualized portrait of Madame X, a provocatively posed American-turned-French aristocrat, showing a bit too much décolletage and atti- tude for Victorian sensibilities. The scandal drove Sargent out of Paris and to Lon- don. There, he set up a studio near Whistler on Tite Street in Chelsea, where in magnificent canvases he captured the beauty and complexity of the Gilded Age. America's nouveau riche—the Rockefellers, the Sears, and the Vanderbilts—just a generation or two removed from their rough-and-tumble past, clamored at his doorstep to be immortalized in oil on canvas by the great artist.

In the sweltering heat of late July, Carey sat for Sargent for six days in full aca- demic regalia. She looked resplendent and regal in her gown—she did not wear the cap—and the final portrait was the antithesis of the painting Madame X that had landed Sargent in hot water in Paris fifteen years earlier. In the portrait, Carey projects a serene, confident, authoritative demeanor, looking every bit assured of her accomplishments and status as America's highest-ranking female educator. The portrait would go on to achieve as much fame as the painting's subject. It was hailed as a milestone in female portraiture, a far departure from the typical de- mure feminine poses, and the portrait traveled to several exhibitions in the United States and Europe. It, along with two other Sargent portraits, won the Grand Prix at the Paris Exposition in 1900. Perhaps as important to Carey, when it was first unveiled at a gala reception at Bryn Mawr in late 1899, the reaction among the alumnae and often-confrontational trustees was one of overwhelming exuber- ance and pride in the college's famous president.

Mary missed the unveiling. She had decided to stay on in Europe and returned to the States the following January. She did not go to Baltimore, still avoiding the family's hostility. She stayed a short time at the Westminster Hotel in New York before turning around and sailing again in February on the North German Lloyd liner the Ems. This time she had new traveling companions, the writer Sarah Orne Jewett and Jewett's longtime companion, Annie Adams Fields. They sailed to Naples and then on to Mary's favorite archaeological sites of Pompeii, Sparta, and Athens.

Mary had gotten to know Jewett and Fields well during the medical school cam- paign a decade earlier. She had recruited them for the Boston committee, and each had contributed fifty dollars, a bit above the average donation. The three women had first traveled together in Italy in 1892, as Mary waited in Rome for the

Hopkins trustees to raise the balance of the endowment. She instantly recognized the women as two additional kindred spirits to bring into her world of intimate friendships. She was drawn to their intellectualism, feminist goals, and talents.

Jewett, born in 1849 in South Berwick, Maine, thrived on the local customs and lore of her hometown. In the 1870s she turned her love of the rugged northeastern region into colorful short stories and eventually novels of quaint New England towns and the craggy and feisty folk who inhabited them. Feminist themes of strong-willed, independent women and the nature of women's relationships to each other often wove through her stories. Jewett gained fame as one of the first women writers to develop the genre of "local color" and later influenced Willa Cather to develop her vivid and poignant depictions of pioneer life on the American prairie.

Fields, fifteen years older than Jewett, by all accounts had been happily married for many years to wealthy publisher James T. Fields. She and her husband shared an outwardly romantic relationship and collaborated on publishing ventures. After her husband's death in 1881, the wealthy Fields took young and aspiring female writers under her wing. Jewett soon proved her extraordinary literary talent, and the two women's relationship moved beyond that of mentor-protégée.

Their relationship became one of the best known of the Gilded Age's "Boston marriages." The Jewett-Fields relationship more than likely inspired novelist Henry James to coin the term in his 1886 novel *The Bostonians*. In it, he satirized women's drive toward equality and wrote of the late-nineteenth-century phenomenon of unmarried women living together. Jewett, too, wrote of the emerging trend of women's same-sex relationships in her first novel, 1877's *Deephaven*, which examines in a sequence of sketches two women's evolving relationship as they vacation in a small coastal town.

From a twenty-first-century vantage point, in our confessional age of telling all, Boston marriages, in which two women cohabited and intimately shared their lives, are difficult to decipher. Victorian women, even liberated New Women, who often wrote highly affectionate and emotional letters to each other did not commit in writing the details of their physical, sexual relationships. Their letters to each other often leave us uncertain of the nature of their relationships. "If only you were here so I could put my arm close around you and feel your heart beating against mine as in lang syne," Antoinette Brown wrote to Lucy Stone shortly before the two women married the Blackwell brothers. In the post–Civil War decades, in which marriageable men were few and career opportunities expanding, women often chose not to marry. Boston marriages usually involved college-educated, career-oriented women who shunned traditional male relationships that would impinge on women's freedom to make their own decisions and stifle their potential. As Jewett wrote in 1887 of women's relationships in *Outgrown Friends*, "Often times our friends seem like rounds of a ladder which help us raise ourselves, our ascent to the level of giving us a wider view."[36]

Boston marriages ran the gamut of emotional and physical attachments. They were generally long-term and committed relationships; some were strictly platonic and companionable, some economic and utilitarian, some, more than likely, sexual and physical. Boston marriages were generally socially accepted as a decorous and appropriate way for two otherwise unattached women to live. Newspaper reports of women companions living or traveling together rarely raised an eyebrow. Mary's travels and visits with friends, for example, were frequently reported in the press. A sexual relationship between two women was not suggested. Most Victorians blanched at the idea that any woman, particularly middle- or upper-class women, could be at all sexual.

Hull House reformers Jane Addams and Ellen Starr, Henry James's sister Alice and Katharine Loring, and Woman's Christian Temperance Union president Frances Willard and her secretary Anna Gordon were among other highly visible partners in Boston marriages. While they lived together in Europe in the 1870s, Carey referred to her relationship with Mamie as a marriage. "The loves of women for each other grow more numerous each day . . . That so little should be said about them surprises me for they are everywhere," Frances Willard observed of the trend in 1889.[37]

Mary often rented a seaside cottage at Dark Harbor, Maine, not far from Jewett's home in South Berwick. There and on her travels with Jewett and Fields, she socialized with their vibrant circle of friends, including Rudyard Kipling, Henry James, and Harriet Beecher Stowe, among a host of other literary stars. John Singer Sargent, during his travels to the United States, often stayed at Fields's Gambrel Cottage, located on Thunderbolt Hill in Manchester by the Sea, Massachusetts.

In turn, Jewett and Fields visited with "our dear friend Miss Garrett, of whom we are both so fond," in Baltimore, with Mary hosting lavish luncheons in her Mount Vernon Place mansion for the two women. On an 1893 trip, Jewett reported that, while staying in Baltimore, "we had some delightful pleasures." The next year, Jewett paid a special compliment to Mary. She wrote *Betty Leicester: A Story for Girls*, an endearing coming-of-age story featuring a fifteen-year-old heroine. She donated the proceeds of the sale of the book to raise funds for the Bryn Mawr School and dedicated the book to Mary, inscribing it "To M.E.G."[38]

Mary, too, would soon intensify her own relationship with Carey, for in June

1904, one of the longest-lived of the Gilded Age's Boston marriages painfully fractured. At age forty-three, Mamie Gwinn, Carey's intimate friend, companion, and housemate of nearly twenty-five years, married former Bryn Mawr faculty member Alfred Hodder. Mamie's marriage to Hodder hardly came as a surprise. She had been passionately in love with him for nine years. Carey had hired Hodder in 1895 to the English faculty, where Mamie also taught, at first describing him to Mary as "a gentleman down to the ground, and more attractive personally, I think, than any other member of the Faculty."[39] William James, the eminent Harvard philosopher and brother of Henry and Alice, had recommended him. Hodder boasted an impressive academic pedigree. He arrived at the college short of his Harvard doctoral dissertation, which eventually was rejected. Within weeks, Jessie, a woman he introduced as his wife, and their child joined him.

The combustion between Hodder and Mamie was palpable. Carey watched angrily but patiently as the relationship heated up. The two lovers were circumspect, often meeting for romantic interludes in the Deanery, where Carey and Mamie had shared an intimate life for a decade. They discreetly exchanged love letters, signed with unsuspicious initials, F. W. and V. W. Within months of Hodder's arrival on campus, Carey was far less enthused about him than when he had arrived. "The Hodders are born to make trouble," she concluded prophetically.[40]

The affair put Carey on shaky ground, personally and professionally. She was losing her intellectual muse, her closest friend and confidante since they had gone to Europe together in the 1870s. They had intimately shared their lives, calling each by their pet names Bunnykins, Rabbitkins, Squirrel, and Mouse. But, as significantly, the Gwinn-Hodder affair was becoming more noticed, particularly by the Bryn Mawr students—with potential leaks back to their wealthy and influential parents. In an era when many parents feared cutting their daughters loose to attend college, the hint of a scandal involving a married male faculty member and the unmarried female companion of the president might reaffirm their wildest fears of the dangers of too much female freedom. Many Bryn Mawr students at the time were fully aware of the affair, finding it quite romantic. A 1904 graduate later recalled, "We were all quite excited about her. Such a scandal. She ran off. It was probably with a professor because how would she have time to go out and meet outside people? She'd have to take one of those professors."[41]

Hodder defused the situation somewhat by leaving Bryn Mawr in 1898 to pursue a writing career in New York. The affair continued, with Mamie remaining on the faculty and living at the Deanery. The inevitable wedding finally took place. Carey noted simply in her journal, "Mamie married Hodder."[42] Unfortunately, the messy situation did not end with a brief journal notation. It got even messier. Within three years, Jessie Hodder filed a bigamy suit against Alfred Hodder, claiming he had not divorced her before marrying Mamie. Her defense was weakened when it became known that her legal marital status with Hodder was ambiguous and more than likely they had never married. She had been Hodder's common-law wife, whom he had taken as a mistress in 1890 after his first wife died. Mamie was prepared to testify that Carey had been aware from the start that Jessie was Hodder's mistress, not his wife, and should have fired Hodder on the spot when she had learned of it. The doubt would linger if Carey condoned the affair or was oblivious to the dangerous liaison taking place in her own home.

A potentially catastrophic legal suit that might have derailed Carey's career and defamed the college was averted before legal action was taken. Hodder died in 1907 of chronic gastritis, possibly brought on by alcoholism. He and Mamie had been married less than three years. After her husband's death, Mamie Gwinn Hodder lived the remainder of her life in Princeton, New Jersey, exonerating her late husband's maligned name and exalting him. "He was a reincarnation of Christ," she once said. Mamie and Carey, companions and intimate friends for twenty-five years, never spoke to each other again after Mamie's marriage. Mamie and Alfred's mother, Mahalia Riley Hodder, found a common bond in spiritualism, often holding séances to contact Alfred from the grave.[43]

While Carey fumed and fretted over the affair, others found the unfolding drama enticing. Gertrude Stein, from her literary vantage point in Paris, was intrigued by the scandal involving her friend Alfred Hodder, whom she had considered one of the most brilliant graduate students at Harvard. Stein knew the Bryn Mawr woman all too well. While attending the Hopkins medical school in the 1890s, she often came in contact with students and graduates of the Seven Sisters colleges, "all activity and no dreaminess," she commented.[44] They intrigued and intimidated her. Although she could more than hold her own intellectually—she, too, had graduated from Radcliff—as a Jew, she felt marginalized by the elite, mostly Protestant women.

In 1904–5, Stein penned a fictionalized version of the scintillating Bryn Mawr *ménage à trois*. Setting her story at a New Jersey college, *Fernhurst: The History of Philip Redfern, a Student of the Nature of Woman*, Stein dissects the affair from the sympathetic perspective of Hodder—Redfern—and his relationship with the brilliant young faculty member, Janet Bruce—Mamie Gwinn. Hovering maliciously and interferingly over their love affair is Carey's fictionalized character—Dean Helen Thorton—"hard-headed, practical, unmoral in the sense that all values give place to expediency and she has a pure enthusiasm for the emancipation of women and a sensitive and mystical feeling for beauty and letters." It is likely that Mary appears in the character of Miss Wyckoff, "a rich spinster of Virginia under the influence of the present Dean," who enabled the dean to "keep the college in a flourishing state."[45]

Stein examines Mamie's latent sexuality and Carey's refusal to understand Mamie's hidden, passionate side and, perhaps, her need to be free of Carey's domination. "The Dean never suspected in this shy, abstracted learned creature a desire for sordid life and the common lot." Stein's assessment of Mamie's relationship with Carey was not inaccurate, for Mamie had often expressed the sentiment that Carey was not her true passion. "I love you dearly, more than anyone else, but I do not love you all I can love," Mamie told Carey. The fiction ends far different than the real-life romance. After Redfern leaves the college, he "failed everywhere," eventually dying alone but never forgetting his great romance. Janet Bruce returns to her uncompromised life with the dean but never fails to ask about her former lover. "Patiently and quietly the dean worked it out and before many years she had regained all property rights in this shy learned creature."[46]

But Carey did not regain all property rights to Mamie—nor did she stay around to witness the painful wedding in June 1904. As Mary had always done when faced with difficulties in her own life, Carey and Mary sailed to Europe. Their trip provided not only the needed diversion from Mamie's wedding, it also was a highlight for Mary. John Singer Sargent had agreed to paint her portrait at his London studio. Mary had first thought of commissioning her own portrait while watching Carey sit for her portrait in Sargent's studio in the summer of 1899. Carey, too, thought the Hopkins trustees should honor Mary with a portrait. While hoping for her own portrait, Mary also began to formulate an idea for another Sargent portrait on a far grander scale—a painting of the founding four doctors of the Hopkins medical school.

In April 1903, Mary saw Sargent at a party at the Boston mansion, "the fairy palace," as she described it, of Isabella Stewart Gardner, one of the country's most ardent supporters of the arts. "Mrs. Jack," as she was called—in reference to her enormously wealthy husband, John L. Gardner—had amassed one of the great art collections of the time and was preparing to open a museum in December to house the collection. Mary quipped that the mansion, with its spectacular double staircase, abundant flowers, and palms—not unlike her own extravagant homes—resembled "a Venetian palace, and a Gothic one at that." Sargent was staying at the mansion, where Gardner provided a large room that he used as a studio. A month earlier, he had tentatively agreed that he might undertake the group portrait of the doctors, but when Mary questioned him at Gardner's about the two paintings, her own and the group portrait, the overcommitted artist hedged. Mary lamented to Carey, "I do so wish there were a possibility of having him paint this group of doctors and surgeons—Welch, Osler, Halsted & Kelly."[47]

Carey wrote to Sargent requesting that he paint Mary. He refused, again citing too many commitments. He telegrammed Mary from the White House, where he was painting President Theodore Roosevelt's portrait: "To Miss Garrett: Sincere regrets cannot undertake commission. Letter follows. Sargent."[48]

"Sargent's telegram was waiting and it is a blow but we might have anticipated that he would be overwhelmed by orders this year," Carey wrote to Mary.[49] Carey pressed on, with Mary joining the letter-writing campaign. Sargent finally acquiesced, agreeing to paint Mary's portrait. But the physicians' portrait would have to wait until Sargent found time. It would be started a year and a half later, in 1905.

Mary had assumed the university would pay the $5,000 cost of her portrait. She was disappointed when she learned the trustees would pay only half, apparently raising the $2,500 through a fundraising drive. Mary paid the other half. She also thought the university should help defray the expenses of the group portrait. "Would it be possible," she queried Carey, "to make the suggestion, do you think, offering to head a subscription with say, $50.00 each? If only he [Sargent] would charge less! It could be like the drive they did for you and for me," referring to the Bryn Mawr alumnae's fundraising drive to finance Carey's painting and the Hopkins trustees' similar campaign to help finance Mary's portrait.[50] Unlike the negotiations for the medical school, this time the trustees won. Mary paid the full amount of the physicians' group portrait, estimated to be $10,000.

Mary began in earnest with the two new portrait projects. Although angered at being overlooked for an invitation to the inauguration of Hopkins' second president, Ira Remsen, in 1902, Mary began writing to the four doctors, asking if they would sit for the group portrait. She maintained close friendships with the famed physicians who had elevated the medical school to national prestige. She especially liked Kelly and Welch, who increasingly showed interest in women's rights, and Halsted was one of her personal physicians.

Their responses to Mary reveal their overwhelming enthusiasm for the idea. "I appreciate more than I can tell you the expression of your wish to have in the possession of the Johns Hopkins Medical School a portrait of my three colleagues and myself, and I should feel highly honored to sit for such a portrait," Welch wrote. "Of course I should be delighted and should be only too pleased to give the time. It is a splendid opportunity. How good and kind of you to think of us!" Osler effused. Kelly and Halsted were equally touched by Mary's offer. Mary's selection of Kelly, Halsted, Osler, and Welch presented a delicate situation for the chosen four, for there were other faculty who were integral to the medical school's success and might feel snubbed. Welch soothed the situation, explaining, "I feel that the other colleagues, especially Drs. Howell, Mall and Abel, have been of the greatest service in the establishment and the development of the Medical School, but I trust that neither they nor others would consider it invidious to be omitted from the group."[51]

Both of the portraits Mary commissioned would prove challenging for Sargent. Mary's sitting for Sargent did not go as easily as Carey's had five years earlier. The artist had difficulty balancing Mary's gentle, dignified features with the primness of her tightly pulled-back hair and wire-rimmed glasses. The first rendering was dim, unexceptional, and worse for a fifty-year-old woman, lifeless and dreary. At middle age, Mary's dark hair was streaked with gray and she had "kindly blue eyes, which can look uncommonly shrewd at times, a strong chin and an amiable mouth."[52] Mary found the portrait unacceptable.

Ever resourceful, Mary and Carey dashed off to a street market near Sargent's studio, where they bought a few props—a white gossamer shawl, leather gloves, and bright red flowers—to brighten up the image. Sargent, who was known for dictating to his clients what to wear, did not get his way with the gloomy portrait. With the added last-minute accessories, the final image was far brighter and more complimentary, capturing the serenity and quiet nature of its subject as Mary sits reposefully next to a stack of her beloved books. Mary's approval must have come as a great relief to Sargent. He later remarked that being in the presence of the two formidable, fussy women made him feel "like a rabbit in the presence of a boa constrictor."[53]

On October 4, 1904, Mary's portrait was unveiled in the rotunda of the Johns Hopkins Hospital, and it was later moved to the main campus's most modern building, McCoy Hall, which boasted electricity and two elevators. Mary wrote to the trustees, thanking them for placing it in a prominent position. The New York Times described the final version of the portrait, made much more acceptable by the last-minute flourishes. The portrait showed "[a] quiet lady, shy and kindly, with a lilt of humor in the eyes clear behind gold-rimmed glasses. Hair plainly dressed, an enveloping fichu [shawl], passive hands, color wan, but enlivened by a flower and a little pile of books, a portrait of a personality bred in gardens of tradition and wholesome refinement."[54] The portrait was later moved to the Welch Library on the East Baltimore campus, where it is now displayed at the medical school Mary had founded a decade earlier.

WINTERS AT BRYN MAWR

Returning from Europe that fall, Mary faced a turning point in her life. She was no longer interested in spending much time in Baltimore. For long months at a time, her grand homes on Mount Vernon Place, at Montebello, and at Deer Park in the Maryland mountains, stood dark. Although absent from Baltimore for much of the time, she had completed yet another major overhaul of 101 West Monument—again, all hopes for economic retrenchment thrown out the window with the old carpets and furniture. She stayed at the nearby Mount Vernon Hotel during the construction upheaval.

It is hard to imagine what she could have improved upon after the massive renovation following her father's death, but the finished product must have been spectacular. "Flowers can justly be called the only fad of Miss Garrett. The conservatories of her townhouse are more magnificent than similar affairs of the kind," the *Washington Post* gushed about her new decor. "In the midst of a bewildering mass of palms, orchids, giant cacti and other tropical plants is a pond filled with wonderful varieties of the water lily. A beautiful fountain throws up spray in the center of the pond, making the whole seem a miniature fairyland." The centerpiece of the glass-domed conservatory was the Roman mosaic floor, a "magnificent reproduction of the days of the Caesars." Mary's renovated mansion was "filled with art treasures, paintings by the best of the modern masters predominating. Her collection of jewels is an exceedingly fine one, although nowadays she rarely wears any ornament of the kind."[55]

Unfortunately, Mary's gloriously refurbished mansion bode misfortune. One of her three private secretaries, thirty-year-old Ida Hoagland, fell forty feet to her death down the elevator shaft in the house. "She was on the third floor and, it is supposed, leaned over and lost her balance, falling headforemost in the basement. Her skull was crushed, and the sound of her body striking the floor of the basement was heard throughout the building." Within four years, "white ants," a wood-boring insect similar to termites, took over, honeycombing their way through the house and causing extensive damage. "Ants Ruin Part of House, Floor in Baltimore residence of Miss Mary Garrett Gives Way," the *New York Times* reported.[56] The library on the second floor caved in and much of the teakwood paneling of John Work Garrett's legendary East Indian Room was ruined.

Mary's other real-estate holdings were equally problematic. The Great Fire, which ravaged much of downtown Baltimore in February 1904, damaged or destroyed several of Mary's lucrative rental properties throughout the city. The Baltimore Trust Company, which held many of Mary's assets, failed. Again, her income plunged. She lamented not having a man in her life to help sort out the difficult aftermath. "It is a time when having no man to even hear news from— much less to expect help or advice from, is hard."[57]

Even her old nemesis, Mary Frick, left the family fold. In 1902, at the age of fifty-one, she married her late husband's forty-three-year-old physician, Dr. Henry Barton Jacobs, who had lived with Robert and Mary Frick for eight years during Robert's prolonged illness. They continued to expand the Mount Vernon Place mansion. When completed, the 39,200-square-foot mansion, with its dramatic Islamic and oriental flourishes, eventually included forty rooms, one hundred windows, sixteen fireplaces, a theater, an art gallery, an elevator, and a musicians' balcony surrounding the grand foyer. Mary Frick Garrett Jacobs had finally brought a bit of elegant New York brownstone to the heart of Baltimore. Dr. Jacobs converted the lower level of the mansion into office space for his medical practice.

Unlike her sister-in-law, Mary was not so firmly entrenched in Baltimore. Mary pondered a move to the Deanery, where much had changed since Mamie's departure in June 1904. While her thirty-year relationship with Carey was complementary and companionable, it was hardly idyllic. Carey often seemed to have two sides, the charming, brilliant, public side that had catapulted her to national fame and prestige, and the temperamental, narcissistic, controlling side that Mary referred to as her "demonic possessions." Despite her unsolicited tirades to Mary about managing fiscal affairs, Carey's own and those of the college were often in the red. Mary generously subsidized her friend's personal coffers and repeatedly helped the college out of financial emergencies, such as paying a $30,000 debt in 1903. Carey often belittled Mary, admonishing her to taking a supporting role to Carey's stardom. In 1902, when Mary attended one of Carey's lectures in New York, Mary sat on the platform with the honored guests. Carey was horrified that Mary would assume such rank and try to upstage her. "I thought you were completely out of place walking in with Professor Harrison . . . I *tried* to insist on you going to the floor but you did not back me up at all," she lashed out.[58]

Mary, too, had her faults. While not given to temperamental outbursts, as Carey often was, she, too, could be imperious, demanding, headstrong, and annoyingly finicky. Carey found her bossy. But Mary did not cower to Carey's rants. She would fire back or simply remove herself from the crosshairs of her friend's fury by setting off on another trip. Should she move to the Deanery, Mary knew theirs would hardly be a marriage—a Boston marriage—made in heaven.

Mary loved being at Bryn Mawr. With Carey's charisma, the college was developing into a hub of invigorating feminist activity and intellectualism that Mary craved for her life. During her campus visits, life at the Deanery with Carey, the faculty, and the students revitalized Mary more than any of her glamorous travels. While abroad in 1902, she wistfully wrote to Carey, "Your little letter made me homesick more than ever for you (and the Deanery, now!)."[59]

Mary wrote to Jewett expressing concern about cohabiting with Carey. Jewett counseled, "Oh Mary dear, I should have no right to give masked opinions on such a serious thing and great change as you speak of making such a move, as that must rest on people's conscience, but I love you very much and it makes me anxious," Jewett cautioned in October 1904. But Jewett realized that living at Bryn Mawr would fill the hollowness of Mary's life and would provide an important step in Mary's work for women's advancement. "After all, it isn't being happy that we ought to ask for, only as Carlyle says, '*the happiness of getting our work done.*'"[60]

Indeed, by the turn of the century, having paid off her six-year pledge to the Hopkins medical school in 1899 and with the Bryn Mawr School thriving, Bryn Mawr College and its president would become Mary's new philanthropic path to "help women." The move to Bryn Mawr, despite its possible emotional landmines, would provide "the happiness of getting her work done."

Caution thrown to the wind, Mary made the move. "Miss Mary Garrett, the famous daughter of the late John Work Garrett, to spend winter at Bryn Mawr," the *Washington Post* announced in November 1904. "She is very intellectual and her greatest interest in the higher education of women has led to a close friendship with Miss Thomas, to whom she has more than once made protracted visits."[61]

The "winter" mentioned in the article would extend for the next eleven winters. But Mary never stayed in one place too long—she had been a nomadic traveler since her days of global treks with her parents, dividing her time between continents. "Residents of her own city are used to her vagaries of travel, for she is just as apt to sail for a six-month tour of Europe at six hours' notice as to remain at home," the *Washington Post* explained. Within a month of moving to Bryn Mawr, she decamped to Jewett's cottage in Maine. But Carey and Bryn Mawr were always in her thoughts. "I woke up often and stayed awake a good deal," Mary wrote from Jewett's home in November of her usual insomnia-plagued nights. "I missed you, my darling."[62]

Mary developed an annual routine of staying at Bryn Mawr for the late fall and winter, sailing abroad in the spring for a long stay through summer, often with Carey or other friends, and returning to Baltimore in early fall for business, all punctuated by extended visits with friends around the country. She continued to visit New York, often going to the theater with Julia de Forest and Lou Knox, now

Mrs. Louis Comfort Tiffany, and continuing her interest in and financial support of the New York Infirmary for Indigent Women and Children.

Mary's extended stays at the Deanery beginning in 1904 proved successful and stabilizing for both women, despite what Mary called Carey's occasional "fits of temper." The two companions were, for the most part, loving and kind with each other and appreciative of the emotional support each gave in times of crisis. They grew increasingly dependent on each other and emotionally intimate. The extent of their physical relationship is unclear, for neither divulged anything more explicit than the usual expressions of love and affection exchanged between two cherished, longtime partners of a Boston marriage.[63]

Mary enjoyed a long period of healthfulness, putting the vicious Garrett family legal battles behind her. In place of her own estranged relatives, she adopted a surrogate family, Carey's big, boisterous extended family of siblings, nieces, and nephews. She threw herself into the rhythms of college life, socializing with the faculty and visiting the students in their dorms. She equally enjoyed the environs west of Philadelphia. First riding in an automobile in 1900, Mary frequently drove along the picturesque road next to the "Main Line" of the Pennsylvania Railroad tracks, from which the bucolic area derived its name. She would stop along the way to gather specimens of leaves, bringing them back to campus to catalogue. She took well to the experience of driving—once she figured out how the car worked. "I assure you the turning around and still more the backing of the thing is a most uncanny experience but while you are going straight ahead it is very nice."[64]

Carey's presidency flourished with her maturity and confidence and Mary's enduring encouragement and abundant patronage. Carey's life settled down and was far calmer than during her years with Mamie. The two women began to take on the familiarity and comfort of a long-married couple, spending quiet, enjoyable evenings at the Deanery. Mary devoured the novels of her favorite authors, Henry James and Edith Wharton, whose tales of oppressed and discontented upper-class women must have held special meaning. By nine each night, Carey and Mary were exhausted, "fit for nothing," from their day's work, as Mary wrote, and dropped off to sleep.[65] They filled the Deanery with cats—Maine Coons being their favorite—and called each other "Pussy."

Carey's niece Mary Worthington, a student at Bryn Mawr, comically captured the volatility and playfulness of the complex relationship. Attending a conference with her aunt and Mary, she wrote:

> Aunt Carey had lost her voice and wasn't allowed to speak & it was funny to see
> Miss Garrett having her revenge when Aunt Carey couldn't answer back. I had

the greatest difficulty restraining my laughter at times. They fought horribly & nearly came to blows at times. Miss Garrett would order Aunt Carey, who was reclining miserably in their drawing room, to do something. Aunt Carey would whisper back hoarsely—"I won't!" Then Aunt Carey would tell Miss Garrett to do something or another, and Miss Garrett quite certainly would say, "Indeed I won't!" And Aunt Carey would almost stamp with anger. But though Aunt Carey was always the most irrational & almost always wrong, you couldn't help taking her side.[66]

In the years leading up to Mary's "winters at Bryn Mawr," the campus began to blossom, bursting with beautiful buildings. In 1901, several Bryn Mawr alumnae wrote to John D. Rockefeller, asking the country's wealthiest industrialist to finance new dormitories. Impressed by the campus and Carey's clout, the senior Rockefeller turned the request over to his son John D. Rockefeller Jr. and philanthropic advisor Frederick T. Gates. Carey met with the men and soon had in hand a gift of $230,000 for a dormitory and power plant. But there was a catch— the amount had to be matched to fund a library building. Like Daniel Coit Gilman in his desperate search for a medical school donor, Carey was forced to take on the role of fundraiser. She did it brilliantly.

The matching gift campaign was a success. By 1902, Carey announced the college had raised slightly more than the required amount. Unfortunately, costs for constructing the huge Gothic stone library building had been grossly underestimated. Construction was well underway, but the money was running out.

Mary, too, dusted off her fundraising skills and stepped in to ask Andrew Carnegie to contribute to the library fund. He declined, as he had done for the medical school campaign. "I realized it was hopeless," Mary wrote to Carey. Four years later, with the failed Carnegie solicitation still on her mind, Mary sailed to Europe on the same ship as Carnegie. She bumped into him on the stairway of the ship and they talked for a while. She lay awake that night, wondering if she should approach him again for another contribution to the college. "I have no doubt I should fail if I did, but at least I could do no harm as he has already definitely refused to consider Bryn Mawr," she wrote to Carey.[67] She did not explain if she asked again.

To help the college's fundraising efforts, in 1903 Mary held a luncheon in honor of Mr. and Mrs. John D. Rockefeller Jr. at her Mount Vernon Place home to thank Rockefeller for his gifts to Bryn Mawr and to cultivate him for future financial support. Her perennial favorites, Drs. Halsted, Remsen, and Welch, rounded out the guest list. Given the importance of the occasion, she fussed endlessly over the details of the day, experimenting with table settings and floral arrangements. She first took the party of twelve to the Walters Gallery, a few doors away, to view her neighbor's extensive art collection. They returned to her home for the luncheon, where "the party of twelve [was] seated at a round table—very nicely with a centerpiece of yellow tulips and daisies." The table talk centered on Bryn Mawr, and Mary took every opportunity to extol Carey, ticking off her many accomplishments. Rockefeller quizzed Mary about the rising construction costs of the library. By the end of the luncheon, Rockefeller, apparently satisfied with Mary's answers to his interrogation, pronounced, "Bryn Mawr is the best woman's college."[68] Mary was delighted with the results. That evening, she excitedly reported the day's events in a letter to Carey, drawing a diagram of the seating arrangements and elaborating on the conversations.

The luncheon might have helped, for Carey again had to solicit Rockefeller for the library building. After tense give-and-take negotiations, the Rockefellers pulled through with $80,000 on Christmas Eve 1905. "The relief was unspeakable," Carey wrote in her journal.[69]

After her move to Bryn Mawr, Mary continued her own building campaign for the college. When the class of 1905 fell short of raising the funds needed to build a campus infirmary, Mary loaned the balance of $15,000, to be repaid if there ever were surplus funds. There never were. She built cottages for two professors, again with the understanding that she would be repaid if the college ever had extra cash. She deposited $36,000 in bonds to cover expenses when the students decided to rebuild the dilapidated College Inn. Aside from Mary's annual $10,000 gifts to the college stated in her offer to the trustees in 1893, Mary's gifts to the college eventually totaled nearly $500,000.

Mary envisioned grand plans to beautify Bryn Mawr College and to enhance Carey's prominence. She repeated a familiar pattern, as she had done with the Bryn Mawr School and the Women's Fund Memorial Building, to erect yet another superb monument to represent women's achievements, this time, Carey's presidency and the college's stature. In 1907, Mary, who was accustomed to living in grand style, made plans to completely overhaul the crowded, outdated, dreary Deanery and transform it into the luxurious locus of campus life.

It was no small vision. Earlier renovations from 1885 and 1896 were expanded or ripped away. The humble five-room Victorian faculty house that Carey and Mamie had shared during Carey's deanship and early presidency eventually evolved into a massive, forty-six-room manor home that, like the college's president, dominated the center of attention. All vestiges of Mary's predecessor were eradicated; Mamie's cramped, dark bedroom was transformed into a deluxe-sized, sunlit room for Mary. A third floor was added for new guest rooms and servants' quarters.[70]

To complete the interior, Lockwood de Forest imprinted his famous Ahmedabad signature throughout, in the brass filigree panels between ceiling beams and the luscious furniture that dominated the rooms. Kurdistan carpets covered the parquet floors. Inlaid tables from Damascus and teakwood tables from China all bore the indelible de Forest imprimatur. He created a beautiful first-floor study befitting the president. It replaced the old living room and gained renown as the "Blue Room," boasting a hand-stenciled ceiling and fireplace and reflecting Carey's love of pre-Raphaelite art. All agreed that de Forest's "decorative genius" permeated throughout the transformed Deanery.[71]

Louis Comfort Tiffany, who had created many pieces for both Mary and Mary Frick in Baltimore, designed the elegant lighting fixtures. The Deanery's rooms were tastefully appointed in the finest of *fin de siècle* elegance. The house was quiet, serene, and serious, with bookshelves lining the hallways and pictures, statuary, Victorian wallpaper, and bric-a-brac covering every available square inch of wall space, much of it transplanted from 101 West Monument Street. To add an exquisite outdoor finishing touch, Frederick Law Olmsted's stepson John created a sumptuous garden to surround the newly expanded building. Mary dotted the garden with her favorite Italian statuary. The finished Deanery, completed in 1909, could accommodate fifty-five houseguests. In many ways it resembled Montebello in its heyday, with its shingled exterior, elaborate gardens, and elegant interior. Not surprisingly, like the Bryn Mawr School with its unanticipated cost overruns, Mary's latest extravagance ended up doubling its original construction estimates, eventually costing more than $100,000.

The college, indebted to her beyond words, made a benevolent gesture. Under Pennsylvania law, the board of trustees created another governing Bryn Mawr board, a hands-on working board, the board of directors, which could include non-Quaker members. For Carey, who had engineered the new plan to distance the college from its Quaker exclusivity, Mary's election to the board broke through the barrier restricting governance to Quakers, at last fulfilling Carey's goal to make the college more secular. No matter the surreptitious reason, Mary was elated. She had finally achieved the academic recognition she had longed for her entire life.

Mary's elegant style and deep pockets transformed the fledging, modest Quaker college into a magnificent work of art, giving it the upper-class panache that Carey wanted and allowing it to attain a high academic standard. Mary's largess brought a polished, elegant look to the college during its formative years, and the college benefited from its association with one of the country's most publicized women.

And she did not just stop with giving scholarships, equipment, books, and buildings. Mary invested as much money and effort into reinventing the college's Quaker president as she did into expanding and enhancing the campus and classrooms. In turn, Carey began to reflect the campus's new elegance and sophistication, affecting her patron's upper-class style and ease in elite social circles. Like Mary, Carey luxuriated in the creature comforts of life.

The magnificent, welcoming campus, with its sturdy stone Gothic architecture, sprawling lawns, and electrifying feminist activism, rolled out the red carpet to an array of luminaries. In November 1905, two guests especially near and dear to Mary's heart, the venerable suffrage leader Susan B. Anthony and Anna Howard Shaw, president of the National American Woman Suffrage Association, visited Bryn Mawr. They met with Carey and Mary to discuss an important event to take place the following February in Baltimore.

—ᶜⁿⁿᵉ—

WISE AND FAR-SIGHTED

THE "FIGHTING BOB" OF WOMAN'S SUFFRAGE

Mary was ignited by suffrage. The movement for women's political enfranchise-ment, equality, and dignity in a society that treated women as second-class citi-zens represented the culmination of everything she had worked for as a philan-thropist and longed for in her own life. In 1894, she wrote to Carey, "I am more and more convicted and conscience-stricken over doing absolutely nothing in connection with Woman Suffrage, when it is so absolutely essential to the ac-complishment of everything we have most at heart. I wish I could think of some way—."[1] Eventually, she did think of a way, although it would take more than a decade before she could make an impact.

In 1894, Mary Putnam Jacobi had presented a paper, "Common Sense Ap-plied to Woman Suffrage," to the New York constitutional committee to argue for the right of women to cast a ballot. Writing in the New York Sun, Jacobi argued the point held by many middle- and upper-class women: that men, including for-mer male slaves and men without property, could vote, while women of all classes were universally excluded from the democratic process. "Never, until the estab-lishment of universal [male] suffrage, did it happen that all the women in a com-munity, no matter how well born, how intelligent, how well educated, how virtu-ous, how wealthy, were counted the political inferiors of all the men, no matter how base born, how stupid, how ignorant, how brutal, how poverty-stricken," Ja-cobi wrote.[2]

Mary, too, felt the sting of political powerlessness. She was incensed that she could not vote in the 1896 election pitting Democratic candidate William Jennings Bryan against Republican William McKinley. Like many Democrats, including incumbent Grover Cleveland, who was serving his second term and would not run again, Mary did not like Bryan and his populist views. Although she could not vote, her male servants could. She encouraged them to vote for McKinley. Later, she watched helplessly as the country veered toward what she felt was a dangerous imperialistic path with the Spanish-American War and the annexation of Hawaii and the Philippines. She resented not being able to cast a dissenting vote.

Mary and many other women wanted more voice in determining the nation's leaders and its future course of events. They also wanted to elect officials who could best protect hearth and home, families and children.

When Susan B. Anthony and Anna Howard Shaw visited Carey and Mary at Bryn Mawr in the fall of 1905, it was more than a social call. As a longtime devotee of suffrage, Mary, along with Emma Maddox Funck, president of the Maryland Suffrage Association, had lobbied to hold the National American Woman Suffrage Association's annual convention in Baltimore. But, that would prove challenging. For the first time, as suffrage historian Ida Husted Harper chronicled in the multivolume *History of Woman Suffrage*, the movement would march straight into "the very heart of conservatism"—Southern, tradition-bound Baltimore. At the meeting with Mary and Carey, Anthony "expressed some anxiety as to its reception in so conservative a city." Once known for its progressivism, in the decades after the Civil War Baltimore had become, according to Funck, "a Southern city, so steeped in conservatism that while its citizens meant well, metaphorically, it had never discarded its ruffles and silver buckles."[3]

By the 1890s, NAWSA struggled to bring life back to the moribund campaign, which over the years had lost steam—and members, with only ten thousand on the rolls. It was in desperate need of a public-relations makeover if it hoped to continue the arduous journey toward the passage of a federal amendment giving women the right to walk into a voting booth.

The movement began humbly, but with unexpected enthusiasm, in 1848, when young Elizabeth Cady Stanton joined older women, especially Philadelphia's Lucretia Mott, in convening a meeting at a church in Seneca Falls, New York. The declared purpose was to discuss "the social, civil and religious condition and rights of women."[4] Most of the three hundred attendees, including many men, were Quakers. Though their feminist ideology was radical, their behavior was quiet and pious. It was not until 1853, when a mob of young men, many of them Irish immigrants, heckled the women at their New York City convention, that the equal rights cause became associated with rabble-rousers.

There was nothing explicit in the United States Constitution that prohibited women from voting. It was simply assumed that women were not equipped with the intellectual ability or emotional stability to participate in the democratic process. The Fifteenth Amendment, ratified in 1870, giving the vote to black men, many of them former slaves, spurred women into even more urgent action.

Building its argument on the Enlightenment ideal of the "natural law" of women to have the right to vote, the movement broadened its scope in the 1850s to include controversial social issues such as divorce reform, experimental dress—such as the baggy, bifurcated "bloomers"—birth control, better education, working women's wages and, perhaps most incendiary, reinterpretations of the Bible. Association with such divisive issues, especially suffragist Victoria Woodhull's unrealistic 1872 presidential bid, added to widespread perceptions that political enfranchisement would not improve women's lives and often alienated leisure-class women.

The movement itself was rife with internal dissent, as well, with two opposing factions splitting off in 1869. Stanton and Anthony formed the militant New York–based National Woman Suffrage Association; Lucy Stone, Julia Ward Howe, and Henry Blackwell responded by establishing the less radical Boston-based American Woman Suffrage Association. Each group employed different tactics to achieve the same goal of suffrage. Finally realizing their opposition to each other was self-defeating, in 1890, the two groups set aside their differences and merged into the National American Woman Suffrage Association. Adding strength to NAWSA's numbers was the powerful Woman's Christian Temperance Union, headed until her death in 1898 by the indefatigable Frances Willard, who coalesced her minions of middle-class women to the cause of women's reform.

But it was not enough. By the last decade of the nineteenth century, NAWSA needed a fresh infusion of ideas and a bit of social élan to bring it respectability and prestige. It was still unpolished and rough around the edges. Suffragists, some thought, needed to abandon their gritty, militant image in favor of one that would provide a safer, more civilized appeal to middle- and leisure-class women who supported the issues but feared association with confrontational tactics.

Suffrage leaders devised a clever strategy, a "society plan" to recruit wealthy, well-connected women to the cause and, as Anthony explained to Mary and Carey during her 1905 visit, to invigorate a younger generation of women, "having a program in some way illustrate distinctly the new type of womanhood—the College woman."[5] Mary's money and Carey's academic stature would serve both purposes perfectly.

Suffrage leaders first introduced the "society plan" in 1893, when they convinced one of Denver's grande dames, Ione Theresa Hanna, to persuade her privileged and influential friends to back the cause. That year, Hanna gained fame at the Congress of Women held at the World's Columbian Exposition in Chicago, where she delivered a stinging speech on "The Ethics of Social Life." It is possible that while at the fair, Mary, Carey, and Mamie heard Hanna's riveting presentation, a speech that no doubt would have held special meaning for Mary. Hanna excoriated the double standard that allowed a son of the elite class to "employ his faculties as he shall choose, receive pecuniary compensation and therefor [sp], and be confident that he is fulfilling what a wise public opinion demands of him." But, "let a young woman of wealth, who is surrounded by sheltering friends, attempt the same career, and she quickly discovers the gates are closed . . . As the customs of society are now, there is nothing for these young women but impatiently waiting for somebody or something to turn up, Micawber-like [sp]."[6]

The endorsement of Hanna and her Denver socialite friends proved to be a turning point for suffrage. "A most marked result," one Denver suffragist wrote, "was that not one paper in Denver said a word of ridicule or even mild amusement concerning the suffragists."[7] Even better than ceasing their mockery of the movement, with the endorsement of Denver's society women, mainstream newspapers started to take the movement and its issues seriously.

But the more open-minded West, where many women were often unmindful of the prohibition against woman suffrage—in Wyoming women had been casting ballots for years—was far removed from the restrictions of the East Coast. Baltimore would be different—and much harder to win over. Mary had recruited the "names of influence" a decade earlier to support the medical school campaign, and suffrage, too, needed elite women to back the cause and give it legitimacy and polish.

Maryland women agitated for and achieved several legal and economic milestones in the closing years of the nineteenth century. Women gained more property rights, a wife was allowed to bring slander charges against her husband, a husband could be imprisoned for nonsupport of his family or wife beating, and the age of consent for girls was raised from fourteen to sixteen years of age. Baltimore women continued to press for suffrage through the Baltimore Suffrage Club, formed in 1894 with Emma Maddox Funck serving as president. They held Sunday afternoon teas to discuss the progress—or lack of it—in the movement and enthusiastically sent petitions to Congress. They wore "bloomers" and bobbed their hair, with one unenthusiastic observer noting of the new style, "a short haired woman and crowing hen are good for neither God nor men."[8] Repeatedly told to go home and tend to their children, suffragists ignored taunts of "queer" and "cracked" and "old crows." Such scoffs only emboldened the already fearless women.

With their economic and legal gains, their impressive accomplishments in education, charity, and public health work, and their brief, but encouraging, foray into suffrage agitation, Maryland women were becoming more confident. It was time to test the waters, to make the quantum leap from organizing state suffrage chapters to holding the highly visible national convention in Baltimore. And to ensure the convention's success, the organizers needed "help in high places," as Baltimore suffragists had noted in 1868.[9]

As one of the country's wealthiest and most publicized women, Mary jumped at the chance to advance suffrage's society plan. She did it wholeheartedly, having lived the suffrage struggle firsthand. Her wealth had not protected her from the societal discrimination women faced; in many ways, her aristocratic status had exacerbated the exclusion from opportunities other women enjoyed, such as Carey and Mamie's freedom to study in Europe in the 1870s. Mary was living testimony to the societal restrictions of upper-class women Ione Hanna had spoken of in her "Ethics of Social Life" speech. As with her crusade for the medical school a decade earlier, Mary became a tireless proselytizer, this time for suffrage. Dr. Lillian Welsh, an early Hopkins medical school graduate, later recalled how Mary had visited with her and Dr. Mary Sherwood, to "convert" them to the cause. "She assumed we were suffragists. In the course of the conversation, she turned to Dr. Sherwood and said: 'Of course, Dr. Sherwood, you believe in suffrage' . . . Dr. Sherwood responded, 'Why, Miss Garrett, I haven't thought much on this subject, but I think I should believe in it.'"[10]

By the time Anthony and Shaw visited Bryn Mawr to talk about the logistics of the 1906 Baltimore convention, Carey, who at first was hesitant about the movement, was as ready as Mary to assure its success. Several Bryn Mawr alumnae already were in the front trenches of the battle, both at the grassroots and national levels. Perhaps best known were Katharine Houghton Hepburn, class of 1899 — mother of another Bryn Mawr alumna, actress Katharine Hepburn, class of 1927 — and her sister Edith Houghton Hooker, class of 1901. Both would go on to become integral to suffrage in the 1910s, with Hooker founding *Maryland Suffrage News*, one of the most respected of the suffrage publications.

Anthony recalled in her autobiography Mary's enthusiasm to help: "I have decided — really I did so yesterday — that I must open my home in Baltimore for that week in order to have the great pleasure of entertaining you and Miss Shaw under my own roof and to do whatever I can to help make the meeting a success," Mary told Anthony.[11]

The convention opened the first week of February 1906. As promised, Mary opened her grand Mount Vernon Place mansion, closed for months at a time after she began spending winters at Bryn Mawr and traveling abroad, to add the glamour and prestige the organizers had hoped for. She made her home available for special meetings, receptions, and dinners and lodged the convention's VIPs.

One by one, the storied old guard of the movement made their way to Baltimore. Anthony arrived two days before the opening ceremony. En route from Rochester, the eighty-six-year-old suffrage veteran, already in failing heath, caught a deathly cold and by the time she arrived at Mary's was frail and exhausted. Anthony bristled at the thought of doctors hovering over her. Nonetheless, Mary immediately summoned her trusted medical advisors. The nurse had to masquerade as a housemaid to mask her identity to Anthony, who fretted about "giving trouble."[12] Next, eighty-seven-year-old Julia Ward Howe, whose "Battle Hymn of the Republic" had made her a national icon during the Civil War, arrived at Mary's. NAWSA president, Rev. Dr. Anna Howard Shaw, who held dual degrees in divinity studies and medicine; Hull House founder Jane Addams; and Carey soon joined Mary's bustling household, to stay for the duration of the convention.

Delegates and guests from around the country stayed at Baltimore's most luxurious hotel, the Belvedere. Holding rank as one of the city's tallest buildings, at twelve stories, its elegant brick-patterned walls and dark-paneled rooms with brass decor typified the Victorian ideal of stately elegance. The Belvedere had entertained kings and presidents and was certainly up to the task of entertaining the "Queens of the home."[13] The convention itself would be held nearby, at the spacious Lyric Theater, where, in an image ironic to the feminist goals of suffrage, each year Baltimore's eighteen-year-old debutantes "came out" to society at the Cotillion Ball, announcing to the world, in their frothy white gowns and elbow-length white gloves, their eligibility for marriage.

The press was starstruck. The city had not seen such a gathering of celebrities since the medical school campaign supporters had descended on Baltimore in 1890 to inspect the Johns Hopkins Hospital and attend Mary's splashy reception. "It is seldom that such a number of notable women gather in one city," the *Baltimore Sun* waxed lyrical. The NAWSA leaders arrived early: Alice Stone Blackwell, Lucy Stone's daughter; Florence Kelley; Carrie Chapman Catt; Dr. Henry Blackwell; Ida Husted Harper; Harriet Taylor Upton; and Elizabeth Hauser; among others. Four of Anthony's family attended, including her sister Mary. "Both [Anthony and her sister] have the same air of some queen who has held sway for a long time. In their bearing there is something which suggests comparison with the late Queen Victoria," the *Baltimore Sun* described.[14]

The 1906 convention proved significant in many ways, not only for breaking the barrier in a Southern, conservative city. Unprecedented numbers of participants attended and more prominent women and men—university presidents and professors, politicians, leaders of other national movements—attended than ever before, a sign of the growing acceptability of the movement.

Perhaps most significantly, the suffrage torch was being passed to a new generation. The old combat veterans of suffrage were getting old and dying out. Anthony had not been well enough to attend the opening ceremony on February 7. A large crowd had gathered to see the country's most recognized woman, "the most famous exponent of the cause," and was disappointed when illness kept her away. Anna Howard Shaw was "getting feeble and was unable to arise when introduced." Clara Barton, the indomitable founder of the American Red Cross, who had bravely nursed the wounded on Civil War battlefields and brilliantly devised the logistics of quickly moving medical supplies from battle to battle, joked that she "was too old to make a speech."[15]

Missing among the impressive lineup was Elizabeth Cady Stanton, who had died in October 1902. Seven years before her death, Stanton published the first volume of the *Woman's Bible*, in which she catalogued passages from the Bible that she felt debased and subordinated women. It immediately hit the bestsellers lists and ignited a firestorm, not least within NAWSA, which was trying to court middle- and upper-class conservative women. The leadership voted to censure her. She died of heart failure two weeks before her eighty-seventh birthday.

Maryland Governor Edwin Warfield, perhaps hoping to downplay Emma Funck's dour description of Maryland, welcomed the august guests: "A man who would not extend a welcome to such a body of women would not be worthy of the name of Maryland, which we consider a synonym for hospitality . . . While I may not agree with all your teachings, I recognize one fact, that there has never been assembled in Baltimore a convention composed of women who have been more useful to this country and who have done more for the uplift of humanity."[16]

Committees convened and delegates debated the issues to be covered during the convention. The agenda was packed. In addition to suffrage, class issues, poverty, child labor, prostitution, pay and working conditions for wage-earning women, and the abolition of war dominated the issues.

As the convention picked up, speakers hammered home the message that women must counteract society's one-dimensional image of them as only homemakers. Careful not to dethrone the "queens of the home," NAWSA president Shaw cautiously crafted her words in her opening address, reinforcing the basic principle of the natural law of women to enjoy the same rights and opportunities as men and to have the right to vote for the representatives who protect the home and its children.

The subject of money made its way into many of the speeches. NAWSA counted a mere $28,000 in its campaign war chest in 1906. "If we had money for all the things we wanted," one delegate noted, "we could enfranchise all the women in half the states in as many years." The attendees, mostly middle-aged and older women, more than likely knew how to roll up their sleeves to raise money. They had done it enough in their own community-based voluntary organizations. But, like for most women's organizations, in suffrage big gifts were the exception and small donations the rule. At every session, the organizers passed the collection basket around. Anthony stepped up to donate the $86 gift that had been raised in Rochester for her eighty-sixth birthday before she had left for Baltimore. Mary followed with a gift of $300 for lifetime NAWSA memberships for herself and Carey. Shaw gave $2,800 representing several state chapters. Even Governor Warfield, taking a moment away from posing for photographers, "tucked a crisp ten dollar bill in among the offerings."[17] By the end of the convention, the organizers added $3,500 to the coffers.

Mary attended most of the sessions, much to the delight of the press, which seldom saw the famous fifty-two-year-old philanthropist in public. She sat quietly each day in her box at the Lyric, wearing her "spectacles" and "absorbed in the presentations." While each day's newspapers were filled with the news of the visiting celebrities and their photographs, Mary had forbidden the newspapers to print any photographs of her. Her name was recognizable, but she, herself, was not. "While Miss Garrett is one of Baltimore's most notable women—perhaps the most notable—she is personally unknown to a great many of her fellow citizens," the Baltimore News reported. "In fact, a large proportion of the audience at the Lyric did not realize that Miss Garrett was in their midst, but when she was pointed out, sitting in a box, all eyes were centered on her. Everyone had heard of Miss Mary Garrett, but few had seen her." In lieu of the forbidden photographs, the press described her as having "a kind, thoughtful face, and a rather literary aspect is added by the spectacles," appearing much like the image John Singer Sargent had captured in her portrait two years earlier. Dr. William Halsted, Governor Warfield, or Major Venable—"a woman's rights man"—usually accompanied her in her box.[18]

Amidst the brilliant speeches and heated debates of the convention, Anthony's "college evening" stole the show. Anthony, who had conceived of the idea of engaging a new generation of college-educated women to endorse the movement, rose from her sickbed at Mary's to attend. "When she appeared on stage and the

great audience realized she was actually with them their enthusiasm was un-
bounded. She was so white and frail as to seem almost spiritual but on her sweet
face was an expression of ineffable happiness; and it was indeed one of the happiest moments of her life for it typified the intellectual triumph of her cause,"
Harper recalled in *History*. The audience was so roused to be in the presence
of their beloved "Aunt Susan" and the accolades flowed so freely that "the 'College Evening' . . . might just as well have been called the 'Susan B. Anthony
Evening,'" the *Baltimore American* noted. One man in the audience—and there
were many men suffragists in attendance—"became so excited when she stood to
speak that he stood right up in the meeting and shouted her name."[19]

Carey drew upon her vast connections in education for the college evening's
speakers and "pretty college girls"—students at Baltimore's Women's College—
"in their caps and gowns, made attractive ushers."[20] Hopkins president Ira Remsen
was part of a stellar lineup that included the country's most renowned women educators: Mary Woolley, president of the country's oldest women's college, Mount
Holyoke; Lucy Salmon, professor of history at Vassar College; Mary Jordon, professor of English at Smith College; Maud Wood Park, of Radcliffe College and
president of the Boston branch of the Equal Suffrage League in Women's Colleges; and Carey, representing Bryn Mawr. The speakers explained how they had
first been energized by suffrage, hoping to incite the younger generation into action. Carey triumphantly closed the college evening with an inspiring speech,
driving home the message of women's need to vote for the right leaders to protect
themselves and their families from hardship.

If Carey held up her end of the bargain to deliver top-tier educators and college women to suffrage, Mary brilliantly did her part to put "society" into suffrage's "society plan." Morning, noon, and night throughout the convention, selected guests dined, brunched, and convened in Mary's home, the social hub of
the convention. To add the dash of elitism the organizers desired—and the press
found irresistible—Mary sent special invitations to the convention's crème de la
crème to attend private meetings to rub elbows with the governor and local VIPs
or, better, with Anthony, Shaw, and Howe.

Following the successful college evening, Mary hosted "one of the largest and
most brilliant receptions of the season," rivaling the fifteen-hundred-guest gala
she had held in November 1890 for the Women's Medical School Fund. It was
held in honor of her houseguests, Anthony, Shaw, and Howe, as well as other convention notables. "The entire first floor, including the famous art gallery, was
thrown open for the occasion, each apartment being lavishly decorated in cut
flowers of a corresponding color tone. In the supper-room, a profusion of Ameri-

can Beauty roses were used with red shaded lights," the *Baltimore American* reported. But the show stopper was the scene of "Miss Anthony and Mrs. Howe sitting side by side on a divan in the large bay window, with a background of ferns
and flowers. At their right stood Miss Garrett and Dr. Thomas, at their left Dr.
Shaw and the line of eminent college women, with a beautiful perspective of
[the] conservatory and the art gallery."[21]

Among the more than four hundred guests was the Friday Night's Bessie King,
who many years earlier had married William Ellicott, heir to a flour mill fortune.
Bessie had faded from the medical school fund campaign as it slowed in the final
year, and she had disagreed about the final terms of Mary's gift. She had transferred her medical school activism to become an outspoken and ardent suffragist.
She was one of the founders of, and eventually president of, the elite Arundell
Club, a group of Baltimore's most prominent women who promoted the eco-
nomical and efficient management of government. Bessie was an important
player in Maryland suffrage and one whom Anthony wanted to court, particularly
to gain entrée to the prestigious Arundell Club.

Jane Addams, famous by the turn of the century for her settlement-house work
for Chicago's immigrants, delivered a stirring speech on "The Modern City and
the Municipal Franchise for Women." Dr. William Welch, dean of the Hopkins
medical school, presided over the session. Addams's presentation at the convention castigated the sorry state of urban affairs in the United States: "[u]nsanitary
housing, poisonous sewage, contaminated water, impure milk . . . ," her list continued. And the reason for the deplorable mess? "City housekeeping has failed
partly because women, the traditional housekeepers, have not been consulted as
to its multiform activities," Addams chastised. By the turn of the century, women's
voluntary groups focused much of the time on improving their communities
through "municipal housekeeping" but often waged an uphill battle against gov-
ernmental policies. "The men have been carelessly indifferent to much of this
civic housekeeping, as they have been indifferent to the details of the household."
Welch heartily agreed, concluding, "the administration of a city was largely
housekeeping on a large scale, and that the more women's influence was felt in
such matters, the better for the people." He later was won over by the suffragists,
declaring that they "are not such a queer lot of people as many suppose."[22]

As the nine-day convention drew to a close, Anthony spoke privately to Mary
and Carey. The movement desperately needed money, the ailing suffragist told
them. The leaders lived hand-to-mouth to meet expenses. Anna Howard Shaw,
in her 1915 autobiography *The Story of a Pioneer*, later recalled how Mary and
Carey "admitted they had sat up throughout the previous night, talking the mat-

ter over and trying to find some way to help us." Carey and Mary, time-tested veterans of several uphill fundraising campaigns, assured Anthony they could "find a number of women like themselves who were unable to take an active part in working for suffrage but sincerely believed in it, and who would be willing to join together in contributing $12,000 a year for the next five years." Shaw later wrote, "The mere mention of so large a fund startled us all. We feared that it could not possibly be raised. But Miss Anthony plainly believed that now the last great wish of her life had been granted. She was convinced that Miss Thomas and Miss Garrett could accomplish anything—even the miracle of raising $60,000 for the suffrage cause—and they did, though 'Aunt Susan' was not here to glory over the result when they achieved it."[23]

The fundraising plan called for a $500 annual contribution from wealthy supporters of the cause. With Mary and Carey's connections, donors lined up to give, a far more enthusiastic response than the women's medical fund campaign fifteen years earlier. It took only three months to raise the $60,000. The *Washington Post* announced that the goal had been met by May 1907, four years ahead of schedule. "The work of securing subscribers to the fund was begun in February of this year [1907] and by April 20 the entire amount was secured, there being twenty-three contributors in amounts of $500, $1,000 and $2,500, and one of $20,000 from 'a friend.'" The "friend" who anonymously gave $20,000 was later revealed to be Olivia Slocum Sage, whose financier husband, Russell, died in 1906, leaving his childless widow with a $65 million fortune and the means to become a renowned and influential philanthropist in her own right. Mary contributed $2,500. The fund was aptly named the Susan B. Anthony Fund and continued to be used until 1912. "It had not seemed possible that such a burden could be lifted from my shoulders," Shaw wrote.[24]

The close of the 1906 convention was especially poignant, for it was obvious to all that Anthony's health was rapidly ebbing. Doctors had long warned her to be more mindful of her health, but she decided she'd rather "die in the harness" than surrender her militancy. Anthony expressed gratitude to the leadership who had kept the dream alive, a critical component of the ultimate success of the movement that can never be overstated. "'There have been others just as true and devoted to the cause—I wish I could name every one—but with such women consecrating their lives'—here she paused for an instant and seemed to be gazing into the future, then dropping her arms to her side she finished her sentence—'failure is impossible!'"[25]

These were the last words Anthony spoke in public. Before returning home to Rochester, she detoured with a large contingency of delegates to Washington,

D.C., to attend the annual hearings of the Senate Committee on Woman Suffrage. But she was too ill to get out of bed. After a difficult, frigid trip back to Rochester, she died of pneumonia a month later in her home. As she lay dying, she said to her sister, "Write to Anna Shaw immediately, and tell her I desire that every cent I leave when I pass out of this life shall be given to the fund which Miss Thomas and Miss Garrett are raising for the cause."[26]

Anthony, once reviled as a troublemaker, would become canonized by the new generation of suffragists, who would revise her militant, combative image into a domesticated, saintly icon as they continued their battle for another fourteen years. On her deathbed, Shaw insisted, Anthony had predicted her immortality. "I may be able to do more for the Cause after I am gone than while I am here."[27]

For NAWSA, the Baltimore convention had been an overwhelming success, "one of the greatest in the history of the movement." The presentations thought-provoking, the participants passionate in their loyalty to the cause, the suffrage torch was handed to a new generation of educated, wealthy women, and the newspapers overflowed with flattery. Mary and Carey emerged as new stars in NAWSA's constellation; Carey for securing the "remarkable representation of Women's Colleges," and Mary for adding "the social prestige which is especially necessary to the success in a southern city."[28]

But the convention had mixed results for women in "the heart of conservatism." Maryland suffragists introduced a bill for the right to vote in the 1906 legislature, but lawmakers "treated it as a joke," Harper wrote.[29] Etta Maddox, Emma Funck's sister and the state's first woman attorney, led a lineup of expert speakers to lobby the Maryland legislature. In 1910, lawmakers finally granted the women a hearing on a suffrage bill. It was voted down sixty-one to eighteen.

Many women supported the Maryland legislators' efforts to keep women out of the voting booth. Not everyone agreed suffrage was a good move for women. The National Anti-Suffrage Association, or "antis," was organized to block the suffrage movement at every turn. Maryland had its own chapter, the Association Opposed to Woman Suffrage, organized in Baltimore in 1911 with many of Baltimore's best-known women throwing their clout and money to stop the enfranchisement of women. Mary Frick Garrett served as president of the Baltimore chapter. The group sent large amounts of money out of state to help defeat the ratification of a federal suffrage amendment.

Mary Frick was as outspoken in her efforts to impede enfranchisement as Mary was in the uphill battle to get the vote. Once again, as in the medical school campaign, the sisters-in-law held polarized views. "I have undertaken this work because I am fully convinced that a large majority of the women of this State do not want the ballot and also because I feel that a number do not realize what having a vote would mean. The use of the ballot is not a right but a privilege and I feel that granting this privilege to women would not be a step to advance womanhood," Mary Frick told the National Anti-Suffrage League in 1912. She fortified her speeches with statistics showing women's lives did not improve after winning the vote. In California, she stated, infant mortality rose after enfranchisement. Suffragists' claims that enfranchisement would improve the lot of the working women were "preposterous," she insisted. She cited statistics "to prove that working women are protected to a greater degree in states where they have no suffrage than in those where they have the voting franchise," as she told the Stenographers Association of Baltimore in the assembly hall of Strayer College.[30]

Of most concern to Mary Frick was that the ideal of womanhood would become tarnished from the association with "unclean politics" and abandoning the home. "A woman can exercise a greater influence in the management of her home than by putting herself on equal political footing with her husband and marching to the polls, deserting her home and doing things in the cause of suffrage." Besides, she argued, women would vote "generally as do the men of the family."[31] As with Mary Frick's efforts to undermine the Women's Medical School campaign, Mary made no public comments about her sister-in-law's oppositional stance on suffrage.

The 1906 convention spurred Mary into greater suffrage activism, in Baltimore and, particularly, at the national level. Following Carey's conversion to suffrage and in the afterglow of the convention, Bryn Mawr emerged as the collegiate nerve center of suffrage. It was the springboard Mary needed, as she gained recognition as one of the first well-to-do, nationally visible women to back the cause. She became treasurer of the National College Equal Suffrage League, started in 1906 by Bostonian Maud Wood Park and presided over by Carey.

Mary often returned to Baltimore during the state suffrage conventions to "order the boards down on her front door, to give some hurried instructions to her chef and fall to entertaining." Suffrage's well-strategized "society plan" soon paid off, as increasing numbers of well-to-do women joined the cause. By 1915, the movement counted one million members.[32]

Once again, the press found the combination of "the country's wealthiest spinster" and activist philanthropist—and now suffragist—to be irresistible. "Miss Mary Garrett of Baltimore. The 'Fighting Bob' of Woman's Suffrage Cause, Comes from Famous Old Family," the *Chicago Daily Tribune* headlined an article. But would her famous old family have been proud of her efforts? "The ancestors of Miss Garrett . . . would have shaken their heads askance if they could have known to what end they were fortune building. Such is the fight that one Puritan woman is putting up in this most modern of battles,"[33] the *Tribune* concluded.

Mary continued the fight. Baltimore made headlines in 1912 with one of the first big suffrage parades, which would come to dominate suffrage activism in its final decade. The Baltimore parade predated the well-known 1913 Washington, D.C., suffrage parade held in conjunction with Woodrow Wilson's inauguration. "Society Aids Suffragists," the *Washington Post* wrote of the planned parade through the heart of Baltimore. "Society girls, business women, college girls, and last, but not least, some well known business and professional men, will take part in the woman suffrage parade . . . There are going to be hundreds of people—some say a thousand—in the parade." The leading participants of the parade gathered at Mary's Mount Vernon Place mansion, where they donned their Joan of Arc costumes and climbed aboard their Roman chariots to ride through the streets of Baltimore to demonstrate "in picturesque effect the progress of the States that have granted votes to women," the *New York Times* reported.[34]

The Maryland state legislature was not impressed. When the Nineteenth Amendment was passed in 1920 giving women the right to vote, Maryland was one of a handful of states that did not ratify the amendment. Not only did Maryland vote down state ratification, but legislators sent the anti-suffrage president to Washington with a resolution threatening to disavow federal ratification in other states as well. No other state took such drastic measures to keep women out of the voting booth.

Despite the flamboyant Joan of Arc costumes, the daring chariot rides through Baltimore, the well-attended conventions, and the countless hours of plotting and agitating, in the end, as Emma Maddox Funck prophesized, Baltimore had never "discarded its ruffles and silver buckles." In Maryland, at least, failure *was* possible.

THE PEACE WHICH COMES WITH YEARS

As Mary closed up her Monument Street mansion after the 1906 convention and returned to her normal routine of dividing her time between Bryn Mawr and travel, she began a quieter, calmer stretch of life than the unsettled, turbulent decade of lawsuits, family estrangement and deaths, and the loss of the B&O. Now in her fifties and "speaking with a voice that must have come to America in that overloaded vessel the *Mayflower*," as the *Chicago Tribune* waxed poetic in

1911, "she was the Priscilla grown older, wealthier, and rosier with the peace which comes with years."[35]

Although she may not have grown wealthier, her finances had stabilized after the final distribution of her father's estate. She accepted the fates, both her losses and gains, and was enjoying the relative "peace which comes with years." While she was still haunted by the rupture of her family, life with Carey steadied her, giving her the ballast she needed. They traveled, she enjoyed the companionship of old friends and the busyness of college life, she remained passionate about suffrage, and she watched with satisfaction the fruits of her labors. The Hopkins medical school gained national fame, the Bryn Mawr School thrived, and suffrage rebounded from the slump of the 1890s. She enjoyed national celebrity as a respected philanthropist and activist.

As she focused on Bryn Mawr College and Carey, Mary untangled and narrowed her complex financial life. Disposing of massive Montebello was a priority. It held only bittersweet memories for her. As a young girl, she had raced across the fields on her father's splendid thoroughbreds. She had enjoyed her parents' many celebrity parties there. The Friday Night had headquartered their Bryn Mawr School meetings there. As children, Mary's nephews had romped through the gardens and ridden their pony carts along the paths; now they no longer spoke to her. Her two oldest brothers had died many years earlier.

The Smith mansion in Lower Montebello had sat unused for decades, and except for occasional stays by her brother Henry in Upper Montebello, her father's once-magnificent country estate served little purpose for her.[36] The house and grounds sat fallow. The estate had followed the fate of John Hopkins's nearby Clifton, falling into a state of dilapidation and disrepair. Mary turned over the unused grounds to the Bryn Mawr School, allowing the students to convert the spacious open areas to athletic fields and to use the gardens to practice their agricultural skills. She renovated her father's once-renowned thoroughbred stables into locker rooms with showers for students.

By the early 1900s, Mary began selling off parcels of the estate. But, like every other business matter in her life, disposing of Montebello, even in bits and pieces, was mired in circumstances beyond her control. John Work Garrett had pieced together his great estate from various parcels of land in northeast Baltimore. For Mary, selling off any one of them was an ordeal. In 1907, the city requested a portion of Lower Montebello for the right of way for a proposed electric railroad to connect Baltimore north to the Susquehanna River. A covenant to the land in question made prior to the Garretts' purchase indicated the land was subject to certain conditions enumerated in the earlier deed. The city held the power to pur-

chase the land for the railroad. "Our view is that a sale of the portion of the property desired by the City would be advantageous to the remainder of your property,
and the offer made is so very close to the value that we would be disposed, were
the property owned by us, to consider the proposition favorably." The city offered
$2,000 an acre. Mary balked at the idea of not selling the land for much more, but
eventually settled. She donated some of the land to Morgan College, now Morgan State University.[37]

That summer, she and Carey met with the purchasing agent to review the electric railroad plans. They carefully walked through the rundown, weed- and
graffiti-covered former home of Revolutionary War hero General Samuel Smith.
The mansion had once been considered to be the most magnificent in the state
and of great sentimental value to Marylanders. Mary and Carey surveyed the
damage from years of neglect and made an on-the-spot decision to tear it down.
The purchasing agent tried to convince them to at least salvage some of the beautiful handcrafted woodwork or the Italian marble fireplace in the oval dining
room. Mary agreed and the ornaments were moved to a nearby shed. Not long
after, the shed burned to the ground, and not a trace of the elegant woodwork remained. The mansion was soon razed.

There were more personal losses. In June 1906, just a few months after Anthony died, Mary's beloved friend and physician, Mary Putnam Jacobi, the muse
who had helped to shape Mary's philanthropies and ideals, who had brought her
through despair and depression thirty years earlier, died of an inoperable tumor.
Always the inquiring scientist to the end, Jacobi documented her disease as it took
her life. Another great friend, Sarah Orne Jewett, had been seriously injured in a
carriage accident in 1902 and remained severely debilitated. Her head injuries essentially ended her brilliant writing career. Mary frequently visited her longtime
friend at her Maine home and, after Jewett's death in 1909, continued her friendship with Jewett's sister Mary, corresponding frequently. Julia de Forest died the
following year.

Mary had lost her ties to her family, as well. On May 1, 1907, Mary's nephew
Robert married Katherine Barker Johnson in a springtime ceremony—"the most
notable in Baltimore in several years"—at the Old St. Paul's Protestant Episcopal
Church. The bride was resplendent in a gown of "ivory chiffon, heavily embroidered with point lace"; the nine bridesmaids "delicate and pretty in white and
pink"; and throngs of onlookers crowded the streets around the church to see the
society guests, which included Woodrow Wilson, then president of Princeton
University.[38] A year later, her other nephew, John Work, married Washingtonian
Alice Warder. By then, John had been working his way up the diplomatic corps

for seven years and was serving as secretary of the American embassy in Rome. He eventually would be appointed ambassador to Italy. The more intimate wedding, held on December 24, 1908, included one hundred family members and friends at St. John's Episcopal Church in Washington, D.C. Mary apparently did not attend either wedding. The newspapers made no mention of her.

A happier event brought Mary back to Baltimore in early 1907. John Singer Sargent had finished the painting Mary had commissioned of the founding physicians of the Hopkins medical school. The portrait was fittingly named *The Four Doctors*. It was nearly eight years from the time Mary first thought of the idea in 1899 until the massive 11- × 14-foot, four-hundred-pound portrait was delivered for the unveiling ceremony.

Sargent had painted large canvases before—his 1882 *El Jaleo*, with its fiery flamenco dancers, being among his most famous—but composing *The Four Doctors* proved difficult. The four physicians traveled to London to sit for Sargent in his Tite Street studio collectively and, on occasion, separately. Sargent struggled mightily with the composition of the portrait, first arranging the subjects in sitting positions, then trying standing positions. When all seemed acceptable, the perfectionist painter panicked. It was all wrong, he insisted, something was missing. "It will not do. It isn't a picture. I cannot see just what to do, but it isn't a picture."[39] He decided to add props, ordering a massive Venetian globe to be brought to the studio. The doorframe had to be removed to allow the globe to fit through.

Despite the difficult logistics, the physicians were very much taken with Sargent. Welch described the artist "as a tall, strong, altogether virile type; very agreeable to meet; a widely cultivated man, able to talk well on any subject that might be brought up."[40]

After working on the painting for a year, Sargent finally exclaimed, "We have got our picture!" Like many of Sargent's paintings, *The Four Doctors* is overwhelmingly dark, with highlights of red and light reflected from the huge globe and the faces and hands of the subjects. He portrayed the famed physicians in their full academic regalia, not in their usual physicians' attire. His reason for doing so is unclear, although Mary may have suggested it after the success of Carey's academic portrait. The academic gowns celebrate the learned achievements of the new age of scientific medicine, which the new Hopkins medical school represented, elevating the physicians to a scholarly status and making them resemble Renaissance scientific gentlemen rather than clinical practitioners. Sargent seamlessly pieced together four large canvases to achieve the overall effect of stature and importance.

The painting was completed in 1906 and shipped from Liverpool on December 15, 1906, insured at a value of $10,000. It arrived at Hopkins' McCoy Hall twenty days later and was hung directly across the room from Sargent's portrait of Mary in the Donovan Room. Mary wrote to university president Ira Remsen, suggesting two versions for the inscription to be placed on the frame. "I should be glad also to know your opinion about inserting the name of the donor. I had not thought of it but Dr. Halsted seemed to think it might be a matter of interest in the future."[41] She suggested the following inscription: "Dr. William H. Welch, Dr. William S. Halsted, Dr. William Osler and Dr. Howard A. Kelly, Professors of Pathology, of Surgery, of Medicine and of Gynecology from the opening of the Medical School of the Johns Hopkins University in 1893 until the painting of this portrait in 1905, to whose eminence as investigators and teachers is due in great measure its fame as a school of scientific medicine. Presented by Mary Elizabeth Garrett." Remsen responded that the frame was too small for such a wordy inscription. Mary, understanding the limitations, suggested that her name be placed on a plaque to hang below the frame, an idea recommended by Sargent. The final inscription was much abbreviated, with simply the names of the four physicians placed in an ornamental oval on the frame. Mary's name, as the benefactor, was omitted.

Another misunderstanding arose over Mary's participation in the unveiling ceremony on January 19, 1907. Remsen had asked Mary to briefly speak, with Osler and New York Tribune art critic Royal Cortissoz giving the main addresses. He had understood that she wanted to make remarks. Mary, mortified at the thought of public speaking, immediately corrected him. "I telegraphed you this morning a receipt of your letter because I feared that we had misunderstood each other about the part you wished me to take in the unveiling of the portrait group." She stated she was "unaccustomed to public speaking . . . I believe donors are usually supposed not to be practiced speakers."[42]

Notwithstanding the absent acknowledgment on the portrait, Remsen was complimentary during the unveiling ceremony. "As long as Johns Hopkins University shall endure you will be remembered for your generous gifts, which made possible the opening of the medical school, which is part of the university."[43]

Within a month of the unveiling, The Four Doctors and Sargent's portraits of Mary and Carey were exhibited at the Corcoran Art Gallery in Washington, D.C. The signage, as well as the newspapers, finally gave Mary her due, acknowledging "the portrait group [was] recently presented to the Johns Hopkins University by Miss Mary Garrett." The Four Doctors achieved much celebrity. Before shipping the portrait to Baltimore, Sargent had agreed to have it serve as the centerpiece at a private showing before the opening of the 138th exhibition of the Royal

Academy in London in 1906. The *New York Sun* reported the painting to be "the noblest work of art that has been hung in the Royal Academy since Sir Joshua Reynolds was president of it, and the most important and impressive of its type that has been painted by any man since the seventeenth century drew its curtain across the art of Holland."[44]

After its 1907 tour, *The Four Doctors* was removed from the exhibition circuit. It now hangs in the Welch Library on the Hopkins medical campus, where Mary's portrait is also exhibited.

To commemorate Bryn Mawr's first quarter of a century in 1910, the trustees gave Carey a much-needed leave of absence. "This is President Thomas' first vacation in the 26 years she has been dean and president of the college," the *Washington Post* reported on New Year's Day, 1911.[45] Carey and Mary sailed to England and traveled on for a three-month stay in Egypt. It was the last major trip the two longtime companions would make together. Not long after their return, Mary would face a much more personal battle, far more difficult than opening the country's most advanced medical school or helping women to get the vote. This time, she would not win.

TO ADVANCE ON THE SAME TERMS AS MEN

A year after her return from Egypt, Mary began to develop health problems far more troubling than the ones that had sent her to health spas for most of her life. Like her father, Mary's years of chronic bad health suddenly turned acute. In late 1911, while living at Bryn Mawr, she consulted a physician, Dr. J. H. Musser, in nearby Philadelphia. Her childhood ankle injury had caused her great pain for more than a year, and her overall health was weakening as well. The physician recommended the usual treatment for the ambiguous aches and pains that might plague a fifty-seven-year-old woman, to "have elimination brought about by sweating, followed by douches."[46]

However, when her symptoms worsened the following April, Mary was hospitalized at the Johns Hopkins Hospital. This time, the diagnosis was more definite—and far more disturbing: leukemia. In the early years of the twentieth century the malignant blood disease baffled pathologists and often was misdiagnosed as pernicious anemia. The disease had only been recognized as a "distinct malady" just a few decades earlier.[47] Carey's brother-in-law Simon Flexner, at the Rockefeller Institute, confirmed Mary's diagnosis. Surgeon William Halsted, Mary's friend and physician, stepped in to supervise her treatment. There were no two places in the country that could better diagnose a disease and collaborate on a course of treatment than Hopkins and "the Rockefeller."

Unfortunately for Mary, there was little doctors could do at the time to stop the progression of the disease. About a decade earlier, x-rays and radiation had been introduced for cancer diagnosis and treatment. The removal of the spleen was also recommended for leukemia patients to remove the body's source of producing the abundant white blood cells that characterize the disease.

Perhaps a lifetime of illness and family tragedy gave Mary the strength to persevere in the face of her latest misfortune. After the diagnosis of what the *Washington Post* called her "puzzling internal illness," Mary carried on, with complaints of a backache, flu-like symptoms, and the malaise of leukemia.[48] She returned from Baltimore to Bryn Mawr, where she continued to handle the business of the Deanery when Carey was traveling. She tended to her own business matters, answering, or ignoring, the endless letters of solicitation for money that arrived daily in the mail, handling lingering issues with the family's B&O divestiture and property settlement, selling timber at Deer Park, supervising housekeeping at her Mount Vernon Place home, or meeting with headmistress Edith Hamilton to discuss Bryn Mawr School business. She managed the care of her invalid brother, Henry.

By the next year, Mary's health was in serious decline. She began a torturous two-year odyssey of ineffective treatments and frequent hospitalizations for medical conditions that, under normal circumstances, would have required little attention. In February 1913, just days after helping Carey to entertain two hundred guests at the annual meeting of the Bryn Mawr Alumnae Association at the Deanery, Mary developed an infection in her left thumb. "It is not expected that she will stay in the hospital more than a few days," the *Baltimore News* reported after she was transported to Johns Hopkins Hospital.[49] The few days stretched into nearly two months. She lay in her bed in Ward 32 of the Hopkins Hospital until April, writing to friends when possible. She was finally able to leave the hospital and travel to her much-loved New York for a few weeks, but her languorous, months-long trips abroad were no longer possible.

Carey was especially attentive during Mary's hospitalizations, writing newsy letters from Bryn Mawr and updating her on the latest campus developments. The college was gaining more fame. Two years earlier, a young alumna, Carola Woerishoffer, class of 1907, had died, leaving a bequest of $750,000 to Bryn Mawr. Carey would soon put it to good use, proposing the country's first graduate school of social work.

Carey put on a brave front as she watched the slow, painful decline of her life-long friend and treasured companion. Carey faced medical problems of her own, undergoing surgery for removal of a tumor and skin grafts on her childhood burn injury. But Carey mended, while Mary worsened.

By 1914, Mary's limited medical options were running out. She was in constant, excruciating pain. She wrote to Dr. Frank Smith of Baltimore, grasping for hope and inquiring about the details of one of his patients, a Miss Huber, with a case similar to her own. His response gave her confidence she could overcome the disease. "It is impossible to make a definitive diagnosis," he responded optimistically, "cancer, I believe, can be outwitted."[50]

Her own physicians were not as optimistic. They recommended the removal of her spleen. Halsted was traveling in Europe for the summer, but concurred with the recommendation, writing his "expression of hope for the operation." Mary shuddered at the thought of major surgery. Her mother's sister, her "Aunt Beebie," comforted her. "I cannot tell you how grieved I am to know how you have suffered," Rebecca Harrison wrote in June 1914, "and that you have to have an operation, but you are in the hands of the best surgeons."[51]

The spleenectomy was successful, but Mary's recuperation was not. Her incision did not heal. She was weak and suffered from debilitating headaches. Halsted returned early from his European trip to attend to her. Drs. Simon Flexner and Henry Thomas, Carey's brother-in-law and brother, frequently treated Mary at Bryn Mawr, where she stayed when not hospitalized in Baltimore.

News of Mary's rapid decline in late 1914 circulated among friends and family. Friends wrote to wish her well. "I think of you and wish good things for you," Mary Jewett, Sarah's sister, with whom Mary had corresponded since Sarah's death five years earlier, wrote. Mary's nephews, Robert III and John Work II, who were not aware of their aunt's serious health problems for the first year, were cordial and conciliatory as her disease progressed, often sending small presents to her. She wrote fewer and fewer letters, her once elegant, embellished handwriting becoming almost indecipherable. In February 1915, she sent a valentine to William Halsted, always one of her favorite people. "I shall prize it & keep it always with the other tokens of your cherished friendship," he responded.[52]

On April 3, as an early-spring snowstorm swept up the East Coast, Mary died peacefully in her sleep at her beloved Deanery at Bryn Mawr, where she had spent the happiest days of her later life. Carey had sat attentively at her side during the last agonizing hours, reciting Elizabeth Barrett Browning's "Little Ellie." Mary simply went to sleep and "never waked again." Carey wrote in her journal,

"Mary died." Mary had turned sixty-one just a month earlier. Carey was inconsolable. "I do not know how I shall pull through Mary's death. It is unlike anything else I have ever been through and leaves me terribly desolate in spite of my dear family. Losing one's daily companion is different from any other loss."[53]

Newspapers that had chronicled Mary's every move for three decades were caught off guard. "Miss Garrett Dies Suddenly, Her Death a Shock," the *Baltimore News* reported the evening of her death. "Miss Garrett Dead," the *Baltimore Sun* announced the next morning. "It [her death] was a great shock to the Garrett connections in Baltimore and to Miss Garrett's many friends in this city and especially to the trustees of the Johns Hopkins University, which institution had benefited on many occasions by Miss Garrett's liberality. Although it was generally known by her relatives and friends here that she was sick, her death was a surprise, no one apparently realizing how sick she was," the *Sun* reported.[54]

Except for occasional visits, Mary had lost contact with Baltimore in the decade before her death. "Though really a Baltimorean and claiming this city as home, Miss Garrett for some time lived at 'The Deanery,' the home at Bryn Mawr of Miss M. Carey Thomas, president of Bryn Mawr College, who was her most intimate friend," a newspaper explained after her death. "She had very few acquaintances in this city and was thoroughly wrapped up in the work being done at the girls' college at Bryn Mawr."[55]

The newspapers seemed compelled to explain her life, reciting her roles in starting the Bryn Mawr School, the Hopkins medical school and hosting the 1906 suffrage receptions. "Essentially a serious-minded woman, Miss Garrett cared little for society or its doings and she devoted her life and her fortune to furthering those things which she believed made for the common good," the *Baltimore Sun* explained of her life's accomplishments. "She was especially interested in educational matters, and particularly the education of girls and women, and was a firm believer in the right of women to suffrage. It was Miss Garrett who made possible the opening of the Johns Hopkins Medical School and was the prime mover in the establishment of the Bryn Mawr School in Baltimore and its principal supporter." Even after her death, the papers did not run photographs of her, perhaps out of deference to her long-standing no-pictures rule. "She had an abhorrence of seeing her photographs in print and newspaper cuts of them are exceedingly rare," the *Baltimore News* explained.[56]

Carey made the funeral arrangements. Mary had left few instructions, except that she wanted to be cremated and requested that the funeral service be conducted by the pastor of the Associated Congregational Church, an outgrowth of her grandfather's and father's Associate Reformed Presbyterian Church. Mary's remains were brought from Bryn Mawr to her Mount Vernon Place home on April 5. A private service, "in accordance with the quiet, retiring habits that characterized Miss Garrett's life," was held the next day in the east parlor. Mrs. Stanley McCormick of Chicago, vice president of the National American Woman's Suffrage Association, led a contingency of suffragists, educators, and physicians, including Drs. Florence Sabin, Florence Welch, and Mary Sherwood, to the funeral. Faculty, university officers, board members, and students from Bryn Mawr College, the Johns Hopkins University, and the Bryn Mawr School also attended. "A number of Miss Garrett's relatives were present," the *Baltimore News* stated, although it is unclear which family members attended.[57]

Following the funeral service at her home, Mary was buried in "a strictly private" ceremony in the family plot on the scenic knoll of Green Mount Cemetery, next to her father and mother and a few steps away from the gravesite of Johns Hopkins. The doctors and educators who had meant the most to her and represented her philanthropies served as the honorary pallbearers.[58]

Carey arranged a memorial service at Bryn Mawr, with Anna Howard Shaw delivering the eulogy. A memorial service was held at McCoy Hall on the Hopkins campus, where Drs. William Welch and Lillian Welsh and Edith Hamilton gave their tributes. Sargent's portrait of Mary stood sentinel in the room.

Carey commissioned Lockwood de Forest to design a memorial plaque for the college. Bereft, he responded that he needed time to do it, given its importance and his many years of friendship with Mary. "I must have time to think it over carefully after I get the wording from you . . . It would be terrible if in our hurry we did this thing wrong, would it not? We need time to think otherwise we may do anything simply to get through," he replied to Carey. The large plaque was erected in the library cloisters at Bryn Mawr. It closed with the statement, "A woman of quiet realized enthusiasms she served her day and her generation well and will long be remembered by those for whom she laboured."[59]

The tributes poured in. From the Bryn Mawr School that she had financed for thirty years: "In 1890, she built the present school building which showed by its size and beauty her conception of what the school should be . . . To stand by the school in those years meant something more than friendly interest and moral support; it meant carrying the financial support of the school to the extent of thousands of dollars each year." From the Johns Hopkins University that she had rescued from national embarrassment twenty-five years earlier by opening the medical school: "The establishment of the 'Mary Elizabeth Garrett Fund' in the Johns Hopkins University, which enabled the University to open its Medical School in 1893, was due mainly to the generous contributions and the efforts of Miss Garrett. How wise and far-sighted were the conditions attached to this endowment and how great was the service thereby rendered to medical education and medical science that have been amply demonstrated by the experience of nearly a quarter of a century." From Bryn Mawr College that she had helped to elevate and enhance through bountiful gifts for three decades: "She had been a member of the Board since 1906 and by the dignity and attractiveness of her personality, her sound judgment and deep interest in the College commanded the personal esteem of each member, while her benefactions, both in gifts for specific purposes and her unique annual contributions, added greatly to the college's efficiency and to the practical convenience of its administration . . . She was a true gentlewoman."[60]

But her family was not quite so effusive. Within a week of her death, Mary's will was made public. Except for a few provisions, Mary had left the bulk of her estate to Carey. Her family was not included, nor even mentioned, save for instructions concerning the care of her brother Henry and her aunt Rebecca Harrison. The estate, which included what was left of her assets of stocks and securities and her homes at Mount Vernon Place, Montebello, and Deer Park, totaled between $525,830 and $1 million.[61] Her philanthropies of $2 million and the B&O losses through the 1880s and 1890s had diminished her once abundant estate to much less than its value when her father died in 1884.

Mary had signed her will on February 27, 1908, witnessed by Drs. William Halsted and Mary Sherwood, John W. Marshall, and George Archer. Carey had first planted the idea of designating herself as legatee and executor as early as 1899, as Mary's ongoing legal battles with her family culminated that year in her second lawsuit. But more than Carey's lobbying to be the primary beneficiary, Mary's overriding reason for excluding her family, notably her two surviving nephews, stemmed back nearly two decades to the distribution and sale of the B&O stocks in the 1880s, when she felt Robert Garrett and Sons had miscalculated her out of nearly $1 million. "In view of the large amounts of money her nephews and her sister-in law Mrs. Robert Garrett received from her estate owing to the transfer of seventeen thousand shares of B&O stock to her father's estate in 1889 and many other similar transactions many of which could not be corrected in the final settlement of the estate, Miss Garrett always felt and frequently stated that her family had profited largely from her estate before her death and that she felt herself entirely free from any obligation to leave any part of it to her nephews," Mary's attorney explained after her death.[62]

She made two changes by codicil in her will after signing it in 1908. She added the first codicil on April 17, 1912. At that time, she changed the beneficiary of her home at 101 West Monument from the Johns Hopkins University to Carey. Article Three of her will originally had bequeathed the mansion to Hopkins, with lifetime occupancy for Carey and any proceeds from the possible sale of the house to be added to her endowment in the medical school. But by 1912, she had changed her mind, designating by codicil that the house go to Carey "to occupy and enjoy in such manner as she may desire and with full power to her at any time in her discretion to sell and convey said house and lot of ground in fee simple or absolutely and to collect and receipt for the purchase money without any obligation."[63] Mary left no explanation for the change. Perhaps by that time she felt more benevolence toward Carey than she did for the university to which she had given so much and from which she had received so little recognition.

She wrote the second codicil just two days before her death, "releas[ing] the said Bryn Mawr School for Girls at Baltimore City from all indebtedness which may be owing to me from it at the time of my death." In her will, she had bequeathed to Bryn Mawr School the building she had built in 1890, providing the school continue in perpetuity as "a school for girls as a college preparatory school exclusively."[64]

If Carey had predeceased Mary, there would have been many other winners. The Bryn Mawr School would have received $100,000; Bryn Mawr College $200,000; and the National American Woman Suffrage Association $10,000. Julia B. de Forest, who had died in 1910, would have inherited Mary's "personal ornaments"—table silver and wardrobe; second in line to inherit Mary's personal ornaments was Sarah Orne Jewett, who had died in 1909. The Thomas kin would have benefited, as well. Helen Thomas Flexner and John Whitall Thomas, Carey's siblings, would have received many of her personal effects, including her valuable books, art collection, and furniture.

Mary's family was furious at their exclusion. Perhaps what most galled them was that she had designated the extended Thomas clan, the surrogate family she had embraced in the wake of the fallout with her own family in the 1890s, to be successive trustees of her estate. She had even made provisions to establish funds for Carey's many nieces and nephews should Carey predecease her, but nothing for her own nephews or Robert III's children.

Within months of Mary's death, the family—including Mary's nephews, their wives, Mary Frick and her husband Dr. Henry Barton Jacobs, and Alice Garrett—brought suit against Carey. Once again, the ghost of the Garrett patriarch haunted the family. The suit asked the court to "construe the will of John Work Garrett." The family questioned Mary's right to bequeath her three houses, claiming that because Mary had no direct heirs, the family should inherit the properties.[65]

The legal suit volleyed back and forth in the courts for months. In January 1916, the court found in favor of the family, stating, "The intention of Mr. Garrett in his will was that Miss Garrett should have possession of the city home, the country home and the cottage at Deer Park only during her lifetime," but did not have the right to dispose of the properties.[66]

By April, a year after her death almost to the day, the court reversed itself, finding that John Work Garrett's will, dated thirty-two years earlier, had given Mary "fee simple" title to the three properties to distribute as she wished. Attorney D. K. Este telegraphed a much-relieved Carey: "Garrett case decree reversed. We have won out completely."[67] Any conciliatory gestures her family might have made during Mary's prolonged illness vanished instantly in the aftermath of the posthumous legal wrangling and their subsequent loss of Mary's valuable and historic Garrett properties.

The *Baltimore Sun* extolled that Mary's will "showed a friendship so complete that it will probably become a classic in the annals of the female movement of this country."[68] But, in hindsight, Mary's will did little to continue the "female movement" she had dedicated her life to promoting. Like her father, who had miscalculated the long-term effects of his binding last will and testament, Mary had misjudged the best steward of her wealth and legacy. It is difficult to know if Mary's decision to leave her fortune to Carey was retaliation against her family, blind obedience to or love for Carey, or what she thought at the time was a sound business decision to carry out her feminist wishes.

Although Mary had astutely finessed many philanthropic coups during her lifetime and became known as a knowledgeable railroad woman for her behind-the-scenes machinations of the B&O, her business judgment lapsed in the final disposition of her estate. She handed over her wealth to Carey with no strings, stating simply in her will, "The said M. Carey Thomas and myself have been closely associated in our work for the higher education of women and I am confident that an appropriate and wise use will be made by her of my gift."[69] Perhaps Mary should have employed her "coercive philanthropy" and attached her usual unambiguous conditions to assure her life's work would continue under Carey's stewardship.

It is unclear how much of Mary's money Carey directed to the causes Mary had been passionate about and had entrusted Carey to continue supporting. Mary had taught Carey too well about grand living. After Mary's death, Carey continued the lifestyle to which Mary had elevated her in their years together. After receiving her abundant inheritance from Mary, plus lifetime income from the estate of about $60,000, Carey frequently traveled abroad, often with Bryn Mawr alumnae. A few years after Mary's death, Carey described her standard of living in the forty-six-room Deanery, made possible through her inheritance: "I have to have eight servants for my entertaining (two waitresses, two house maids, cook, laundress, seamstress and ironer, lady's maid) and [a] housekeeper and they have very little to do. There is also Charles [the chauffer] and two cars, one open and one closed, Franklin and a Ford."[70]

Carey spent through most of her inheritance. At the time of her death at age seventy-eight in 1935, all that remained of Mary's estate were 77 acres of Montebello property and the ruins of the mansion and outbuildings, 1,077 acres of forest land near Deer Park, two paintings, and three rugs. Carey established funds and prizes in her name and Mary's, leaving an estate valued at $104,900.[71]

Today, there are few physical traces of the shy, elusive woman whose "munificent" philanthropies from a century ago continue to affect our lives in countless ways. The beautiful homes that represented her life are gone. In 1929, her Mount Vernon Place mansion, after serving as the first venue of the Baltimore Art Museum six years earlier, was torn down and replaced with an apartment building. The thirty-room mansion with its conservatory, sunken pool, and mosaic floor, its expansive art gallery, its grand foyer with a spiral staircase, numerous Tiffany windows, and John Work Garrett's renowned de Forest Teakwood Room, lay in a heap of rubble on the corner of Cathedral and West Monument streets. Months later, the remaining mansion at Montebello burned to the ground under suspicious circumstances.[72] A decade later, the Deer Park cottage also went up in flames.

Similarly, the memorial that Mary insisted be built to celebrate women's hard-fought battle to revolutionize American medicine is gone. The Women's Fund Memorial Building, "the building that nurtured Hopkins glory," was torn down in 1979.[73] The Preclinical Sciences Building now stands in its place.

While the continued success of her philanthropies attests to Mary Elizabeth Garrett's enduring legacy, little concrete evidence remains of the woman who knew the importance of memorializing in bricks and mortar women's struggles for equality and opportunities. She understood firsthand, through her countless battles to "help women" and from thirty years of giving bountiful philanthropic gifts, how easily women's contributions to society could be diminished and eventually forgotten.

Always the "persuasive" philanthropist—even posthumously—Mary left one tantalizing clue of how she might have used her wealth to continue her crusades. In her final will and testament she had not completely forgotten about the medical school she funded. Midway through her twenty-page will—after she had outlined her conditions for leaving her estate to Carey and other non–family members—

Mary wrote a clause that, had it been enacted, would have stirred even greater controversy. If Carey had predeceased her, the Johns Hopkins University would have been offered the bulk of her estate—but only under Mary's usual nonnegotiable conditions.

In "Article Eleventh," almost reiterating the terms of her December 22, 1892, letter to initiate the medical school, Mary notched up the requirements in her will. No longer focused on women medical *students*—they had been given the opportunity for equal consideration in her 1893 gift—her will instead emphasized women medical *faculty*. A century ago, women physicians could hardly hope to break through to the higher ranks of medical faculty—a "glass ceiling" that is now just beginning to crack as women represent only 4 percent of top faculty ranks compared to male faculty's representation of 21 percent of senior faculty.[74]

When she wrote her will, Mary fully understood what Mary Putnam Jacobi had cited as "the habitual exclusion of women." Mary wanted to increase the odds of success. In order to accept the bequest, the Johns Hopkins University would have had to agree to promote women faculty proportionate to the number of women students at the medical school, and the university trustees would have to assure that women faculty received every opportunity to advance on the same terms as male faculty.[75] In Mary's "wise and far-sighted" equation, with women students now comprising more than 50 percent of medical students, women faculty today would comprise the majority of senior faculty positions.

Had the Johns Hopkins medical school been in a position to receive her estate in 1915, had the university trustees once more been bribed by her trademark coercion, Mary Elizabeth Garrett again would have forever changed American medicine by ensuring women's leadership at the highest levels. Perhaps once again a beneficiary of Mary Elizabeth Garrett's "coercive philanthropy" would have expressed Dr. William Osler's long-ago sentiment that it is a "pleasure to be bought."

The twenty members of the class of 1879 of the Woman's Medical College of Pennsylvania provide a snapshot of the diverse backgrounds of women medical students and their course of study.[1] The cost of their three-year education was $265, which included the commencement ceremony. They paid $15 per ticket to attend a lecture; students who intended to work as medical missionaries received discounts. Aside from class work and clinical rounds, students were required to complete a thesis, as was required in European medical study. Demographically, the class of 1879 represented an ethnic mosaic. They were Baptists, Jews, Quakers, and Lutherans and hailed from nine states. Slightly over 50 percent had American-born parents. The majority of their fathers were tradesmen or from the working class, and most of the students had graduated from normal schools, female seminaries, or public schools. Prior to entering medical study, six students had been teachers, and five had worked as domestics. When entering medical study, six students were between nineteen and twenty-five years old, eleven were twenty-six to forty, and three were over forty years of age. Nine were married with children, two divorced, and nine had never married. At commencement, on March 13, 1879, the class of 1879 was sent off with stern advice: "The woman of society is too often its slave. You should be wise enough and shrewd enough to make society serve you."[2]

The graduates proved to be not only wise and shrewd but healthy as well. In 1881, three physicians, Emily and Augusta Pope and Emma Call, published one of the first longitudinal studies on the effects of practicing medicine on women physicians. They concluded, "We do not think it would be easy to find a better record of health among an equal number of women, taken at random, from all over the country."[3] The class of 1879 verified the study. Seven died before reaching sixty, and most of the class survived well past the life expectancy.

The *Report of the Women's Fund for the Medical School of the Johns Hopkins University*, dated May 26, 1891, lists the donors—"subscribers"—and the committee members who raised $111,300 to endow the medical school. Although more than seven hundred donors eventually contributed to the fund, the campaign faltered and would not have reached its original goal of $100,000 without Mary Elizabeth Garrett's gift of $47,787.50. The Women's Medical School Fund exemplifies the challenges nineteenth-century women faced in raising large amounts of cash. Women's fundraising campaigns a century ago were much different than the massive direct-mail and billion-dollar major gift campaigns that characterize modern fundraising. The WMSF campaign was conducted through intense letter writing, national networking, word of mouth, social events, tapping into women's voluntary groups, and several well-placed articles arguing for the need for better medical education and, specifically, coeducational medical education.

The fund's fundamental weakness lay in the lack of major contributions from the wealthy regional committee members. Overall, fewer than half of the members solicited early in the campaign to serve on fundraising committees ever contributed to the fund. In Boston, for example, only fourteen of the thirty-one committee members made a donation. In Washington, D.C., only twenty of forty-four committee members contributed. They lent their highly visible names to the campaign but not their financial support.

The report lists each contributor to the campaign. Baltimore subscribers gave the largest amount, $68,882.56, with Mary Elizabeth Garrett giving $47,787.50 of that amount. Contributions from other regions totaled: Boston, $20,231.07; Philadelphia, $8,075.77; New York, $5,400; Pacific Coast (San Francisco), $2,142; Washington, D.C., $2,087; Chicago, $1,140; Essex County (MA), $649; Milwaukee, $610; Springfield (MA), $608; St. Louis, $550.70; Port Deposit (MD), $500; Madison (WI), $129.50; Annapolis, $180.75; The Kennebec (ME), $88.65; and Buffalo, $25.

Most contributors gave between $10 and $50, a typical amount at the time for a woman to contribute to a voluntary cause, with the average gift to the fund between $5 and $10. The largest contributor to the overall campaign, aside from Mary, was Marian Hovey of Boston. Thirteen years after she offered $10,000 to Harvard to make its medical school coeducational, Hovey contributed that amount to the Hopkins campaign. Without Mary's gift of nearly $48,000 or Marian Hovey's $10,000 contribution, the national campaign would have raised little more than $43,000.

Despite the lack of large gifts from wealthy and well-known committee members, it appears the campaign had broad appeal. It was well publicized in newspapers, and readers of various socio-economic backgrounds might have been aware of it. Several contributors gave a dollar, fifty cents, or twenty-five cents. Presumably, these were not the "names of influence," but rather contributors interested in the cause who could not give larger amounts. Boston counted 123 donors, including Miss K. Clifton, who contributed $1.50 "for eleven working women," Henry Redman, who gave ten cents, and Catharine Hasey, who contributed twenty-five cents. In Washington, D.C., the Ladies of the "Newport" collectively gave $17. Some donors gave anonymously, listing themselves as "a friend" or "a woman." The *Baltimore American* noted, "One of the first contributions received was the sum of $2,000 from Liverpool [England]."[1] This gift is listed as coming from Mr. William Johnston, who was connected to the Baltimore Committee. More than likely he was the president of William Johnston and Company, a Liverpool-based shipping line affiliated with the B&O's merchant fleet. Mary might have solicited him for the gift.

Perhaps the most intriguing outcome of the campaign was the failure of all but a handful of women physicians to endorse it. We have no way of knowing how many women physicians overall were solicited to give contributions to the fundraising campaign or to serve on the regional committees. Mary had asked her own physician, Dr. Mary Putnam Jacobi, to rally women physicians of the Association for the Advancement of the Medical Education of Women to join the campaign. It is unclear whether the members of this group were widely solicited.

Although the fund organizers felt that women physicians would eagerly support the cause, this was not the case. Only thirty-three of the seven hundred contributors were listed as doctors, and many of them were men. Only twenty women physicians (identified as medical doctors on the roster) served on the regional committees. We can speculate that either the fund's organizers did not solicit enough women physicians or, more interesting, that women physicians—beyond Drs. Jacobi and Emily and Elizabeth Blackwell and other supporters of the women's medical movement—did not align themselves with the issue of coeducation or did not support the WMSF specifically. Almost all women physicians at the time of the campaign would have been graduates of women's medical colleges. It is possible that their failure to support the WMSF campaign was a reflection of their satisfaction with their own all-female medical education, their lack of interest in being educated with men, or their ambivalence about opening a coeducational medical school at Hopkins. Also, it is possible that many women physicians felt that medical coeducation was more of a feminist goal for equal rights than a medical goal for better education for women physicians. And in the late nineteenth century, not all women endorsed the controversial goal of equal rights for women.

Notes

ABBREVIATIONS

AMC	Alan Mason Chesney Medical Archives
BMC	Special Collections Department, Bryn Mawr College Library
BMS	Bryn Mawr School
JHU	Johns Hopkins University
JWG	John Work Garrett
JWG II	John Work Garrett II
LOC	Library of Congress
MCT	M. Carey Thomas
MEG	Mary Elizabeth Garrett
MHS	Maryland Historical Society

INTRODUCTION. QUIET REVOLUTIONARY

1. John Work Garrett was often referred to as the "Railroad King." See, e.g., the *Pittsburg Dispatch*, September 26, 1884. The anecdotal statement attributed to John Work Garrett about his daughter has long been part of Baltimore oral history and is documented in several Baltimore historical accounts. Frank Shivers, *Walking in Baltimore: An Intimate Guide to the Old City* (Baltimore: Johns Hopkins University Press, 1995), 206: "I have often wished . . . that Mary was a boy . . . I know she would carry on my work after I am gone." Also, Elizabeth Fee, Linda Shopes, and Linda Zeidman, eds., *The Baltimore Book: New Views of Local History* (Philadelphia: Temple University Press, 1991), 27, cite John Work Garrett's statement: "If the boys were only like Mary, what a satisfaction it would be to me. I have always wished in these last few years that Mary was a boy. I know she could carry on my work after I am gone."

2. *Chicago Tribune*, July 30, 1896; *New York Times*, July 24, 1888; *Baltimore News*, April 13, 1915.

3. *New York Times*, February 24, 1891.

4. *Baltimore News*, April 13, 1915.

5. *Baltimore American*, December 30, 1892.

6. Margaret W. Rossiter, *Women Scientists in America: Struggles and Strategies to*

1940 (Baltimore: Johns Hopkins University Press, 1982), 91, explains that "coercive" or "creative" philanthropy was a strategy employed "for changing institutional policies." While such a tactic was not always successful, "a very astute and vigilant donor (like Mary Garrett) would enforce unpopular conditions to a gift."

7. Letter from Miss Garrett to the Trustees of the University, Baltimore, December 22, 1892, Daniel Coit Gilman Papers, ms. 1, Special Collections, Sheridan Libraries, JHU; unidentified Chicago newspaper, January 3, 1893, Mary Elizabeth Garrett Collection, AMC, JHU.

8. *Baltimore Sun*, September 27, 1884.

9. *Baltimore Sun*, April 14, 1915.

10. MEG to Charles Mayer, February 13, 1894, Mary Elizabeth Garrett Collection, Box: The Garrett Estate, Folder: 1–11, BMC.

11. Association of American Medical Colleges statistics quoted in *Washington Post*, November 4, 2003.

CHAPTER 1. GARRETT'S ROAD

1. Garrett Family Genealogy, Evergreen House Foundation at Evergreen Museum and Library, JHU; Mary Elizabeth Garrett Collection, MEG inventory of jewelry, 1895, Box: Mary Garrett Business Papers, Folder: F5, BMC.

2. *Philadelphia Record*, September 27, 1884; eulogy read by Jonathan Leyburn at Rachel Garrett's funeral, November 18, 1883. Miscellaneous document, Garrett Family Papers, Box 137, Manuscript Division, LOC; gifts are noted in MEG jewelry inventory, 1895.

3. *Baltimore Sun*, November 16, 1883; Marjorie Luckett, ed., *Maryland Women* (Baltimore: King Brothers Press, 1942), 123.

4. *Ladies' Garland* 1, no. 1 (April 15, 1837): 19; *New York Tribune*, September 28, 1884.

5. Genealogical information and quotations taken from Garrett Family DNA and Genealogical Research Project, directed by Donald Garrett Dickason, Princeton, N.J.

6. Ibid.

7. Ibid. Move west noted in Clayton Coleman Hall, ed., *Baltimore: Its History and Its People*, biographical vol. 2 (New York: Lewis Historical Publishing Co., 1912), 452.

8. Dickason, Garrett Family Project.

9. Ibid.

10. Francis F. Beirne, *The Amiable Baltimoreans* (New York: E. P. Dutton and Co., 1951), 14; Edward Hungerford, *The Story of the Baltimore & Ohio Railroad, 1827–1927* (New York: G. P. Putnam's Sons, 1928), 1:12.

11. Hungerford, *Story of the Baltimore & Ohio Railroad*, 1:12; *Baltimore Sun*, February 19, 1928.

12. J. Thomas Scharf, *History of Western Maryland, Being a History of Frederick, Montgomery, Carroll, Washington, Allegany and Garrett Counties from the Earliest Period to the Present Day Including Biographical Sketches of Their Representative Men* (Philadelphia: Louis H. Everts, 1882), 2:1512.

13. For sentimental reasons, while possibly eyeing a future profit, the family also held on to Garrett Farm in West Middletown near the National Road. Noted in 1895 inventory of John Work Garrett estate, Box: Mary Garrett Business Papers, Folder: F2, BMC.

14. Scharf, *History of Western Maryland*, 2:1512.

15. John C. French, *A History of the University Founded by Johns Hopkins* (Baltimore: Johns Hopkins University Press, 1946), 11.

16. William Bruce Catton, "How Rails Saved a Seaport," *American Heritage* 8, 2 (1957): www.americanheritage.com/articles/magazine/ah/1957/2/1957_2_26.shtml.

17. *Baltimore Sun*, February 7, 1857; George W. Howard, *The Monumental City, Its Past History and Present Resources* (Baltimore: J. D. Ehlers, 1873), 34.

18. *Baltimore: Its History and Its People*, 2:454.

19. Dickason, Garrett Family Project. Robert Garrett married for the first time at age twenty-eight in 1811 to Martha Hanna of Baltimore. She gave birth to a daughter, Sara Margaret, the same year and died in 1812. Sara Margaret died in 1840 at the age of twenty-nine.

20. Scharf, *History of Western Maryland*, 2:1512.

21. John Work Garrett did not graduate from Lafayette College but is recorded as a nongraduate, class of 1838. *Baltimore: Its History and Its People*, 2:456. In 1865, the college awarded him an honorary master of arts degree.

22. Harold A. Williams, *Robert Garrett & Sons, Incorporated: Origin and Development, 1840–1965* (Baltimore: Press of Schneidereith & Sons, 1965), 8–9; *Baltimore Sun*, September 26, 1884.

23. *Baltimore: Its History and Its People*, 2: 455; Scharf, *History of Western Maryland*, 2:1513; *Baltimore Sun*, September 26, 1884; *Services and Address at the Funeral of the Late Henry S. Garrett*, October 12, 1867 (Baltimore: Kelly & Piet, Printers), Cincinnati Museum Center.

24. Quoted in Roderick N. Ryon, *West Baltimore Neighborhoods: Sketches of Their History, 1890–1960* (Baltimore: Institute for Publications Design at the University of Baltimore, 1993), 80.

25. *Baltimore American*, June 9, 1888. The precise year of the house fire is not clear. The *Baltimore American* reported that it occurred when Harry was about three years of age, which would have been 1852. However, the city directories list John Work Garrett as living in that house in 1854, the year Mary was born. West Point–educated George Hume Steuart would later gain fame as a Confederate general.

26. The Garretts lived at 27 Calhoun Street, sometimes called "Delaware Row." It is possible that the house occupied the area where Franklin Square Hospital is now located. City directories of the late 1850s alternately list John Work Garrett as living at 27 Calhoun and "Delaware Place."

27. Mary Ellen Hayward and Charles Belfoure, *The Baltimore Rowhouse* (Princeton University Press, 1999), 60.

28. Not much is known about the Landsdowne property. It is noted in Williams, *Robert Garrett & Sons* and is also listed in the 1895 inventory of John Work Garrett's estate, Box: Mary Garrett Business Papers, Folder: F2, BMC.

29. MEG memoir, Box: Mary Garrett Diaries, Etc., Folder: F1–89–1, BMC.

30. *Baltimore Sun*, March 6, 1854; the College of Medicine of Maryland was chartered in 1807 and later rechartered as the University of Maryland.

31. MEG memoir.

32. Ibid.

33. Ibid.

34. *American and Commercial Daily Advertiser*, July 7, 1828.

35. Hungerford, *Story of the Baltimore & Ohio Railroad*, 1:14; H. W. Brands, *Andrew Jackson: His Life and Times* (New York: Doubleday, 2005), 393.

36. James D. Dilts, *The Great Road: The Building of the Baltimore & Ohio, the Nation's First Railroad, 1828–1853* (Stanford, Calif.: Stanford University Press, 1993), 38.

37. Ibid., 46.

38. Hungerford, *Story of the Baltimore & Ohio Railroad*, 1:324, 326.

39. *Baltimore Sun*, November 18, 1858.

40. Eric L. Holcomb, *The City as Suburb: A History of Northeast Baltimore Since 1660* (Santa Fe: Center for American Places, 2005), 106.

41. *Baltimore Sun*, November 18, 1858.

42. Ibid.

43. Hungerford, *Story of the Baltimore & Ohio Railroad*, 1:330.

44. Catton, "How Rails Saved a Seaport"; Fee, Shopes, and Zeidman, *Baltimore Book*, 21–22.

45. Catton, "How Rails Saved a Seaport."

46. "Railroad King" noted in Scharf, *History of Western Maryland*, 2: 1514; "before Garrett" quoted in Beirne, *Amiable Baltimoreans*, 69.

47. John F. Stover, *History of the Baltimore and Ohio Railroad* (West Lafayette, Ind.: Purdue University Press, 1987), 95, 99.

48. Ibid., 100; Ele Bowen, *Rambles in the Path of the Steam-Horse* (Philadelphia: William Bromwell and William White Smith, Publishers, 1855), Cincinnati Museum Center.

49. Hungerford, *Story of the Baltimore & Ohio Railroad*, 1:334, 330 (quote on steamship line); Scharf, *History of Western Maryland*, 2:1511.

50. Hungerford, *Story of the Baltimore & Ohio Railroad*, 1:330.

51. Shivers, *Walking in Baltimore*, 226.

52. James Dixon, *Personal Narrative of a Tour through Part of the United States and Canada with Notices on the History and Institutions of Methodism in America* (New York: Lane & Scott, 1850), quoted in William C. Chase, ed., *Descriptions of Maryland: A Miscellany*, 41. wwwfac.mcdaniel.edu/History/miscellany.html.

53. The address at the time of construction was 77, but it was changed in 1892 to 101 West Monument Street. For clarity and consistency, the current addresses of the Garrett homes are used here.

54. *Baltimore Sun*, February 5, 1857.

55. Ibid.

56. *Baltimore Sun*, February 7, 1857.

57. Value of Garrett mansion taken from 1860 federal census, 11th ward, 98.

58. Information presented here about the interior is compiled from descriptions of similar mansions of the era and miscellaneous references to the Garrett mansion.

59. The fence was removed in 1877 after Baltimoreans had complained for years that their tax dollars maintained an exclusive park that was off-limits to them.

60. According to City directories, the John Work Garretts still lived on Franklin Square in 1860. The directories were not published between 1861 and 1862, but by 1864, John Work Garrett's address was listed as 50 (now #12) Mount Vernon Place.

61. Nikolaus Pevsner, An Outline of European Architecture (Baltimore: Penguin Press, 1966), 441.

62. On Thomas's house, Mount Vernon Cultural District Walking Tour, www.wam .umd.edu/~jlehnert/highlights.htm; on Pratt's house, Beirne, Amiable Baltimoreans, 51.

63. MEG memoir.

64. Quoted in Marion E. Warren and Mame Warren, Baltimore: When She Was What She Used to Be (Baltimore: Johns Hopkins University Press, 1983), 38, 40; Beirne, Amiable Baltimoreans, 103.

65. Robert H. Bremner, American Philanthropy (Chicago: University of Chicago Press, 1988), 104.

66. John Robert Godley, Letters from America (London: John Murray, 1843), quoted in Chase, Descriptions of Maryland: A Miscellany, wwwfac.mcdaniel.edu/ History/miscellany.html.

67. Catherine C. Lorber, "The Garretts of Baltimore: Collectors and Patrons," Evergreen House Foundation at Evergreen Museum and Library, JHU; Baltimore Sun, July 18, 1877; on Association for the Improvement and Condition of the Poor, Baltimore: Its History and Its People, 2:454.

68. Jessica I. Elfenbein, The Making of a Modern City: Philanthropy, Civic Culture and the Baltimore YMCA (Gainesville: University Press of Florida, 2001), 10.

69. Sermon of Jonathon F. Stearns, "Discourse on Female Influence," 1837. Reprinted in Aileen S. Kraditor, ed., Up from the Pedestal: Selected Writings in the History of American Feminism (Chicago: Quadrangle Books, 1968), 47–48.

70. Compiled from Anne Firor Scott, Natural Allies: Women's Associations in American History (Urbana: University of Illinois Press, 1991) and Philanthropy in Baltimore: A Timeline for Benevolent Giving and Humane Goodness, 1623–1900 (Baltimore: Friends of Clifton, 2000).

71. 1860 federal census, MEG Collection, Box 1–4, Folder: 6–4, BMC; Mount Vernon Cultural District, www.wam.umd.edu/~jlehnert/highlights.htm.

72. Hungerford, Story of the Baltimore & Ohio Railroad, 1:378.

CHAPTER 2. ASCENSION

1. MEG memoir; Anthony Trollope, North America, vol. 1 (New York: J. B. Lippincott & Co., 1863), quoted in Chase, Descriptions of Maryland: A Miscellany, www fac.mcdaniel.edu/History/miscellany.html.

2. MEG memoir.

3. Stover, *History of the Baltimore and Ohio Railroad*, 101; Hungerford, *Story of the Baltimore & Ohio Railroad*, 1:350.

4. Quoted in Williams, *Robert Garrett & Sons*, 39

5. Ibid., 41; MEG memoir.

6. MEG memoir.

7. Ibid.

8. Ibid.

9. Ibid.

10. Hungerford, *Story of the Baltimore & Ohio Railroad*, 1:348.

11. Ibid., 19.

12. Robert I. Cottom Jr. and Mary Ellen Hayward, *Maryland in the Civil War: A House Divided* (Baltimore: Maryland Historical Society, 1994), 32.

13. "In Memory of John Work Garrett," *Sketch of John Work Garrett*, MEG Collection, Box: Mary Garrett, Folder, F1, BMC, 5.

14. Quoted in Scott Sumpter Sheads and Daniel Carroll Toomey, *Baltimore during the Civil War* (Baltimore: Toomey Press, 1997), 14.

15. Quoted in Stover, *History of the Baltimore and Ohio Railroad*, 104; on rebels, Hungerford, *Story of the Baltimore & Ohio Railroad*, 1:350.

16. *Services and Address at the Funeral of Henry S. Garrett*.

17. MEG memoir.

18. Robert J. Brugger, *The Maryland Club: A History of Food and Friendship in Baltimore* (Baltimore: Johns Hopkins University Press, 1998), 27. John Work Garrett was not listed as a member of the Maryland Club.

19. Beirne, *Amiable Baltimoreans*, 30; Williams, *Robert Garrett & Sons*, 43, 44–45.

20. MEG memoir.

21. Stover, *History of the Baltimore and Ohio Railroad*, 106, 109.

22. Ibid.

23. MEG to Charles F. Mayer, February 13, 1894, MEG Collection, Box: Mary Garrett Business Papers, Folder: F4, BMC.

24. MEG memoir.

25. "Clash Comes to Symbolize Civil War," www.cnn.com/2004/US/06/25/gettysburg/.

26. MEG memoir.

27. MEG to Charles F. Mayer, February 13, 1894.

28. Ibid.

29. MEG memoir.

30. Luckett, *Maryland Women*, 124.

31. Williams, *Robert Garrett & Sons*, 43; Abraham Lincoln to JWG, January 10, 1865, Garrett Family Collection, Box 124, LOC.

32. Abraham Lincoln, Second Inaugural Address, March 4, 1865, www.loc.gov/exhibits/treasures/trt053.html.

33. Hungerford, *Story of the Baltimore & Ohio Railroad*, 1:61.

34. Quoted in Carl Bode, *Maryland: A Bicentennial History* (New York: Norton, 1978), 133.

35. Hungerford, *Story of the Baltimore & Ohio Railroad*, 1:61.

36. Ronald C. White Jr., *Lincoln's Greatest Speech: The Second Inaugural* (New York: Simon & Schuster, 2002), excerpted in "Absence of Malice" in *Smithsonian Magazine* (April 2002): 111.

37. Speech by John Work Garrett presented to the Merchants and Business Men of Baltimore on September 22, 1865. Noted in *Sketch of John Work Garrett*, 8.

38. Bremner, *American Philanthropy*, 73.

39. MEG memoir.

40. *Baltimore: Its History and Its People*, 2:452.

41. Hungerford, *Story of the Baltimore & Ohio Railroad*, 1:330; Stover, *History of the Baltimore and Ohio Railroad*, 161; *Baltimore Sun*, November 18, 1858.

42. *Services and Address at the Funeral of Henry S. Garrett*.

43. *Baltimore Sun*, October 14, 1867.

44. Ibid.; *Services and Address at the Funeral of Henry S. Garrett*.

45. *Baltimore Sun*, October 11, 1867.

46. 1895 jewelry inventory, Box: Mary Garrett, Folder: F5, BMC; The Milk and Honey and Kindness farms were later purchased by John Work Garrett and became part of his large Western Maryland holdings: 1895 Garrett Estate Inventories, Box: Mary Garrett Business Papers, Folder: F2, BMC.

47. MEG memoir.

48. Robert J. Brugger, *Maryland: A Middle Temperament, 1634–1980* (Baltimore: Johns Hopkins University Press in association with the Maryland Historical Society), 312.

49. Fee, Shopes, and Zeidman, *Baltimore Book*, 21.

50. Ibid. (quote appears on 21–22).

51. For more on Garrett City, see www.rootsweb.com~indekalb/other/garrett.html.

52. Martin Ford, "Alien Nation? Immigration Here and There, Then and Now," *Maryland Humanities* (September 2002): 4.

53. MEG 1895 jewelry inventory, BMC. Mary's memoir also alludes to Miss Kummer's as the school she attended, and she notes that at one time she wanted to study with her former teacher who offered French lessons in Paris, where Kummer later moved. In 1870, Mary identified her school as "Miss K's."

54. Barbara Landis Chase, "M. Carey Thomas and the 'Friday Night': A Case Study in Female Social Networks and Personal Growth" (master's thesis, Johns Hopkins University, 1990), 16.

55. "Third Annual Circular," Miss D. T. Kilbourn's Academy, Baltimore, 1854, Maryland Ephemera Collection, MDX EP8, Enoch Pratt Free Library.

56. "Circular," Franklin Square Female Seminary, n.d., Maryland Department, Ephemera Collection, MDX EP21, Enoch Pratt Free Library; literary journal: *The Literary Budget*, edited by the Young Ladies of the Academy of Miss D. T. Kilbourn, May 4, 1853, Maryland Ephemera Collection, MDX-ED1, Enoch Pratt Free Library.

57. MEG memoir.

58. Ibid.; dissection noted in French, *History of the University Founded by Johns Hopkins*, 111.

59. MEG memoir.

60. Ibid.; 1870 Diary, Box: Mary Garrett Diaries, Etc., Folder: F2, BMC; miscellaneous journals, Box: Mary Garrett Diaries, Etc., Folder: F2, BMC.

61. MEG memoir.

62. Ibid.; physician quote from Carroll Smith Rosenberg, *Disorderly Conduct: Visions of Gender in Victorian America* (New York: Oxford University Press, 1985), 184.

63. MEG memoir.

64. Personal Accounts Ledger, Box: Mary Garrett Diaries, Etc., Folder: F2, BMC.

65. MEG Correspondence Diary 1873–1883, Box: Mary Garrett Diaries, Etc., Folder: F2, BMC; journal, Box: Mary Garrett Diaries, Etc., Folder: F2, BMC.

66. Elizabeth Schaaf, "George Peabody: His Life and Legacy, 1795–1869," *Maryland Historical Magazine* 90, no. 3 (Fall 1995): 270.

67. John Work Garrett, *Address Delivered on the 30th of January, 1883, Before the Young Men's Christian Association of Baltimore on the Occasion of the Thirtieth Anniversary* (Baltimore: News Steam Printing Office, 1883); reprinted in *Baltimore Sun*, January 31, 1883.

68. Ibid.

69. The exact date of the meeting between Hopkins and Peabody at the Garrett home is uncertain, although Franklin Parker in *George Peabody: A Biography* (Nashville: Vanderbilt University Press, 1971), 201, speculates that it was April 25, 1867. While staying with the Garretts, Peabody wrote several letters using the Garrett stationery, indicating possible dates when the meeting might have taken place: October 24–30, 1866, November 12–13, 1866, February 3, 1867, and April 25, 1867.

70. *Address Delivered on the 30th of January, 1883*.

71. Ibid.

72. Stover, *History of the Baltimore and Ohio Railroad*, 123.

73. Kevin Phillips, "The New Face of Another Gilded Age," *Washington Post*, May 26, 2002.

74. *Baltimore: Its History and Its People*, 462.

75. MEG 1895 jewelry inventory, Box: Mary Garrett, Folder: F2, BMC.

76. Stover, *History of the Baltimore and Ohio Railroad*, 128, 129.

77. Ibid., 134; *Sketch of John Work Garrett*, Appendix.

78. Stover, *History of the Baltimore and Ohio Railroad*, 161; Scharf, *History of Western Maryland*, 2:1515.

79. *Baltimore Sun*, September 25, 1884.

80. MEG to Elizabeth Barbara Garrett, August 23, 1873, Box 128, Garrett Family Papers, Manuscript Division, LOC.

81. Robert Garrett to JWG, October 23, 1873. Box 128, Garrett Family Papers, Manuscript Division, LOC.

82. 1873–1874 Travel Itinerary, Box: Mary Garrett Diaries, Etc., Folder: F2, BMC; MEG to Elizabeth Barbara Garrett, November 7, 1873, Box 128, Garrett Family Papers, Manuscript Division, LOC. "The Old Lady" is the term Londoners use to refer to the Bank of England, located in the heart of London on Threadneedle Street; MEG to Elizabeth Barbara Garrett, August 23, 1873, Box 128, Garrett Family Papers, Manuscript Division, LOC.

83. JWG to Elizabeth Barbara Garrett, September 18, 1873, Box 128, Garrett Family Papers, Manuscript Division, LOC.

84. Scharf, *History of Western Maryland*, 2:1514.

85. JWG to Elizabeth Barbara Garrett, September 16, 1873, Box 128, Garrett Family Papers, Manuscript Division, LOC.

86. MEG to Elizabeth Barbara Garrett, April 1874 [exact date unclear], Box 128, Garrett Family Papers, Manuscript Division, LOC.

87. JWG to Elizabeth Barbara Garrett, September 16, 1873, Box 128, Garrett Family Papers, Manuscript Division, LOC; MEG to Elizabeth Barbara Garrett, November 7, 1873, Box 128, Garrett Family Papers, Manuscript Division, LOC.

88. MEG to Elizabeth Barbara Garrett, September 16, 1873. Box 128, Garrett Family Papers, Manuscript Division, LOC.

89. MEG to Elizabeth Barbara Garrett, April 1874 [exact date unclear], Box 128, Garrett Family Papers, Manuscript Division, LOC; MEG 1896 jewelry inventory, Box: Mary Garrett, Folder: F5, BMC.

90. Robert Garrett to Elizabeth Barbara Garrett, July 11, 1874, Box 128, Garrett Family Papers, Manuscript Division, LOC.

91. Harry and Alice's first child, Elizabeth, died at the age of eight months in 1871. Their fifth and last child also died.

92. MEG to Elizabeth Barbara Garrett, August 23, 1873, Box 128, Garrett Family Papers, Manuscript Division, LOC.

93. Katharine B. Dehler, "Mount Vernon Place at the Turn of the Century: A Vignette of the Garrett Family," *Maryland Historical Magazine* 69, no. 3 (Fall 1974): 290; at the time of Elizabeth's death in 1877, the other surviving founder of the Society for the Relief of the Indigent Sick was Mrs. E. R. Harney. Noted in *Baltimore Sun*, July 18, 1877.

94. *Baltimore American*, September 27, 1884.

95. On annual pay, Stover, *History of the Baltimore and Ohio Railroad*, 135; on suicide, Fee, Shopes, and Zeidman, *Baltimore Book*, 5.

96. Brugger, *Middle Temperament*, 344; Hungerford, *Story of the Baltimore & Ohio Railroad*, 2:149.

97. Scene described in Catton, "How Rails Saved a Seaport."

CHAPTER 3. EXPANSION AND RESTRICTION

1. Holcomb, *The City as Suburb*, 106.

2. Ibid., 109.

3. Joanne Giza and Catharine F. Black, *Great Houses of Baltimore* (Baltimore: Maclay & Associates, 1982), 56; Holcomb, *City as Suburb*, 110.

4. Ibid., 111.

5. J. Gilman and D. Paul, "Montebello, Home of General Samuel Smith," *Maryland Historical Magazine* 42, no. 4 (December 1947): 258.

6. Williams, in *Robert Garrett & Sons*, estimates that at some point John Work Garrett's holdings in the area might have totaled three thousand acres. Its boundaries

today include Homestead Village on the south end, Hillen and Old York roads to the east and west, and Joppa Road on the north.

7. Gilman and Paul, "Montebello," 428; Holcomb, *City as Suburb*, 115–16.

8. Ibid., 116–17.

9. MEG to Elizabeth Barbara Garrett, August 23, 1873, Box 128, Garrett Family Papers, Manuscript Division, LOC; JWG to Elizabeth Barbara Garrett, September 16, 1873, Box 128, Garrett Family Papers, Manuscript Division, LOC.

10. Damascus noted in Williams, *Robert Garrett & Sons*, 55, and also cited in *Baltimore American*, September 27, 1884; JWG, *Catalogue of Trotting Stock* (Baltimore: Press of Isaac Feldman, 1881, 1882, 1883, 1884), Maryland Ephemera Collection, MDX EP8, Enoch Pratt Free Library, Baltimore; Garrett, *Catalogue of Trotting Stock* (Baltimore: Press of Isaac Feldman, 1885), 3.

11. JWG to Elizabeth Garrett, August 23, 1873, Box 128, Garrett Family Papers, Manuscript Division, LOC.

12. *Baltimore Sun*, September 26, 1884.

13. Andrew Carnegie, *Autobiography of Andrew Carnegie, 1835–1919* (Boston: Northeastern University Press, 1986), 123.

14. *The National Cyclopedia of American Biography* (New York: James T. White Publishers, 1913), 7; a Garrett family servant told the anecdote about the lodged bullet many years later to a writer for the *Glade Star* 4, no. 6 (September 1970). Quoted in "John Work Garrett: Mr. Baltimore and Ohio Railroad."

15. Helen Lefkowitz Horowitz, *The Power and Passion of M. Carey Thomas* (New York: Alfred A. Knopf, 1994), 91.

16. "History of Coldstream-Homestead-Montebello," Live Baltimore Home Center, www.livebaltimore.com/nb/list/coldstr/history/.

17. J. W. Garrett, *Address Delivered on the 30th of January, 1883*.

18. Ibid.

19. Stephen Schlosnagle and the Garrett County Bicentennial Committee, *Garrett County: A History of Maryland's Tableland* (Parsons, W.Va.: McClain Printing Co., 1978), 279–80.

20. *Washington Post*, December 11, 2002; on exclusivity, Brugger, *A Middle Temperament*, 366.

21. Alison K. Hoagland, "Deer Park Hotel," *Maryland Historical Magazine* 73, no. 4 (December 1978): 342.

22. Schlosnagle et al., *Garrett County*, 281.

23. MEG to Rachel Garrett, June 6, 1882, Box: Mary Garrett to her Mother, 1882–1883, Folder: F1, BMC; Garrett County Historical Society, *Deer Park Then and Now* (Parsons, W.Va.: McClain Printing Co., 1994), 9.

24. Technically, Robert Garrett and Sons purchased Evergreen.

25. Elizabeth Cady Stanton, Susan B. Anthony, and Matilda Joslyn Gage, eds., *The History of Woman Suffrage (1861–1876)* (New York: Source Book Press, 1970), 2:82.

26. *New York Evangelist*, September 28, 1882.

27. Sara M. Evans, *Born for Liberty: A History of Women in America* (New York: Simon & Schuster, 1997), 147.

28. Joseph Hill, *Women in Gainful Occupations, 1870–1920,* 1929; repr., Westport, Conn.: Greenwood Press, 1978), 16.

29. Candace Wheeler, *Yesterdays in a Busy Life* (New York: Harper and Brothers, 1918), 222.

30. The women interchangeably called their group the "Friday Evening" or the "Friday Night." Mary usually referred to it as the "Friday Night" or the "F.N."; Mamie Gwinn Hodder interview with Logan Pearsall Smith, exact date unknown, early 1938, File 45, AMC.

31. Chase, "M. Carey Thomas and the Friday Night," 7.

32. MEG to MCT, August 18, 1879, M. Carey Thomas Papers, reel 42, BMC.

33. MEG Diary, 1872, Box: Mary Garrett Diaries, Etc., Folder: F2; Mamie Gwinn Hodder interview with Logan Pearsall Smith, 8 [exact date unknown], File 45, AMC; Chase, "M. Carey Thomas and the Friday Night," 55.

34. Mamie Gwinn Hodder interview with Logan Pearsall Smith; MEG Diary, June 14, 1870, Box: Mary Garrett Diaries, Etc., Folder: F2, BMC.

35. MEG to Charles F. Mayer, February 13, 1894; noted in MEG Correspondence Journal, 1873–1883, Box: Mary Garrett Diaries, Etc., Folder: F2, BMC (none of the letters are extant); Horowitz, *Power and Passion,* 91, and also MCT to MEG, Feb 19, 1880, reel 15, BMC.

36. Mamie Gwinn Hodder interview with Logan Pearsall Smith.

37. This scene is described in Horowitz, *Power and Passion,* 85–86.

38. Jealousies noted in Chase, "M. Carey Thomas and the Friday Night," 18; MCT to Mary Whitall Thomas, Aug. 23, 1880, reel 31, BMC; Horowitz, *Power and Passion,* 179.

39. Ibid., 178.

40. Quoted in Horowitz, *Power and Passion,* 78; Mamie Gwinn Hodder interview with Logan Pearsall Smith.

41. MEG to MCT, January 6, 1880, reel 42, BMC.

42. Miscellaneous document, "Social Questions," Box: Mary Garrett Diaries, Etc., Folder: F2, BMC.

43. MEG letter to Charles Mayer, February 13, 1894. It is unclear if in this letter Mary, from the vantage point of several years later, was rationalizing her own decision not to marry or if her father had, indeed, forbidden her to marry; MEG to Elizabeth Barbara Garrett, August 23, 1873, Box 128, Garrett Family Papers, Manuscript Division, LOC.

44. Horowitz, *Power and Passion,* 91, notes "The exam did not lead to entrance to the university, but certified accomplishment. For some women who studied privately, it emerged as an important marker of educational attainment."

45. From a letter of Alice Garrett to Rachel Garrett, June 2, 1879, Box: The Garretts, Folder: F3, BMC.

46. MEG to MCT, June 7, 1879, reel 42, BMC; MEG to MCT, June 10, 1879, reel 42, BMC.

47. MEG to MCT, June 18, 1879, reel 42, BMC; MEG to MCT, June 10, 1879, reel 42, BMC.

48. MEG to Charles F. Mayer, February 13, 1894.

49. MEG to MCT, October 24, 1879, reel 42, BMC; MEG to MCT, January 4, 1879, reel 42, BMC; MEG memoir.

50. MEG to Rachel Garrett, February 12, 1882, Box: From Mary Garrett to Her Mother, 1882–1883, Folder: F1, BMC.

51. Chase, "M. Carey Thomas and the Friday Night," 17.

52. MCT to MEG, November 5, 1879, reel 15, BMC.

53. JWG to unnamed doctor, September 16, 1880, Box 128, Garrett Family Collection, LOC.

54. Lizzie Garrett to Rachel Garrett, Aug 1, 1873, Box 128, Garrett Family Papers, Manuscript Division, LOC; MEG to Rachel Garrett, June 1882 [exact date unclear]. Box: From Mary Garrett to Her Mother, 1882–1883, Folder: F1, BMC.

55. MEG to MCT, July 10, 1880, reel 42, BMC.

56. MEG to MCT, September 11, 1880, reel 42, BMC.

57. MEG to MCT, May 4, 1880, reel 42, BMC.

58. MEG to MCT, September 27, 1880, reel 42, BMC; MEG to MCT, September 11, 1880, reel 42, BMC; MEG to MCT, September 26, 1880, reel 42, BMC.

59. JWG to unnamed doctor, September 16, 1880, Box: The Garretts, Folder: F8, BMC; MCT to Mary Whitall Thomas, Aug 23, 1880, reel 31, BMC.

60. Carolyn Heilbrun, in *Writing a Woman's Life* (New York: Ballantine Books, 1988), 49, explains Erik Erikson's theory as a maturation phase that occurs before the age of thirty, when the individual "appears to be getting nowhere, accomplishing none of his aims, or [is] altogether unclear as to what those aims might be. Such a person is, of course, actually preparing for the task that, all unrecognized, awaits."

61. National Institutes of Health, "The Changing Face of Medicine" website: www .nlm.nih.gov/changingthefaceofmedicine/physicians/biography_163.html.

62. Ibid.

63. MEG to MCT, June 13, 1878, Unnumbered Box, Folder: 39–3, BMC; MEG to MCT, June 13, 1878, reel 42, BMC.

64. MEG to MCT, May 18, 1876, reel 42, BMC. Of Mexican descent, Romualdo Pacheco was born in Santa Barbara, California, and served as governor from February to December 1875, when he lost the election.

65. MEG to MCT, July 21, 1878, reel 42, BMC.

66. Jane Austen, *Emma*, www.online-literature.com/austen/emma/1/; MEG to MCT, July 1879 [exact date unclear], reel 42, BMC.

67. MEG to MCT, November 23, 1880, reel 42, BMC.

68. MEG to Rachel Garrett, June 11, 1878, Box: Mary Garrett to Her Mother 1882–1883 (also contains unnumbered folder for letters to 1881), BMC.

69. Noted in letter to her mother, February 4, 1882, Box: Mary Garrett to Her Mother 1882–1883, Folder: F1, BMC.

70. MEG to Rachel Garrett, June 4, 1879, Garrett Family Papers, Manuscript Division, Box 128, LOC.

71. MEG to Rachel Garrett, April 15, 1882. Box: Mary Garrett to Her Mother,

1882–1883, Folder: F1, BMC; MEG to Rachel Garrett, February 4, 1882, Box: Mary Garrett to Her Mother, 1882–1883, Folder: F1, BMC.

72. Ibid.

73. MEG to Charles F. Mayer, February 13, 1894.

74. Ibid.

CHAPTER 4. AFTER GARRETT

1. John C. Schmidt, *Johns Hopkins: Portrait of a University* (Baltimore: Johns Hopkins University, 1986), 4.

2. Hugh Hawkins, *Pioneer: A History of the Johns Hopkins University, 1874–1889* (Ithaca, N.Y.: Cornell University Press), 1960, 3.

3. A. McGehee Harvey et al., *A Model of Its Kind: A Centennial History of Medicine at Johns Hopkins*, vol. 1 (Baltimore: Johns Hopkins University Press, 1989), 7, 8.

4. Hawkins, *Pioneer*, 9.

5. Ibid., 328–31.

6. Schmidt, *Johns Hopkins*, 5.

7. www.krieger.jhu.edu/about/history.html.

8. Hawkins, *Pioneer*, 69.

9. Ibid., 10.

10. Harvey et al., *A Model of Its Kind*, 11.

11. *New York World*, April 13, 1890.

12. MEG to Julia Rogers, September 15, 1876, quoted in Chase, "M. Carey Thomas and the Friday Night," 18.

13. Hawkins, *Pioneer*, 11; Eliot quote: Julia Morgan, "The Women of Johns Hopkins University: A History" (1986), 1:1. www.library.jhu.edu/collections/specialcollections/archives/womenshistory/index.html; www.hopkinsmedicine.org/history.html.

14. Angell quote: www.hopkinsmedicine.org/history.html; Gilman quote: Francesco Cordasco, *The Shaping of American Graduate Education: Daniel Coit Gilman and the Protean Ph.D.* (Leiden, Netherlands: E. J. Brill, 1960), 51.

15. Morgan, *Women of Johns Hopkins University*.

16. Cordasco, *Shaping of American Graduate Education*, 54.

17. Hawkins, *Pioneer*, 317.

18. Ibid.

19. Ibid., 145; French, *History of the University Founded by Johns Hopkins*, 59.

20. *New York Times*, January 1, 1893.

21. F. B. Mayer to JWG, April 26, 1882, Box 134, Garrett Family Collection, LOC.

22. Ibid.

23. *Baltimore Sun*, January 31, 1883. Garrett's speech was reprinted in this edition of the *Sun*.

24. Ibid.

25. Ibid.

26. *Baltimore Sun*, January 31, 1883.

27. *Baltimore American*, September 27, 1884, except horses "in high spirits," *Baltimore Sun*, October 13, 1883.

28. Florence Harrison to Rachel Garrett, August 26, 1882, Box 128, Garrett Family Papers, Manuscript Division, LOC; *Baltimore American*, September 27, 1884.

29. Luckett, *Maryland Women*, 123.

30. MEG to Mr. Andrews, December 20, 1883. Box 137, Garrett Family Papers, Manuscript Division, LOC; MEG to MCT, March 18, 1884, reel 42, BMC.

31. MEG to MCT, June 15, 1884, reel 42, BMC.

32. Ibid.

33. *Baltimore Sun*, September 26, 1884.

34. Joseph Drexel to JWG, Box 137, Garrett Family Papers, LOC.

35. *Baltimore American*, September 27, 1884; JWG to Robert Garrett, January 30, 1884, Box 137, Garrett Family Papers, Manuscript Division, LOC.

36. MEG to Andrew Anderson, Box 137, Garrett Family Papers, LOC.

37. *Sketch of John Work Garrett*, Appendix, 14.

38. *Baltimore Sun*, September 25, 1884; "dying in inches," *Baltimore American*, September 27, 1884; MEG to MCT, September 21, 1884, reel 42, BMC.

39. *Baltimore American*, supplement, September 27, 1884; *New York Tribune*, September 28, 1884.

40. *Sketch of John Work Garrett*, Appendix, 14–15.

41. *Pittsburg Dispatch*, September 26, 1884. The spelling reflects the older spelling of the city's name.

42. *Baltimore Sun*, September 27, 1884; Stover, *History of the Baltimore & Ohio Railroad*, 162.

43. *Baltimore Sun*, September 27, 1884; The B&O stock price at Garrett's death varies according to different sources. Hungerford, *Story of the Baltimore & Ohio Railroad*, 2:152, notes it was valued between $167 and $178; John Work Garrett Collection, Smithsonian Institution Archives Center (http://americanhistory.si.edu/archives/d8171.htm) estimates stock price in 1884 as $200; and the *Baltimore American*, September 27, 1884, states that on the day of Garrett's death the stock was valued at $175; on growth of B&O, *Sketch of John Work Garrett*, Appendix, 13; on largest monthly revenue, *Baltimore Sun*, September 25, 1884.

44. *Baltimore Sun*, September 29, 1884.

45. Ibid.; *Baltimore American*, September 28, 1884; on Central Headquarters Building, *Baltimore Sun*, September 28, 1884.

46. MEG to MCT, December 1884 [exact date unclear], reel 42, BMC.

47. MEG to Charles F. Mayer, February 13, 1894. This letter, written a decade after John Work Garrett's death, provides important insight into how Mary later recalled the events surrounding her father's death and her inheritance; *New York Tribune* quoted in Bremner, *American Philanthropy*, 103.

48. *Baltimore American*, September 27, 1884; "Garrett Estate, Inventories and Assets and Accounts," Box: Mary Garrett Business Papers, Folder: 2-J, BMC.

49. *Baltimore American*, October 2, 1884.

50. Last Will and Testament of John Work Garrett, signed August 8, 1884, Ever-

green House Foundation at Evergreen Museum and Library, JHU. The will uses the old street numbers: 77 is now 101; 71 Mount Vernon Place is Robert's house, which is now 11; 50 Mount Vernon Place is now 12.

51. The rental properties are listed on the "Garrett Estate Inventories and Assets, 1895," Box: Mary Garrett Business Papers, Folder: F2, BMC.

52. JWG Last Will and Testament.

53. *Baltimore American*, September 27, 1884.

54. Ibid.

55. Charles F. Gross, *Cincinnati, The Queen City* (Cincinnati: S. J. Clarke Publishing, 1912), 1:227.

56. *Baltimore American*, September 27, 1884.

57. JWG Last Will and Testament.

58. *Baltimore American*, September 27, 1884.

59. *Baltimore Sun*, July 30, 1896.

60. MEG to Charles F. Mayer, February 13, 1894.

61. Ibid.

62. *Baltimore Sun*, September 27, 1884.

63. Charles F. Mayer to W. F. Frick, esq., July 2, 1889, "Garrett Estate, Settlement of Estate: Losses incurred by Miss Garrett." Box: The Garrett Estate, Folder: F1, BMC.

64. Rev. J. W. Wilson to MEG, February 1, 1892. Garrett Collection, Box: Mary Garrett, Folder: F3, BMC; Austen Brown to MEG, November 1913, Garrett Collection, Box: Mary Garrett, Folder: F3, BMC; undated letter, Mary Garrett Collection, Box 15, Correspondence to M. E. Garrett, Garrett Family Papers, MS979, H. Furlong Baldwin Library, MHS; MEG to A. B. Crane, November 2, 1889, Box 14, Correspondence to M. E. Garrett, Garrett Family Papers, MS979, MHS.

65. *American Architect and Building News* (January 6, 1886): 21.

66. *New York Times*, November 16, 1890.

67. *Baltimore Sun*, September 27, 1884; *Baltimore American*, September 28, 1884.

68. *Baltimore Sun*, September 27, 1884; *American Architect and Building News* (January 6, 1886): 21.

69. Warren Wilmer Brown, "The Baltimore Museum of Art: Its Evolution and Future" *Art and Archeology: The Arts through the Ages* (Archeological Society of Washington, 1925).

70. From "Inventory of Furniture, etc. in Miss Garrett's Cottage, Deer Park." Box: Mary Garrett Business Papers, Folder F2, BMC.

71. *American Architect and Building News* (January 6, 1886): 20.

72. Giza and Black, *Great Baltimore Houses*, 86.

73. *Baltimore American* (July 30, 1888): 2; *Chicago Tribune*, March 5, 1896.

74. Carlos P. Avery, *E. Francis Baldwin, Architect: The B&O, Baltimore, and Beyond* (Baltimore: Baltimore Architecture Foundation, 2003), 123; Garrett Power, "High Society: The Building Height Limitations on Baltimore's Mt. Vernon Place," *Maryland Historical Magazine* 79, no. 3 (Fall 1984): 202.

75. Katharine Dehler, "Mount Vernon Place at the Turn of the Century: A Vignette of the Garrett Family," *Maryland Historical Magazine* 69, no. 3 (Fall 1974): 289.

76. Giza and Black, *Great Houses of Baltimore*, 61. Many commentators theorize that economist and social critic Thorstein Veblen had the Garretts of Baltimore in mind when he captured the excesses of the Gilded Age and coined the term "conspicuous consumption" in his 1889 *The Theory of the Leisure Class* (New York: Dover Publications, 1994). According to Faith M. Holland, "What a Difference a Year Made: John Work Garrett Finds a Diplomatic Career," *Maryland Historical Magazine* 91, no. 3 (Fall 1996): 285, Veblen's work is a "mordant critique of the Garretts' world." Also noted in Power, *High Society*, 201; *Chicago Daily Tribune*, November 29, 1890. See also Evergreen House website: www.jhu.edu/evergreen.

77. *Baltimore: Its History and Its People*, 463.

78. *Baltimore American*, September 27, 1884.

79. Annie Nathan Meyer, ed., *Woman's Work in America* (New York: Henry Holt and Co., 1891), 287.

80. Page Smith, *The Rise of Industrial America: A People's History of the Post-Reconstruction Era* (New York: McGraw Hill, 1984), 668.

81. Amzi Crane to MEG, March 17, 1894, Box 15, Folder 1891–95, Correspondence to M. E. Garrett, Garrett Family Papers, MS979, H. Furlong Baldwin Library, MHS; causes supported noted in Joan Margaret Fisher, "A Study of Six WomenPhilanthropists of the Early Twentieth Century" (Ph.D. diss., Union Institute, 1992), 196.

82. 1886 *Annual Report*, Baltimore Woman's Industrial Exchange.

83. Heather E. Erst, "In Aid of Ladies in Reduced Circumstances: The Decorative Arts Society and the Woman's Industrial Exchange in Baltimore," presentation, Garrett-Jacobs Mansion Symposium "Rich in Vision, Catalysts of Change: Women in 19th Century Baltimore," April 21–23, 2006.

84. Elizabeth Cady Stanton, "To Find Our Own Sphere," quoted in Sue Heinemann, *Timelines of American Women's History* (New York: Berkley Publishing Group, 1996), 173.

85. MEG memoir.

CHAPTER 5. THE PRACTICAL HEAD OF THE GARRETT FAMILY

1. MEG to "Dear Girls," August 1, 1885, reel 42, BMC.

2. Horowitz, *The Power and Passion*, 144.

3. MEG to "Dear Girls," August 1, 1885, reel 42, BMC.

4. Ibid.

5. Howard Zinn, *A People's History of the United States* (New York: Harper-Perennial, 1990), pp. 116–17.

6. Sue Heinemann, *Timelines of American Women's History* (New York: Berkley Publishing Group, 1996), 172.

7. Similarities not differences noted in Andrea Hamilton, *A Vision for Girls: Gender, Education and the Bryn Mawr School* (Baltimore: Johns Hopkins University Press, 2004), 25; E. H. Clarke, *Sex in Education: A Fair Chance for Girls* (1873), quoted in Ruth J. Abram, ed., *"Send Us a Lady Physician": Women Doctors in America, 1835–1920* (New York: W. W. Norton & Co., 1985), 64.

8. MEG memoir; BMS 1896 Catalogue, BMS.

9. MEG to Mamie Gwinn, undated, BMS, quoted in Hamilton, *Vision for Girls*, 21.

10. MEG to MCT, July 10, 1880, reel 42, BMC.

11. From Carey Thomas, "A Brief Account of the Founding and Early Years of the Bryn Mawr School," *Bryn Mawrter* 1931 (BMS Yearbook), 84–88, quoted in Hamilton, *Vision for Girls*, 33.

12. MEG to "Dear Girls," July 24, 1885, reel 42, BMC; Amzi Crane to MEG, 1889 [exact date unknown], MS979, Box 15, Folder 1889, M. E. Garrett Correspondence, Garrett Family Papers, MHS.

13. MEG to "Dear Girls," July 20, 1885, reel 42, BMC; Rosamond Randall Beirne, *Let's Pick the Daisies: The History of Bryn Mawr School, 1885–1967* (Baltimore: Bryn Mawr School, 1970), 5.

14. Amzi Crane to MEG, 1889 [exact date unknown], MS979, Box 15, Folder 1889, M. E. Garrett Correspondence, Garrett Family Papers, MHS.

15. MEG to "Dear Girls," October 15, 1886, reel 42, BMC.

16. Beirne, *Daisies*, 5, 6–7.

17. MEG to MCT, May 9, 1886, reel 42, BMC; Mamie Gwinn Hodder to MCT, April 4, 1884, quoted in Horowitz, *Power and Passion*, 481n35.

18. MCT to MEG, June 12, 1886, reel 15, BMC, quoted in Horowitz, *Power and Passion*, 231.

19. Horowitz, *Power and Passion*, 231.

20. *Baltimore Sun*, June 4, 1886; Schlosnagle et al., *Garrett County*, 282.

21. Stover, *History of the Baltimore and Ohio Railroad*, 169.

22. *Baltimore Sun*, July 31, 1896.

23. *Chicago Tribune*, July 30, 1896.

24. MEG to Elizabeth Barbara Garrett, undated, probably summer 1887. Box 137, Garrett Family Papers, LOC.

25. *Chicago Daily Tribune*, July 20, 1888.

26. An account of Mary's meetings with Gilman was published by W. T. Barnard in the *Baltimore & Ohio Company, Office of the President: Service Report on Technical Education, with Special Reference to the Baltimore & Ohio Railroad Service* (1887) noted in Hawkins, *Pioneer*, 318n5; Hawkins, *Pioneer*, 319.

27. Ibid., 318.

28. Ibid., 319; *New York Times*, January 1, 1893.

29. Paul Winchester, *Graphic Sketches from the History of the Baltimore & Ohio Railroad* (Baltimore: Maryland County Press Syndicate, 1927), 197.

30. Stover, *History of the Baltimore and Ohio Railroad*, 167.

31. *Chicago Tribune*, July 30, 1896.

32. *Baltimore: Its History and Its People*, 2:461.

33. MEG to MCT, October 31, 1887, reel 42, BMC; MEG to MCT, November 6, 1887, reel 42, BMC.

34. MEG to MCT, December 13, 1887, reel 42, BMC.

35. Itinerary cited in *Baltimore Sun*, July 30, 1896.

36. *Baltimore American*, June 9, 1888.

37. Ibid.

38. Ibid.

39. *Baltimore American*, June 11, 1888; *Baltimore Sun*, June 12, 1888.

40. *Baltimore Sun*, June 14, 1888; *Baltimore American*, June 13, 1888.

41. *Baltimore Sun*, June 14, 1888.

42. *Chicago Tribune*, July 30, 1896.

43. *Baltimore Sun*, July 30, 1896.

44. *Washington Post*, August 23, 1888; *Baltimore American*, July 30, 1896.

45. *Chicago Daily Tribune*, July 20, 1888.

46. MEG to MCT, July 22, 1888, reel 42, BMC.

47. *Chicago Daily Tribune*, December 21, 1888; Stover, *History of the Baltimore and Ohio Railroad*, 169.

48. *Chicago Daily Tribune*, December 21, 1888. The statement refers to Garrett factions and not a member of the Garrett family.

49. *New York Times*, July 14, 1888; *Chicago Daily Tribune*, July 20, 1888.

50. *Chicago Tribune*, July 20, 1888; *Springfield (IL) Republican News*, undated, BMS.

51. Charles F. Mayer to W. F. Frick, esq., July 2, 1889, "Garrett Estate, Settlement of Estate: Losses incurred by Miss Garrett," Box: Mary Garrett Business Papers, Folder: F7, BMC.

52. Beirne, *Daisies*, 8.

53. *Baltimore Sun*, January 7, 1972.

54. MEG to "Dear Girls," October 2, 1889, reel 42. BMC; *Baltimore Sun*, January 12, 1889.

55. *New York Times*, January 16, 1889; MEG to MCT, January 17, 1889, reel 42, BMC.

56. *New York Times*, January 16, 1889.

57. Unidentified and undated newspaper clipping, BMS; *Harrisburg Patriot*, January 23, 1889; *Richmond State*, undated, probably early 1889, BMS; *New York Times*, January 16, 1889.

58. Untitled and undated newspaper clipping, probably 1889, BMS; *Kitchen Magazine*, April 1889; *Baltimore Sun*, January 7, 1972.

59. *The Cincinnati Enquirer*, 1889 [exact date unknown], BMS; *New York Times* [exact date unknown, probably 1889], BMS.

60. Morris Homans to MEG, October 29, 1889, Box: Mary Garrett Business Papers, Folder: F2–3–2, BMC; MEG to MCT, November 12, 1889, reel 42, BMC.

61. Avery, *E. Francis Baldwin*, 88; Beirne, *Daisies*, 12–13.

62. Noted in Edith Finch, *Carey Thomas of Bryn Mawr* (Harper & Brothers Publishers, 1947), 196; MEG to MCT, February 1889 [exact date unclear], reel 42, BMC.

63. Beirne, *Daisies*, 14.

64. Ibid., 16.

65. Descriptions taken from 1907 inventory of classroom, BMS Archives, and

Beirne, *Daisies*, 16; Lucy Bull, "A Model School in Baltimore," *Critic*, December 3, 1894, BMS.

66. Newspaper article quoted in Beirne, *Daisies*, 10–11; Luckett, *Maryland Women*, 15.

67. *Baltimore American*, September 23, 1890.

68. Mary H. Cadwalader, "No Carpet and No Red Door; Bryn Mawr School Stood for Brains," *Evening Sun*, date unknown, BMS.

CHAPTER 6. THE SCHEME

1. Regina Markall Morantz-Sanchez, *Sympathy and Science: Women Physicians in American Medicine* (New York: Oxford University Press, 1985), 5; on Lester: http://womenshistory.about.com/library/prm/blwomeninmedicine1.htm.

2. Mary Roth Walsh, *"Doctors Wanted: No Women Need Apply": Sexual Barriers in the Medical Profession, 1835–1975* (New Haven, Conn.: Yale University Press, 1977), 14.

3. Morantz-Sanchez, *Sympathy and Science*, 68; Paul Starr, *The Social Transformation of American Medicine* (New York: Basic Books, 1982), 83; Ruth J. Abram, ed., *"Send Us a Lady Physician": Women Doctors in America, 1835–1920* (New York: W. W. Norton & Co., 1985), 18.

4. Abram, *"Send Us a Lady Physician,"* 17.

5. Ibid., 53; www.hopkinsmedicine.org/abouthistory6.html.

6. Morantz-Sanchez, *Sympathy and Science*, 67.

7. Quoted in Walsh, *"Doctors Wanted,"* 109.

8. Ibid., xv; Harvey et al., *A Model of Its Kind*, 138.

9. Abram, *"Send Us a Lady Physician,"* 99.

10. Harvard University School of Medicine Joint Committee on the Status of Women, "The Matriculation of Women at Harvard Medical School 1871–1920" timeline: www.hms.harvard.edu/jcsw/matriculation2.htm.

11. Ibid.

12. Morantz-Sanchez, *Sympathy and Science*, 164.

13. Jill Jones, "Opening Days: Joy and Relief," in special issue, "The Medical Centennial," *Johns Hopkins Magazine* (June 1989): 30.

14. Charles Rosenberg, "What It Was Like to Be Sick in 1884," *American Heritage* (October/November 1984): 31.

15. Harvey et al., *A Model of Its Kind*, 16.

16. *American Architect and Building News*, February 6, 1886.

17. "Records of the Development Programs before 1950: The Johns Hopkins University," http://ead.library.jhu.edu/rg11–002.xml; *Chicago Journal*, April 20, 1891; Hawkins, *Pioneer*, 320.

18. "Sources of the Original $500,000," File 50, AMC.

19. Daniel Coit Gilman to Charles Gwinn and George Dobbin, "Dear Sirs," November 9, 1888, Box 507277, AMC.

20. Ibid.

21. Bert Hansen, "America's First Medical Breakthrough: How Popular Excitement about a French Rabies Cure in 1885 Raised New Expectations for Medical Progress," *American Historical Review* 103, no. 2 (April 1998).

22. Records of the Development Programs before 1950: The Johns Hopkins University, http://ead.library.jhu.edu/rg11–002.xml.

23. *Baltimore Sun*, May 8, 1889.

24. *St. Louis Republic*, April 5, 1891.

25. Descriptions taken from Jill Jones, "Opening Days," 30, and Harvey et al., *A Model of Its Kind*, 23–24; *Hospital Plans*, quoted in Harvey et al., *A Model of Its Kind*, 9; *A Model of Its Kind*, 29.

26. *Baltimore Sun*, May 8, 1889.

27. Jones, "Opening Days," 32.

28. MCT to MEG, December 7, 1888, reel 15, BMC.

29. MEG to MCT, December 4, 1888, reel 42, BMC.

30. Ibid.; MCT to MEG, December 31, 1888, reel 15, BMC.

31. MCT to MEG, April 15, 1890, reel 15, BMC.

32. Ibid.; "General Circular," Women's Medical School Fund Papers, File 21, AMC.

33. MEG to MCT, December 4, 1888, reel 42, BMC; MCT to MEG, April 15, 1890, reel 15, BMC.

34. MEG to MCT, December 4, 1888, reel 42, BMC; MCT to MEG, December 7, 1888, reel 15, BMC.

35. MEG to MCT, August 14, 1889, reel 42, BMC.

36. MCT to MEG, September 24, 1889, reel 15, BMC.

37. *Nation*, March 30, 1890.

38. MEG to MCT, April 14, 1890, reel 42, BMC.

39. Ibid.

40. MEG to MCT, April 15, 1890, reel 42, BMC.

41. MEG to "Dear Girls," undated. Quoted in "Dear Girls," *Celebrating the Philanthropy of Mary Elizabeth Garrett*, www.medicalarchives.jhmi.edu/garrett/deargirls.htm.

42. MEG to "Dear Girls," May 13, 1890, reel 42, BMC.

43. MEG to MCT, April 14, 1890, reel 42, BMC.

44. MEG to MCT, April 18, 1890, reel 42, BMC.

45. MCT to MEG, April 16, 1890, reel 16, BMC.

46. MEG to MCT, April 15, 1890, reel 42, BMC.

47. *Washington Post*, November 3, 1890; *Chicago Daily Tribune*, June 2, 1890; MEG to "Dear Girls," May 22, 1890, reel 42, BMC.

48. Mamie Gwinn Hodder to Alan Mason Chesney, January 29, 1939. Women's Medical School Fund Papers, File 21, AMC.

49. MEG to "Dear Girls," May 22, 1890, reel 42, BMC.

50. MEG to MCT, April 20, 1890, reel 42, BMC.

51. MEG to MCT, April 18, 1890, reel 42, BMC.

52. MCT to MEG, April 20, 1890, reel 16, BMC.

53. MCT to MEG, April 19, 1890, reel 16, BMC.

54. Ibid.

55. It is unclear exactly when the women adopted this name for the campaign, although the May 2 meeting seems likely. The name does not appear in early drafts of fundraising circulars, publicity, or letters. The name is identified in the "Resolutions Adopted by the Board of Trustees on October 28, 1890," in which the trustees accepted the fund's offer of $100,000: "The fund so contributed shall be invested and known as 'The Women's Medical School Fund' . . . It is also called the 'Women's Medical Fund Campaign.'"

56. MEG to "Dear Girls," May 13, 1890, reel 42, BMC.

57. Daniel Coit Gilman to Trustees, August 13, 1890, Box 507277, AMC; Judge George W. Brown to Daniel Coit Gilman, August 16, 1890, Box 507277, AMC.

58. MEG to MCT, August 23, 1890, reel 42, BMC.

59. Nancy Morris Davis, Chairman of the Baltimore Committee, to the JHU Board of Trustees, October 28, 1890, Women's Medical School Fund Papers, File 21, AMC; "Resolutions Adopted by the Board of Trustees on October 28, 1890," Women's Medical School Fund Papers, File 21, AMC.

60. "Noble act," *Baltimore American*, November 4, 1890; *Report of the Women's Fund for the Medical School of the Johns Hopkins University* (May 26, 1891), 3, AMC.

61. "Resolutions Adopted by the Board of Trustees on October 28, 1890."

62. *Baltimore American*, November 15, 1890; *Baltimore Sun*, November 15, 1890.

63. *Baltimore Sun*, November 15, 1890.

64. *Baltimore Sun*, quoted in Lavinia Edmunds, "The Price of Admission," *Johns Hopkins Magazine* (June 1989): 64; *Washington Post*, November 15, 1890.

65. *Baltimore Sun*, November 15, 1890.

66. *Baltimore American*, November 15, 1890.

67. Ibid.; *Washington Post*, November 15, 1890.

68. *Century Illustrated Magazine*, February 1891.

69. MEG to MCT, March 5, 1890, reel 42, BMC.

70. Edmunds, "The Price of Admission," 125.

71. MEG to MCT, February 12, 1891, reel 42, BMC; MEG to MCT, February 28, 1891, reel 42, BMC.

72. Ibid.

73. MEG to MCT, February 19, 1891, reel 42, BMC; MCT to MEG, October 1891 [exact date unknown], reel 16, BMC.

74. MEG to MCT, February 28, 1891, reel 42, BMC.

75. "Kate Field's Washington," *National Independent Review*, March 11, 1891.

76. Ibid.; *Century Illustrated Magazine*, February 1891.

77. Mary E. Garrett to Hon. George W. Dobbin, April 27, 1891, Women's Medical School Fund Papers, File 21, AMC. In her letter to Dobbin, Mary listed the final amount as $109,000. The committee raised only an additional $11,300 between the time the offer was presented to the trustees in October 1890 and when the money was

handed over in May 1891; The university's share included $67,480.42 from the original funding, plus accrued interest of $14,242.58 for a total of $81,723. See "Records of the Development Office before 1950," http://ead.library.jhu.edu/rg11–002.xml.

CHAPTER 7. A PLEASURE TO BE BOUGHT

1. *Baltimore American,* May 4, 1891.

2. MEG to Hon. George Dobbin, President of the Board of Trustees of the Johns Hopkins University, April 27, 1891. Women's Medical Fund Campaign Papers, File 21, AMC.

3. *Sunday Herald,* May 3, 1891; *Baltimore American,* April 29, 1891.

4. *New York Telegraph,* May 2, 1891; *Sunday Herald,* May 3, 1891; *Cincinnati Enquirer,* May 8, 1891; *Baltimore American,* May 3, 1891.

5. *St. Louis Republic,* May 4, 1891.

6. MEG to MCT, July 16, 1891, reel 42, BMC.

7. MEG to Charles Stewart, January 15, 1892, reel 43, BMC; *Baltimore Sun,* February 8, 1892.

8. Charles Stewart to MEG, February 9, 1892, reel 173, BMC; MEG to MCT, September 24, 1891, reel 42, BMC; MEG to MCT, January 24, 1892, reel 43, BMC.

9. MEG to MCT, February 21, 1892, reel 43, BMC.

10. Ibid.

11. MCT to MEG, November 29, 1892, reel 17, BMC.

12. MEG to MCT, December 9, 1892, reel 43, BMC.

13. Letter from Miss Garrett to the Trustees of the University, December 22, 1892, Daniel Coit Gilman Papers, ms. 1, Sheridan Libraries, JHU.

14. Ibid.

15. Ibid.

16. Ibid.

17. Hawkins, *Pioneer,* 108; Edmunds, "The Price of Admission," 65.

18. MCT to MEG, December 23, 1892, reel 17, BMC.

19. *Action of the Trustees,* December 24, 1892, Daniel Coit Gilman Papers, ms. 1, Sheridan Libraries, JHU.

20. Edmunds, "The Price of Admission," 65.

21. "An Account of the Negotiations with Miss Mary E. Garrett Concerning the Terms of Her Gift to the Medical School" [no date]. Daniel Coit Gilman Papers, ms. 1, Sheridan Libraries, JHU.

22. Edmunds, "The Price of Admission," 65.

23. MEG to Board of Trustees, January 30, 1893, Daniel Coit Gilman Papers, ms. 1, Sheridan Libraries, JHU.

24. MEG to MCT, February 7, 1892, reel 43, BMC; MCT to Hannah Whitall Smith, March 11, 1894, reel 29, BMC, noted in Horowitz, *Power and Passion,* 237.

25. "Account of the Negotiations with Miss Mary E. Garrett Concerning the Terms of Her Gift to the Medical School."

26. *Baltimore Herald,* February 11, 1893.

27. Daniel Coit Gilman to MEG, December 23, 1892. Daniel Gilman Papers, ms. 1, Sheridan Libraries, JHU; Osler quote, Harvey et al., *A Model of Its Kind*, 28.

28. "Preliminary Announcement of the Johns Hopkins Medical School," File 41, AMC.

29. *Chicago Herald*, December 20, 1892. All newspaper clippings in MCT Subject Files, Reels 172/173, BMC; *San Francisco Examiner*, February 14, 1893; *Baltimore Sun*, January 2, 1893; *Baltimore American*, December 30, 1892.

30. *Baltimore Sun*, December 15, 1892.

31. *Philadelphia Call*, January 5, 1893.

32. *Review of Reviews*, February 1893; *Philadelphia Ledger*, January 7, 1893.

33. *Wilmington Journal*, January 4, 1893.

34. William Osler to Ira Remsen, September 1, 1911, quoted in Harvey et al., *A Model of Its Kind*, 140. Osler was referring to the Women's Medical School Fund.

35. Harvey et al., *A Model of Its Kind*, 30.

36. *St. Louis Post Dispatch*, July 25, 1891.

37. Morantz-Sanchez, *Sympathy and Science*, 233.

38. MEG to MCT, January 22, 1893, reel 43, BMC.

39. Gerri Kobren, "The Building That Nurtured Hopkins Glory," *Sunday Sun* (Baltimore), May 13, 1979.

40. Richard Bridgman, *Gertrude Stein in Pieces* (New York: Oxford University Press, 1970), 55; Osler quote, Harvey et al., *A Model of Its Kind*, 140.

41. www.hopkinsmedicine.org/about/history/history6.html.

42. Jane Sellman, "Pioneers of Excellence," *Gazette* 25 (Johns Hopkins University, January/March 1996), www.jhu.edu/~gazette/janmar96/mar2596/womsom.html.

43. Janet Farrar Worthington, "Concrete Ceiling," *Hopkins Medicine* (Fall 2005), www.hopkinsmedicine.org/hmn/F05/annals.cfm.

44. Ibid.

45. Ibid.; Sellman, "Pioneers of Excellence."

46. Morantz-Sanchez, *Sympathy and Science*, 123.

47. Bridgman, *Gertrude Stein in Pieces*, 35, 36.

48. Morantz-Sanchez, *Sympathy and Science*, 234.

49. Ibid., 232.

50. MEG to Daniel Coit Gilman, December 31, 1894, Daniel Coit Gilman Papers, ms. 1, Sheridan Libraries, JHU; MEG to Daniel Coit Gilman, January 2, 1895, Daniel Coit Gilman Papers, ms. 1, Sheridan Libraries, JHU.

51. MCT to Hannah Smith, March 11, 1894, quoted in Horowitz, *Power and the Passion*, 237.

52. Harvey et al., *A Model of Its Kind*, 28, 50.

53. Edmunds, "The Price of Admission," 125.

54. Helen Lefkowitz Horowitz, *Alma Mater: Design and Experience in the Women's Colleges from their Nineteenth Century Beginnings to the 1930s* (New York: Alfred A. Knopf, 1984), 111, 110.

55. Ibid., 106.

56. Ibid., 113.

57. Ibid., 114, 115.

58. Ibid., 6; Brenda Wineapple, *Sister Brother: Gertrude and Leo Stein* (Baltimore: Johns Hopkins University Press, 1996), 145.

59. Horowitz, *Power and Passion*, 203.

60. Ibid., 249.

61. MEG to MCT, August 30, 1892, reel 43, BMC.

62. MCT to MEG, January 17, 1892, reel 16, BMC, quoted in Horowitz, *Power and Passion*, 249–50.

63. Minutes of trustees' meetings, vol. 1A2, 1890–1895, BMC.

64. MEG to MCT, March 11, 1893, reel 43, BMC.

65. Mamie Gwinn Hodder to Logan Pearsall Smith, early 1938 [exact date unknown], Box 45, AMC.

66. MEG to MCT, March 23, 1893, reel 43, BMC.

67. Ibid.; on Mammon, Horowitz, *Power and the Passion*, 258.

68. BMC *Financial Report* (1889–1890), 7, 1QT, BMC.

69. Minutes of trustees' meeting, April 14, 1893, BMC; letter quoted in Edith Finch, *Carey Thomas of Bryn Mawr* (New York: Harper & Brothers Publishers, 1947), 209.

70. Minutes of trustees' meeting, April 14, 1893, BMC.

71. Horowitz, *The Power and the Passion*, 258.

72. Finch, *Carey Thomas*, 211; *Bryn Mawr College Quarterly* (January 1917), 128, BMC.

73. William D. Andrews, "Women and the Fairs of 1876 and 1893," *Hayes Historical Journal* (Spring 1977), 179; Henry Adams, *The Education of Henry Adams: An Autobiography* (New York: Oxford Classics, 1999), 273.

74. Beirne, *Daisies*, 20.

75. MEG to MCT, February 18, 1893, reel 43, BMC.

76. Minutes, Board of Trustees, November 17, 1893, BMC.

77. Horowitz, *Power and the Passion*, 263; Minutes, Board of Trustees, December 8, 1893, BMC.

78. List compiled from annual financial reports and donors lists 1885–1936, 1QT, BMC.

79. MCT to MEG, December 13, 1894, reel 18, BMC, quoted in Horowitz, *Power and the Passion*, 278.

80. MEG to MCT, April 17, 1895, reel 44, BMC.

CHAPTER 8. THE HAPPINESS OF GETTING OUR WORK DONE

1. MEG to MCT, March 23, 1893, reel 43, BMC.

2. Ibid.

3. Holland, "What a Difference a Year Made," 281–83.

4. MEG to Robert de Forest, November 20, 1895; MEG to Robert de Forest, September 27, 1895; Robert de Forest to William Frick, December 26, 1895. All in Box: The Garrett Estate, Folder: F1–11, BMC.

5. Stover, *History of the Baltimore and Ohio Railroad*, 182.

6. *Chicago Daily Tribune*, April 21, 1896.

7. Stover, *History of the Baltimore and Ohio Railroad*, 186–87.

8. MEG to JWG II, April 8, 1896, Box: The Garrett Estate, Folder: F1–11, BMC.

9. Ibid.

10. Charles Mayer to William Frick, May 20, 1889, Box: Mary Garrett Business Papers, Folder: F7, BMC.

11. *Baltimore American*, November 4, 1890.

12. MEG to MCT, April 17, 1895, reel 44, BMC; MEG to Charles Mayer, February 13, 1894, Box: The Garrett Estate, Folder: F1–11, BMC.

13. MEG to MCT, July 22, 1895, reel 44, BMC.

14. Holland, "What a Difference a Year Made," 281. John II was an avid natural historian. His collection of natural objects can be seen in his childhood room at Evergreen.

15. In 1974, Robert Garrett & Sons merged with Alex Brown Incorporated, which in 2008 is known as Deutsche Banc Alex. Brown.

16. MEG to MCT, April 18, 1895, reel 45, BMC.

17. Ibid.; MEG to MCT, April 4, 1895, reel 45, BMC; MEG to MCT, April 18, 1895, reel 45, BMC.

18. MEG to Mrs. Rowland, January 28, 1895, Henry A. Rowland Papers, ms. 6, Sheridan Libraries, JHU.

19. Amzi Crane to MEG, March 17, 1893; A. B. Crane to MEG, April 21, 1893. Both in Box 15, Garrett Family Papers, MHS.

20. *Washington Post*, September 13, 1896.

21. MEG to Robert de Forest, September 27, 1895, Box: The Garrett Estate, Folder: F1–11, BMC; JWG II Diary, 1896, Evergreen House Foundation at Evergreen Museum and Library, JHU.

22. Memo for Conference with C.F.M. (Charles Mayer), September 26, 1895, Box: The Garrett Estate, Folder: 1–11, BMC; the inventory is contained in the document "Estate of John Work Garrett: Summary of Accounts from September 25th, 1884 to September 30th, 1895," Box: Mary Garrett Business Papers, Folder: F2, BMC.

23. *Chicago Tribune*, July 30, 1896; *Philadelphia Telegraph*, July 29, 1896; *Baltimore Sun*, July 30, 1896.

24. *Chicago Tribune*, July 30, 1896; *Baltimore Evening News*, July 29, 1896; MEG to MCT, July 30, 1896, reel 46, BMC.

25. *Baltimore Sun*, August 1, 1896; MEG to MCT, August 2, 1896, reel 46, BMC; *Chicago Tribune*, July 30, 1896.

26. *Louisville Courier Journal*, August 1, 1896; *Chicago Tribune*, July 30, 1896; *Baltimore American*, July 30, 1896; *Chicago Tribune*, July 30, 1896.

27. MEG to MCT, July 30, 1896, reel 46, BMC.

28. *Chicago Tribune*, December 22, 1896.

29. *New York Times*, June 24, 1898. The figure of $10 per share might have been misreported. The B&O's historic low was $13 in March 1896, according to Stover, *History of the Baltimore and Ohio Railroad*, 183.

30. Stover, *History of the Baltimore and Ohio Railroad*, 191.

31. Robert Garrett II to MEG, February 12, 1899, Evergreen House Foundation at Evergreen Museum and Library, JHU.

32. Ibid.; Robert Garrett II to MEG, June 1899 [exact date unknown], Evergreen House Foundation.

33. *Washington Post*, June 18, 1899; *Syracuse Standard*, June 19, 1899; *Washington Post*, June 18, 1899.

34. Finch, *Carey Thomas*, 240.

35. MCT to MEG, January 5, 1899, reel 21, BMC, quoted in Horowitz, *Power and the Passion*, 285.

36. Sarah Orne Jewett, *Outgrown Friends*, 1887, www.public.coe.edu/~theller/soj/una/outgrown.html, quoted in Gail Collins, *America's Women: Four Hundred Years of Dolls, Drudges, Helpmates and Heroines* (New York: William Morrow, 2003), 256.

37. Horowitz, *Power and the Passion*, 253; Collins, *America's Women*, 257.

38. Sarah Orne Jewett to Louisa Dresel, August 18, 1896, www.public.coe.edu/~theller/soj/let/dresel.html; Sarah Orne Jewett to Louisa Dresel, March 10, 1893, www.public.coe.edu/~theller/soj/let/dresel.html.

39. Horowitz, *Power and Passion*, 292.

40. Ibid., 204.

41. Quoted in Kristen Ikola, "Scandal at the Deanery" (unpublished student paper), May 3, 1993, based on a 1977 interview by Caroline Smith Rittenhouse with Franny Travis Cochran, Oral History Collection, BMC. Mamie Gwinn Papers, 3H/Gwinn, BMC.

42. Horowitz, *Power and the Passion*, 368.

43. On "reincarnation of Christ," ibid., 372; on séances, "Alfred and Mary Gwinn Hodder papers, A Finding Aid," Manuscripts Division, Department of Rare Books and Special Library Collections, Princeton University Library (1992), 3. Mamie died in the 1940s.

44. Leon Katz, "Introduction," in Gertrude Stein, *Fernhurst, Q.E.D., and Other Early Writings* (New York: Liveright, 1971), xii.

45. Stein, *Fernhurst*, 5, 15, 18.

46. Ibid., 32; Horowitz, *Power and the Passion*, 280; Stein, *Fernhurst*, 49.

47. MEG to MCT, April 21, 1903, reel 49, BMC; MEG to MCT, December 8, 1902, reel 49, BMC.

48. John Singer Sargent to MEG, February 19, 1903, Box: Mary Garrett, Folder: F9, BMC.

49. "The Four Doctors, Material Culture Collections Files," Ready Reference File, AMC.

50. MEG to MCT, December 8, 1902, reel 49, BMC.

51. William H. Welch to MEG, March 4, 1903; William Osler to MEG, Feb 24, 1903; William H. Welch to MEG, March 4, 1903. All in Box: Mary Garrett, Folder: F9, BMC.

52. *Washington Post*, September 13, 1896.

53. "The Sargent Portrait: M. Carey Thomas and John Singer Sargent," www
.brynmawr.edu/Library/Exhibits/sargent/portrait2.html.

54. *New York Times*, March 4, 1923.

55. *Washington Post*, 1896 [exact date unclear]; *Baltimore Sun*, September 22,
1928; *Washington Post*, 1896 [exact date unclear].

56. *Chicago Daily Tribune*, January 8, 1897; *New York Times*, November 29, 1900;
New York Times, January 10, 1897.

57. MEG to MCT, February 8, 1904, reel 50, BMC.

58. MEG to MCT, September 3, 1909, reel 51, BMC; Horowitz, *The Power and
the Passion*, 362.

59. MEG to MCT, 1902 [exact date unknown], reel 49, BMC.

60. Sarah Orne Jewett to MEG, October 1904 [exact date unclear], Box: Mary
Garrett, Folder: F1, BMC.

61. *Washington Post*, November 6, 1904.

62. Ibid.; MEG to MCT, November 29, 1904, reel 51, BMC.

63. MEG to MCT, September 3, 1909, reel 51, BMC. "The many hundreds of
thousands of pages that Carey Thomas wittingly or unwittingly left for posterity con-
tain no clear, unambiguous statement revealing that her physical expressions of lovemaking with Mary (or Mamie) included genital contact. Absence of evidence, however, proves nothing at all. Testimony to the most private pleasures of lovemaking does
not usually rest in archives." Horowitz, *Power and the Passion*, 290.

64. MEG to MCT, February 12, 1900, reel 48, BMC.

65. Horowitz, *Power and Passion*, 376.

66. Diary of Mary Whitall Worthington, October 2, 1908, Scrapbook Collection,
9LS, #30, BMC.

67. MEG to MCT, April 29, 1902, reel 49, BMC; MEG to MCT, May 19, 1906,
reel 51, BMC.

68. MEG to MCT, February 3, 1903, reel 50, BMC; MEG to MCT, February 17,
1903, reel 50, BMC.

69. Horowitz, *Power and Passion*, 332.

70. Remodeling details taken from Ruth Levy Merriam, "A History of the Deanery" (Bryn Mawr College: Deanery Management Committee, 1965).

71. Quoted in Merriam, "History of the Deanery," 5.

CHAPTER 9. WISE AND FAR-SIGHTED

1. MEG to MCT, May 1, 1894, reel 44, BMC.

2. *New York Sun*, April 1894 [exact date unknown].

3. Ida Husted Harper, ed., *History of Woman Suffrage* (New York: J. J. Little &
Ives Co., 1922), 5:151, 167; *Baltimore Sun*, August 24, 1930.

4. Harper, *History of Woman Suffrage*.

5. Marjorie Spruill Wheeler, ed., *One Woman, One Vote: Rediscovering the
Woman Suffrage Movement* (Troutdale, Ore.: NewSage Press), 14; Harper, *History of
Woman Suffrage*, 5:157.

6. Ione T. Hanna, "Ethics of Social Life," in Mary Kavanaugh Oldham Eagle, ed., *The Congress of Women: Held in the Woman's Building, World's Columbian Exposition, Chicago, U. S. A., 1893* (Chicago: Monarch Book Co., 1894), 53–57. "A Celebration of Women Writers" website: http://digital.library.upenn.edu/women/eagle/congress/hanna.html.

7. Wheeler, *One Woman, One Vote*, 162.

8. *Baltimore Sun*, August 30, 1930.

9. Elizabeth Cady Stanton, Susan B. Anthony, and Matilda Joslyn Gage, eds., *The History of Woman Suffrage* (Rochester: Charles Mann Printing Co., 1886), 3:815.

10. Lillian Welsh, M.D., LL.D., *Reminiscences of Thirty Years in Baltimore*, quoted in Marion Warren, *Baltimore: When She Was What She Used to Be*, 98.

11. Harper, *History of Woman Suffrage*, 5:167.

12. Shaw, *The Story of a Pioneer* (chapter 10), 5.

13. *Baltimore Sun*, February 8, 1906.

14. *Baltimore Sun*, February 6, 1906; *Baltimore Sun*, February 7, 1906.

15. *Baltimore Sun*, February 8, 1906.

16. Harper, *History of Woman Suffrage*, 5:153.

17. *Baltimore News*, February 8, 1906.

18. Ibid.; *Baltimore Sun*, February 11, 1906.

19. Harper, *History of Woman Suffrage*, 5: 167, 168; *Baltimore American*, February 9, 1906; *Baltimore News*, February 9, 1906.

20. *Baltimore News*, February 9, 1906.

21. *Baltimore American*, February 9, 1906; Harper, *History of Woman Suffrage*, 5:182.

22. Ibid., 179; Fee, Shopes, and Zeidman, *Baltimore Book*, 30.

23. Shaw, *The Story of a Pioneer* (chapter 10), 6; Doris Weatherford, *A History of the American Suffragist Movement* (Santa Barbara: ABC: CLIO, 1998), 179.

24. *Washington Post*, May 10, 1907; Shaw, *The Story of a Pioneer* (chapter 13), 9.

25. "Not for Ourselves Alone: The Story of Elizabeth Cady Stanton and Susan B. Anthony," www.pbs.org/stantonanthony/resources/index.html?body=biography.html; on gratitude, Harper, *History of Woman Suffrage*, 5:192.

26. *New York Times*, March 13, 1906.

27. Wheeler, *One Woman, One Vote*, 174.

28. Luckett, *Maryland Women*, 142.

29. Harper, *History of Woman Suffrage*, 6:255.

30. *Baltimore Sun*, January 22, 1912; *Baltimore Sun*, February 14, 1913.

31. *Baltimore Sun*, February 14, 1913.

32. *Chicago Daily Tribune*, November 12, 1911; Jean Baker, "Getting It Right with Suffrage," *Journal of the Gilded Age and Progressive Era*, 5, no. 1, www.historycooperative.org/journals/jga/5.1/baker.html.

33. *Chicago Daily Tribune*, November 12, 1911.

34. *Washington Post*, June 20, 1912; *New York Times*, June 29, 1912.

35. *Chicago Daily Tribune*, November 12, 1911.

36. Henry Garrett died in 1917.

37. Real Estate Officer, Safe Deposit and Trust Company of Baltimore to MEG, November 26, 1907, Box: Mary Garrett Business Papers, Folder: F22, BMC; Holcomb, *City as Suburb*, 114.

38. *Baltimore Sun*, May 2, 1907.

39. "The Four Doctors, Material Culture Collections Files," Ready Reference File, AMC.

40. "The Johns Hopkins University Circular, Commemoration Day, Sargent's Painting of the *Four Doctors*, Enumeration of Classes." MCT subject files, reels 172, BMC.

41. Ibid.

42. Ibid.

43. *Baltimore Sun*, April 14, 1915.

44. *New York Sun*, February 7, 1907; "JHU: Chronology": http://webapps.jhu.edu/jhuniverse/information_about_hopkins/about_jhu/chronology/index.cfm.

45. *Washington Post*, January 1, 1911.

46. J. H. Musser to "The Physician in Charge," December 20, 1911, Box: Mary Garrett 1–5 to MG Misc., Folder: F5, BMC.

47. Some of Mary's obituaries, in fact, mention "progressive anemia" as the cause of death, e.g., *Baltimore Sun*, April 4, 1915; on "distinct malady," Emil J. Freireich and Noreen A. Lemak, *Milestones in Leukemia Research and Therapy* (Baltimore: Johns Hopkins University Press, 1991), 7–8.

48. *Washington Post*, February 25, 1913.

49. *Baltimore News*, February 26, 1913.

50. Dr. Frank R. Smith to MEG, May 18, 1914, Box: Mary Garrett 1–5 to MG Misc., Folder: F4, BMC.

51. William Halsted to MEG, June 14, 1914, Box: Mary Garrett 1–5 to MG Misc., Folder: F6, BMC; Rebecca Harrison to MEG, June 12, 1914, Box: Mary Garrett 1–5 to MG Misc., Folder: F4, BMC.

52. Mary Jewett to MEG, September 14, 1914. Mary Garrett 1–5 to MG Misc., Folder: F4, BMC; William Halsted to MEG, February 1915 [exact date unknown], Mary Garrett 1–5 to MG Misc., Folder: F6, BMC.

53. Horowitz, *Power and Passion*, 408, 409.

54. *Baltimore News*, April 3, 1915; *Baltimore Sun*, April 4, 1915.

55. Unidentified newspaper article, "Miss Mary E. Garrett Dies at Bryn Mawr," date unknown, Evergreen House Foundation at Evergreen Museum and Library, JHU.

56. *Baltimore Sun*, April 4, 1915; *Baltimore News*, April 3, 1915.

57. *Baltimore News*, April 4, 1915; *Baltimore News*, April 6, 1915.

58. *Baltimore News*, April 4, 1915; *New York Times*, April 4, 1915. Honorary pallbearers included R. Brent Keyser, president of the Board of Trustees of the Johns Hopkins University; James Wood of Mt. Kisco, New York, president of the Board of Trustees of Bryn Mawr College; Dr. William Halsted; Dr. Henry Thomas of Baltimore; Mary and Carey's attorney, D. K. Este Fisher of Baltimore; Dr. Thomas Branson of Bryn Mawr; Warren Delano of Baltimore; and Dr. Simon Flexner.

59. "The Very Best Woman's College There Is: M. Carey Thomas and the Making of the Bryn Mawr Campus," BMC, www.brynmawr.edu/Library/exhibits/thomas/details3.html (September 21–December 20, 2001); *Bryn Mawr Quarterly* (January 1917).

60. "Minutes of the Bryn Mawr School" [undated]; Trustees of the Johns Hopkins University to MCT, April 8, 1915; Minutes of the Directors of Bryn Mawr College. All in Box 1, Business Papers, BMC.

61. *Washington Post*, December 17, 1915. Horowitz, *Power and Passion* (426), notes that tax assessors in 1915 valued the estate at $1 million.

62. Garrett Estate, Settlement of Estate, Losses Incurred by Miss Garrett [date unknown, probably 1915–1916], Box: Mary Garrett Business Papers, Folder: F7, BMC.

63. MEG Last Will and Testament, signed February 27, 1908, and codicil signed April 17, 1912 and filed with Register of Wills for Baltimore City on April 8, 1915.

64. MEG Last Will and Testament, signed February 27, 1908, and codicil signed April 1, 1915, and filed with Register of Wills for Baltimore City on April 8, 1915; MEG Last Will and Testament signed February 27, 1908, and filed with Register of Wills for Baltimore City 1915.

65. *Washington Post*, December 17, 1915; *New York Times*, January 8, 1916.

66. *Washington Post*, January 8, 1916.

67. *Washington Post*, April 9, 1916; Horowitz, *Power and Passion*, 425.

68. Beirne, *Daisies*, 30.

69. MEG Last Will and Testament, signed February 27, 1908.

70. Horowitz, *Power and Passion*, 426.

71. Ibid., 454.

72. In 2008, the Peabody Court Hotel stands on the lot once occupied by the Garrett mansion; on Montebello fire, *Baltimore Sun*, April 4, 1929.

73. *Baltimore Sun*, May 13, 1979.

74. "Women in U.S. Academic Medicine: Statistics and Medical School Benchmarking 2004–2005," American Association of Medical Colleges, www.aamc.org/members/wim/statistics/stats05/start.htm.

75. Article Eleventh of Mary's will states "that women shall be eligible as professors and teachers of every grade in all departments of the Medical School and that all such opportunities, privileges, prizes, dignities and honors shall not only be open to women aforesaid on equal terms but that every effort shall be made by the Trustees administering the trust to ensure that the proportion of the same to be enjoyed by women shall at no time be less than that which would fall to their share if due regard were paid to the relative numbers of men an[d] women studying in the Medical School at any given time and to the maintenance of a high standard of scholarship; And in like manner that women shall not only be eligible, but that every effort shall be made by the Trustees administering the said School to ensure that the proportion of the professors chairs and of other teaching posts held by Women shall at no time be less than the proportions that would fall to them or to their share, due regard being had to the relative numbers of Men and Women studying in the medical School at any given time and to the maintenance of a high standard of Scholarship."

APPENDIX A. CLASS OF 1879, WOMAN'S MEDICAL COLLEGE OF PENNSYLVANIA

1. Study profile taken from Abram, *"Send Us a Lady Physician,"* 131–224.
2. Ibid., 164.
3. Ibid., 65.

APPENDIX B. ANALYSIS OF THE WOMEN'S MEDICAL SCHOOL FUND CAMPAIGN

1. *Baltimore American*, November 3, 1890.

Fortunately for this writer and, it is hoped, for the reader, Mary Elizabeth Garrett's rich and complex life provides an engaging intersection of biography and history. Many topics converged in her life, from the development of railroads and American medicine to education, suffrage and, not least, a woman's quest for purpose and self-identity. Recounting her life's story required a broad, sweeping historical narrative supported by recent theories of feminist biography.

Starting in the 1970s, when women's history and social history marched together to claim a prominent place in historical scholarship, women's biography also gained importance and credibility. But writing the biography of a "nontraditional" woman, who did not always play by the rules and conform to expected models of behavior for an upper-class woman, would prove challenging. I found three works to be helpful in understanding the psychological progression of Garrett's life: Carolyn G. Heilbrun, *Writing a Woman's Life* (New York: Ballantine Books, 1988); Sara Alpern, Joyce Antler, Elizabeth Israels Perry, and Ingrid Winther Scobie, eds., *The Challenge of Feminist Biography: Writing the Lives of Modern American Women* (Urbana: University of Illinois Press, 1992); and Carol Gilligan's seminal *In a Different Voice: Psychological Theory and Women's Development* (Cambridge, Mass.: Harvard University Press, 1993).

"When the subject is female," the editors note in *The Challenge of Feminist Biography*, "gender moves to the center of the analysis" (7). This idea became fundamental as I formulated Garrett's life's story. How did her philanthropic motivations and techniques differ from those of her male counterparts? Would a male philanthropist have faced similar personal consequences for his activism? Moreover, as Heilbrun notes, when the "marriage plot" of a woman's life drama is removed, events other than marriage and motherhood become pivotal in a woman's life. The biographer must use other benchmarks to assess the woman's life (121). Such was the case with Garrett as she struggled for identity and eventually found her life's work in removing for others those obstacles that had thwarted her.

In addition, Gerda Lerner's 1997 *Why History Matters: Life and Thought* (New York: Oxford University Press) is important in understanding the primary reasons for researching women's history: to not only uncover long-lost or long-subsumed women's historical events, but to give ownership of women's history back to its lawful proprietors. Lerner writes, "When women discover their history and learn their connectedness to the past and to the human social enterprise, their consciousness is dramatically transformed. Their experience enables them to fully understand the impact women have had on building societies" (210).

Mary's life exemplifies what women's historians have long suspected—that women want their stories to be told for future generations. Perhaps knowing their history would be forgotten or not recorded in official documents and accounts, they instead left to posterity an endless array of letters and diaries, meeting minutes and ledgers so that we, today, can better understand the issues of most importance to them. Archives and libraries across the country are filled with such valuable accounts. When women are brought into the historical equation, Gilligan notes, it changes "how the human story is told" (xi). Mary's thirty-year record of philanthropy and activism, articulated through her personal and family papers and the meticulous records she and her associates kept to document their campaigns, shows she wanted the human story, at least women's part in it, to be told very differently—and in women's own voices.

Before the age of sixteen, Mary left few personal accounts, and there is little record of her childhood—not unusual for a girl of her era. Consequently, her earliest years are reconstructed within the context of her family, Baltimore, the B&O, and the maelstrom of the antebellum years. Later in life, possibly in her fifties, Mary penned a brief memoir, a short autobiography identified here as the MEG memoir. It is most helpful in piecing together her early childhood. In it, she recalls her earliest memories and, particularly, her relationship with her father. Her memory may have been selective at this point, but the memoir is valuable for understanding Mary's developing ideas. Many of the events and impressions she describes are corroborated in other sources.

By late adolescence, Mary began to correspond with friends, family, doctors, and new acquaintances, leaving behind more personal insight into her developing personality and revealing the early influences on her philanthropy. In her mature years, after her father died and she began an independent life, the volume of her correspondence and legal papers greatly increased, adding more dimensions to the record of her life. The sum of these documents, augmented by Garrett family papers and abundant press coverage, provide balanced views of her private and public lives.

To gain perspective on the wide range of topics examined in this historical biography, I found the following sources to be of major importance:

MANUSCRIPT COLLECTIONS

Special Collections Department, Bryn Mawr College Library. Mary's bequest to M. Carey Thomas in 1915 included the bulk of her personal papers and small artifacts. The Mary Elizabeth Garrett Collection comprises diaries and travelogues; her memoir; official Garrett family papers, including deeds and legal papers relating to her frequent disagreements with her family about the settlement of her father's estate; expense accounts; gift lists; travel itineraries; telegrams; documentation of her commissioning of John Singer Sargent for the *Four Doctors* portrait and her own portrait done by Sargent; miscellaneous other correspondence with Daniel Coit Gilman and other Hopkins officials; invitations; personal health journals; many personal letters to her mother and other family members; and documents relating to her estates at Montebello, Mount Vernon Place, and Deer Park.

Also at the Bryn Mawr Library, in the M. Carey Thomas Papers, are the original letters (also on microfilm) between Thomas and Garrett, from the time of their first meeting in 1877 until Garrett's death in 1915, and other relevant Thomas papers relating to Garrett. The two women engaged in a lively, often daily, correspondence for thirty-five years. Their letters record their developing personal relationship, which strengthened and grew more intimate over time, as well as documentation of Mary's activities as conveyed to Thomas when they were not together. Though thousands of letters passed between them, the volume diminishes after 1904 when Garrett began spending more time at Bryn Mawr College.

Of particular importance in this collection are letters Mary wrote to the "Dear Girls," Carey Thomas and Mamie Gwinn, in the mid-1880s to early 1890s. The letters chronicle the formation of the Bryn Mawr School and Women's Medical School Fund campaign.

The Johns Hopkins University. Several important relevant collections are held by the university: the Daniel Coit Gilman Papers (the Sheridan Libraries, Department of Special Collections and Archives), the Mary E. Garrett Collection (Alan Mason Chesney Medical Archives), and the papers relating to the Garretts, particularly T. Harrison and his descendants, at Evergreen House Foundation at Evergreen Museum and Library, the Johns Hopkins University. The documents in these collections include private correspondence between Mary and various members of the Hopkins community; letters recounting the negotiations concerning her gift to establish the School of Medicine; public announcements about the gift; and the establishment and activities of the Women's Medical School Fund. The Evergreen House provides a firsthand look at the grand lifestyle of wealthy Baltimoreans such as the Garretts, as does the Garrett-Jacobs Mansion, now owned by the Engineers Club.

Bryn Mawr School. The school archives hold extensive records and correspondence concerning the initiation of the school in 1885 and the planning and building of the 1890 school building. The collection includes newspaper articles, which are especially helpful in articulating the founders' expectations for the new school and gauging public reaction to the concept of the new school.

The H. Furlong Baldwin Library of the Maryland Historical Society. The Garrett Family Papers include a collection of Mary Elizabeth Garrett's correspondence, primarily to Amzi Crane, John Work Garrett's personal secretary and, later, Mary's personal secretary. Many of these papers relate to the management of properties; the building of the new Bryn Mawr School; personal charitable solicitations from people in Maryland; and the management of the Garrett mansions and estates. Crane often vetted applications for students and faculty at Bryn Mawr School, and his correspondence with Mary sheds light on the selection process and the standards the founders set for the school.

The Library of Congress Manuscript Division. The Garrett Family Papers include extensive documentation on the development of Baltimore, the B&O, and the Garrett family enterprises. The collection also is valuable for its comprehensive documentation of American business and railroading in the nineteenth century. Within the collection are letters written by Mary and John Work Garrett during their travels. Of most importance are the files covering the Garretts' many travels abroad, particularly their year-long trip to Europe (1873–74) for John Work Garrett's convalescence. During this time, Mary first became "Papa's secretary," drafting correspondence and sitting in on business meetings. These documents reveal a great deal about her exposure to and developing interest in the B&O beginning at the age of nineteen.

Garrett Family DNA and Genealogical Research Project, directed by the late Donald Garrett Dickason, Princeton, New Jersey. For many years, Dickason delved into the background of his extended family and discovered valuable information about the family's life in Northern Ireland prior to their immigration to the United States in 1790 and about their early years of settlement in Pennsylvania and Maryland. This work was very helpful in providing the details of Robert Garrett's early life and the influence of his adolescence in Western Pennsylvania in shaping the Garretts' commercial empire.

Cincinnati Museum Center. The Baltimore and Ohio Collection provides valuable supplemental information not found elsewhere on the expansion of the B&O into the Midwest, background on John Work Garrett and his brother Henry, and the B&O's enticement of Midwesterners to the resort area of Garrett County.

PUBLISHED PRIMARY SOURCES

Although she always sought privacy, Mary's philanthropic and reform activities made her a public personality in the last half of her life, from 1885 to 1915. Newspaper articles from this time period offer a rounded perspective of her life not found in her private letters. In addition, the press regularly reported on other members of the Garrett family.

The early history of Baltimore and its commercial links to the West are described in Thomas Scharf's 1882 *History of Western Maryland, Being a History of Frederick, Montgomery, Carroll, Washington, Allegany and Garrett Counties from the Earliest Period to the Present Day, Including Biographical Sketches of Their Representative Men* (Philadelphia: Louis H. Everts); the two-volume *Baltimore: Its History and People* (New York: Lewis Historical Publishing Co., 1912); and William Chase's (ed.) *Descriptions of Maryland: A Miscellany,* www.fac.mcdaniel.edu/history/dom.html, an entertaining and insightful compilation of travelogues and testimonials of nineteenth-century visitors to Maryland, with their comments on Mount Vernon Place, slavery, and the Civil War, among other topics.

Writers and historians have long been intrigued by the colorful, complex history of the B&O. I found Edward Hungerford's two-volume *The Story of the Baltimore & Ohio Railroad 1827–1927* (New York: G. P. Putnam's Sons, 1928) to be especially helpful in offering not only background about the company, but also useful anecdotes on Maryland, Baltimore, and Robert and John Work Garrett. Also, Ele Bowen's 1855

Rambles in the Path of the Steam-Horse (Philadelphia: William Bromwell and William White Smith Publishers, 1855) provides understanding of the B&O's early history and unique position in the years leading up to the Civil War. John Moody's 1919 *The Railroad Builders: A Chronicle of the Welding of the States* (New Haven, Conn.: Yale University Press), offers a critical perspective on John Work Garrett's management of the B&O that counterbalances some newspaper articles published during his lifetime.

Mary's twenty years of suffrage activism are represented through her correspondence as well as newspaper accounts of her activities, particularly the play-by-play accounts of the 1906 suffrage convention in Baltimore. Suffrage volumes augment these records. Suffragists were compulsive chroniclers, and there is no shortage of information on the topic. Of most relevance to this work were the various *History of Woman Suffrage* volumes (New York: J. J. Little and Ives Company, 1922), edited by Ida Husted Harper, Elizabeth Cady Stanton, Susan B. Anthony, and Matilda Gage, and Anna Howard Shaw's 1915 autobiography *The Story of a Pioneer* (reprinted, Cleveland, Ohio: Pilgrim Press, 1994).

Similarly, the medical school campaign garnered much public attention during its four years and is covered in private documents and also copious newspaper accounts and magazine articles. The articles are valuable not only for tracking the progression of the campaign but, more important, for revealing the organizers' manipulation of the press, what we today would call putting a positive public-relations spin on a difficult fundraising campaign.

Of most interest is the *absence* of information about Mary Elizabeth Garrett and the medical school campaign in published books. The early scholarly histories of the Johns Hopkins University have deconstructed and diminished women's roles in starting the medical school and reforming American medicine. In his 1906 autobiography *The Launching of a University* (New York: Dodd, Mead, and Company), Daniel Coit Gilman devoted only passing reference to Mary: "It was not until Mary E. Garrett came forward years later . . . with a gift of nearly a half-million dollars supplementing a large contribution from friends of the medical education of women that the organization of the medical school was perfected" (123). Similarly, Fabian Franklin's 1910 biography *The Life of Daniel Coit Gilman* (New York: Dodd, Mead, and Company) summarized the women's contributions in a short paragraph. It is unknown whether Mary read either book, for she did not comment on them.

SECONDARY SOURCES

For background on Baltimore, the B&O, and the development of Robert Garrett and Sons, James D. Dilts's *The Great Road: The Building of the Baltimore and Ohio, the Nation's First Railroad, 1828–1853* (Stanford, Calif.: Stanford University Press, 1993); John F. Stover's *History of the Baltimore and Ohio Railroad* (West Lafayette, Ind.: Purdue University Press, 1987); Harold Williams's *Robert Garrett & Sons, Incorporated* (Baltimore: Press of Schneidereith & Sons, 1965); and Bruce Catton's "How Rails

Saved a Seaport," published in *American Heritage*, www.americanheritage.com/articles/magazine/ah/1957/2/1957_2_26.shtml were indispensable sources. Francis F. Beirne's *The Amiable Baltimoreans* (New York: E. P. Dutton and Company, 1951) has long been a favorite among readers for its solid history and charming anecdotal details of "Old Baltimore."

There is no dearth of sources on the Civil War and Baltimore's role in it, but I found Scott Sumpter Sheads and Daniel Carroll Toomey's *Baltimore during the Civil War* (Baltimore: Toomey Press, 1997), Robert I. Cottom Jr. and Mary Ellen Hayward's *Maryland in the Civil War: A House Divided* (Baltimore: Maryland Historical Society, 1994), and Robert J. Brugger's *The Maryland Club: A History of Food and Friendship in Baltimore, 1857–1997* (Baltimore: Maryland Club, 1998) helpful in understanding Baltimore's dual alliances and secessionist activities during the war. George M. Frederickson's *The Inner Civil War: Northern Intellectuals and the Crisis of the Union* (New York: Harper & Row Publishers, 1965) helped to explain the irrational nature of the Civil War and the eagerness with which young elite men like Robert Garrett succumbed to the seduction of war to break with parental authority and traditional expectations.

The history of the Johns Hopkins University as the country's first graduate-level research university and of its equally original medical school similarly has a rich scholarship. Laurence R. Veysey's *The Emergence of the American University* (Chicago: University of Chicago Press, 1965) and Francesco Cordasco's *The Shaping of American Graduate Education: Daniel Coit Gilman and the Protean PhD* (Leiden, Netherlands: E. J. Brill, 1960) offered perspective on the unique concept of the university, and Hugh Hawkins's *Pioneer: A History of the Johns Hopkins University 1874–1889* (Ithaca, N.Y.: Cornell University Press, 1960) added descriptions of the Garretts' early involvement and Mary's subsequent financial offers to the university. Paul Starr's Pulitzer- and Bancroft-prize-winning *The Social Transformation of American Medicine* (New York: Basic Books, 1982) is most helpful in explaining Hopkins' role as an early prototype of modern American medicine. A. McGhee Harvey et al., in the two-volume *A Model of Its Kind* (Baltimore: Johns Hopkins University Press, 1989), provide an overview of the development of the Johns Hopkins Hospital in relation to the university and the medical school.

The history of women in medicine has long been of interest to scholars, and several general histories provide a comprehensive view of the victories and defeats women encountered in their efforts to be accepted in the profession. Regina Markall Morantz-Sanchez, *Sympathy and Science: Women Physicians in American Medicine* (New York: Oxford University Press, 1985); Mary Roth Walsh, *Doctors Wanted: No Women Need Apply: Sexual Barriers in the Medical Profession* (New Haven, Conn.: Yale University Press, 1977); and Ruth Abram, ed., *"Send Us a Lady Physician": Women Doctors in America, 1835–1920* (New York: W. W. Norton & Company, 1985) carefully chronicle the evolution of women as physicians. Also of great help in understanding the WMSF's fundraising campaign was Nancy McCall's "The Savvy Strategies of the First Campaign for Hopkins Medicine," *Hopkins Medical News* 8, no. 6 (Fall 1984).

As the leading proponent of women's education in the nineteenth and early twentieth centuries, M. Carey Thomas has been the subject of two notable biographies. In 1947, Edith Finch penned *Carey Thomas of Bryn Mawr* (New York: Harper and Brothers, 1947), and in 1994, Helen Lefkowitz Horowitz in *The Power and Passion of M. Carey Thomas* (New York: Alfred A. Knopf) closely examined the voluminous papers of Thomas to create a deeper understanding of the brilliant, controversial academician. Horowitz's work is especially valuable to this biography for the insight it provides about the Garrett-Thomas personal relationship as well as the women's shared campaigns to open the Bryn Mawr School and the Hopkins medical school and their mutual interest in suffrage. In addition, Horowitz's *Alma Mater: Design and Experience in the Women's Colleges from Their Nineteenth Century Beginnings to the 1930s* (New York: Alfred A. Knopf, 1984) is an important source on the development of women's higher education. Rosamond Randall Beire's *Let's Pick the Daisies: The History of the Bryn Mawr School, 1885–1967* (Baltimore: Bryn Mawr School, 1970) offers a detailed history of the school's philosophy and founding, and Andrea Hamilton's *A Vision for Girls: Gender, Education and the Bryn Mawr School* (Baltimore: Johns Hopkins University Press, 2004) provides new insight into the founding and development of the school within the context of theories of women's education in the nineteenth century.

Women's philanthropy and voluntarism are integral components of women's history, as researchers acknowledge the myriad voluntary organizations that women formed throughout the nineteenth century as sources of empowerment and effective paths for moving into the public sphere. There are many notable trailblazers in this field. Kathleen McCarthy, Kathryn Sklar, Karen Blair, Carroll Smith Rosenberg, Aileen Kraditor, Barbara Berg and Suzanne Lebsock, Anne Firor Scott, Nancy F. Cott, and Ruth Crocker, among many others, have vastly expanded our knowledge of the importance of women's groups in forming a strong women's culture and providing social and economic alternatives for disenfranchised women. This biography incorporates the important scholarship of these historians. They have shown us that, above all else, women have wanted to tell their own story.

Index